"As a lifelong proponent of healthy living, I know that the earlier you start, the better off you are. In this solidly researched new book, the authors present an effective scientific program that puts kids on the right health track from day one."

—Kenneth H. Cooper, M.D., M.P.H., author of
The Aerobics Program for Total Well-Being

"Drs. Roberts and Heyman meld the best of contemporary nutritional science with a wealth of practical experience. This book is for every new parent."

—Walter Willet, M.D., Professor and Chair, Department
of Nutrition, Harvard School of Public Health

"*Feeding Your Child for Lifelong Health* provides up-to-the-minute, scientifically sound, and easy-to-read answers to the ever-growing galaxy of nutrition questions facing the parents of young children. Don't leave the maternity ward without it."

—Bonnie Liebman, M.S., Director of Nutrition,
Center for Science in the Public Interest

"A wealth of up-to-date information for parents. Even health professionals who want a quick reference on pediatric nutrition would find it a welcome addition to their library!"

—Ann M. Coulston, M.S., R.D., Past President, The American Dietetic Association

"Well-researched and thoroughly practical . . . Roberts and Heyman have a reassuring and sensible answer for every imaginable question. I wish their book had been available when my children were young."

—Marion Nestle, Ph.D., Professor and Chair, Department
of Nutrition and Food Studies, New York University

"This remarkable book should be read by any parent interested in the latest guidance that nutrition science can provide."

—Rudolph L. Leibel, M.D., Professor of Pediatrics, Columbia
University College of Physicians and Surgeons

"Excellent! The advice on how to encourage eating a variety of foods . . . is extremely positive. The age-specific recommendations, sample menus and recipes are a strong feature of the book."

—Connie M. Weaver, Ph.D., President,
American Society of Nutritional Sciences

"Timely and authoritative, this book delivers a highly innovative and easy-to-follow food guide for children's lifelong health."

—George L. Blackburn, M.D., Ph.D., Past President,
American Society of Clinical Nutrition

"Engaging and highly impressive . . . an absolutely first-rate piece of work. The sections on how to deal with toddlers' eating idiosyncrasies are delightful as well as informative."

—Peter J. Jones, Ph.D., Professor and Director, School
of Dietetics and Human Nutrition, McGill University

"Very user-friendly, with a wealth of practical information . . . Must reading for parents who have children up to six years of age."

—John N. Udall, M.D., Ph.D., Professor of Pediatrics and Chief, Gastroenterology and Nutrition, Louisiana State University, New Orleans

FEEDING YOUR CHILD FOR

Lifelong Health

BIRTH THROUGH AGE SIX

Susan B. Roberts, Ph.D.
and Melvin B. Heyman, M.D.
with Lisa Tracy

FOREWORD BY
Irwin H. Rosenberg, M.D.

BANTAM BOOKS
NEW YORK · TORONTO · LONDON · SYDNEY · AUCKLAND

FEEDING YOUR CHILD FOR LIFELONG HEALTH

A Bantam Book / August 1999

All rights reserved.
Copyright © 1999 by Susan B. Roberts, Melvin B. Heyman, and Lisa Tracy.
Introduction copyright © 1999 by Irwin H. Rosenberg.
Cover art copyright © 1999 by The Image Bank and The Stock Market.

ILLUSTRATIONS BY WENDY WRAY.

Library of Congress Cataloging-in-Publication Data

Roberts, Susan B. (Susan Barbara).
Feeding your child for lifelong health : birth through age six / Susan B. Roberts and Melvin B. Heyman with Lisa Tracy ; foreword by Irwin H. Rosenberg.
          p.   cm.
Includes bibliographical references and index.
ISBN 0-553-37892-9
1. Infants—Nutrition.   2. Children—Nutrition.   I. Heyman, Melvin B.   II. Tracy, Lisa.   III. Title.
RJ206.R663   1999
813.2'083—dc21   99-20253
                                                          CIP

Published simultaneously in the United States and Canada

Bantam Books are published by Bantam Books, a division of Random House, Inc. Its trademark, consisting of the words "Bantam Books" and the portrayal of a rooster, is Registered in U.S. Patent and Trademark Office and in other countries. Marca Registrada. Bantam Books, 1540 Broadway, New York, New York 10036.

PRINTED IN THE UNITED STATES OF AMERICA

BVG   10   9   8   7   6   5

For Diana, who inspired this book,
and John, who gave invaluable help and advice at every step of the way

—SBR

And Jody, for numerous invaluable contributions,
and Brahm, Will, and Ben, whose boundless energy and consequent
food intake provided the best encouragement

—MBH

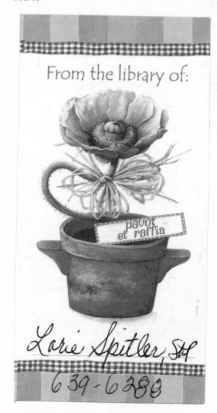

From the library of:

pavot
et raffia

ACKNOWLEDGMENTS

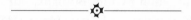

This book would not have been possible without the efforts of a great many people. First we would like to thank the scientists whose work has helped inspire our own, and led to the framework of our advice in this book. In particular, Alan Lucas (who first proposed "metabolic programming"), Leanne Birch, Barbara Rolls, and Kay Dewey have all conducted studies that really made us stop and think. We are also very grateful to the NIH, the USDA, Ross Laboratories, Mead Johnson, and other funding institutes who have supported independent nutrition research in our laboratories and others. Without you, the scientific progress described in this book would not have been possible.

We also thank all the individuals who so generously gave their expert advice, help, and support during the writing of this book. From Tufts University: Helen Armstrong, Lynne Ausman, Gretchen Beherrell, Jeff Blumberg, Paul Fuss, Richard Grand, Nick Hays, Megan McCrory, Moshen Meydani, Miriam Nelson, Gail Peronne, Abbey and Ronenn Roubenoff, Ed Saltzman, Jacob Selub, Angela Vinken, and Richard Wood. From the University of California at San Francisco: Maria Melko, Bob Pantell, and Richard Shames. Also Rita Tsay from the Massachusetts Institute of Technology, David Ludwig, Mary Pickett, and Elizabeth Thiele from Harvard Medical School, Marc Masor and Bridget Barrett Reis from Ross Laboratories, Margaret Neville from the University of Colorado, Boston psychiatrist Edward Hallowell, Boston lactation consultant Naomi Bar-Yam, and our knowledgeable friends and relatives Bart and Val Broadman, David Bjornsson, Carol Borman, Jonah and Ben Detofski, Nancy Doyne, Cara Flanagan, Dennis Flanagan, Geraldine Lux Flanagan, Vivian Golden, Susan Greatorex, Mary Klaus, Lonnie Tait, and Barbara Williams. Thanks also to Henry Roberts for introducing SBR to the joys of both good food and the science of nutrition, and Jody Heyman for sharing her extensive professional expertise on food and menus.

We are deeply grateful to our agents, Nancy and Herb Katz, for their many invaluable suggestions and help and support along the way. We also owe the utmost appreciation to Toni Burbank, our tremendously gifted editor at Bantam, whose vision and extraordinary skills made the critical difference. It has been a privilege to work with her, from the day we showed her our proposal to the day the book went to press.

And finally, we also thank the many families who shared their experiences with us and whose voices appear throughout the book. We hope this book helps you as much as your wisdom and stories helped us.

CONTENTS

———————◆———————

FOREWORD
by Irwin H. Rosenberg, M.D., Dean, School of Nutrition, Tufts University xiii

part one
THE POWER OF FOOD IN YOUR CHILD'S LIFE

I. METABOLIC PROGRAMMING
What It Is, and What It Can Do for Your Child 3

Metabolic Programming: The Power of Childhood Feeding · *How* You Feed Your Child Is Just as Important as *What* You Feed · Programming Your Child's Future Food Preferences

2. INSIDE YOUR CHILD'S HEAD
Why Children Eat the Way They Do—Starting from Day One 14

Who Needs Smart Strategies? · Building on Your Child's Instincts

3. THE KEY EIGHT NUTRIENTS 29

Fat, Fiber, and Calories · Three Essential Minerals: Iron, Calcium, and Zinc · Folate and B Vitamins (B_6 and B_{12}) · Antioxidants: Vitamins A, C, and E · What About Supplements? · A Word About Water

part two
YOUR BABY ARRIVES

4. FOOD FOR THOUGHT
Preparing to Feed Your New Baby 53

Harness Instincts—Your Newborn's and Yours—for a Trouble-free Start

5. BREAST-FEEDING MADE EASY 59

Getting Started · From Three Days to Four Weeks · Nutrition and Your Milk Supply · From Four Weeks On · Special Concerns

6. NEW OPTIONS IN FORMULA FEEDING 86

Six Formula Types: Which Is Best for Your Baby? · Your Baby's First Feedings · How Much Formula Does Your Baby Need? · Common Problems with Formula Feeding

7. FEEDING A PREMATURE INFANT 101

Getting Started Breast-feeding a Premature Infant · Formula Options for Premature Infants · After You Leave the Hospital

part three
FOOD TRANSITIONS: FOUR MONTHS TO SIX YEARS

8. THE FAMILY BALANCING ACT 113

Balance for the Whole Family · How Safe Is Our Food? · Vegetarian and Macrobiotic Diets · Foods to Avoid or Strictly Limit · Helping Baby-sitters to Feed Your Child Right

9. FOUR TO TWELVE MONTHS
The Big Transition to Solid Food 133

Opportunities and Goals · When Should You Start? · Moving on to a Mixed Diet · Smart Strategies for Feeding Babies Four to Twelve Months Old · Common Problems

10. TWELVE TO TWENTY-ONE MONTHS
A Nine-month Window of Opportunity 159

Opportunities and Goals · What Your Child Eats · Good Foods to Try · Food Traps to Avoid · Smart Strategies for Feeding Toddlers · Common Problems and Frequently Asked Questions

11. TWENTY-ONE MONTHS TO THREE YEARS
Feeding Your Terrific "Terrible Two" 185

Opportunities and Goals · What to Feed Your Child · Smart Strategies for Keeping a Basically Good Eater on Track · Handling Food Jags and Extreme Fussiness · Coping with Constipation · Common Problems and Frequently Asked Questions

12. THREE TO SIX YEARS
Moving into the Outside World 206

Meet Your Preschooler, the Social Animal · Opportunities and Goals ·
What to Feed Your Child · Smart Strategies: Maintaining Great Eating
Habits—or Establishing Them · Preschool · Talking About Nutrition
and Health · Your Child's Body Image · Frequently Asked Questions

part four
FOOD SOLUTIONS FOR COMMON PROBLEMS

13. FEEDING YOUR SICK CHILD
Diarrhea, Vomiting, and Other Common Illnesses 231

Diarrhea, Vomiting, and Fever · Colds and Other Illnesses That
Primarily Reduce Appetite · Frequently Asked Questions

14. FOOD, SLEEP, AND YOUR BABY 241

Encouraging Your Baby to Sleep Through the Night · Getting Your Baby
to Sleep · Cow's Milk Sensitivity as a Cause of Chronic Sleep Problems

15. PROBLEMS WITH WEIGHT
The Spectrum from Obesity to Anorexia and Bulimia. 249

Does Your Child Weigh Too Much? · Why Some Children Become
Overweight · How to Normalize a Weight Problem · Eating Disorders:
Every Child Is at Risk · Frequently Asked Questions

16. ABOUT ALLERGIES, FOOD INTOLERANCES, AND COLIC 275

Routine Prevention of Food Allergies · Additional Steps for Allergy
Prevention in High-risk Infants · When Your Child Develops a Food
Allergy or Intolerance · Colic · Common Problems and Frequently
Asked Questions

17. FOOD, HYPERACTIVITY, AND
ATTENTION DEFICIT HYPERACTIVITY DISORDER 299

Does My Child Have a Problem? · Do Some Foods and Chemicals in
Foods Cause Hyperactivity or ADHD? · Your Decision: Will a Special
Elimination Diet Help Your Child with ADHD?

APPENDIX 1: *Good Food Sources of Key Nutrients* 312

APPENDIX 2: *Growth Charts* 318

BIBLIOGRAPHY 331

INDEX 346

FOREWORD

Susan Roberts started her career as a scientist long before I met her, researching infant nutrition and lactation in England and Africa in the late 1970s and early 1980s. By 1986, when we first met, she was already one of the brightest young scientists of her generation. She subsequently came to work at Tufts University, bringing fresh ideas and a new perspective to our work on obesity and aging.

With her characteristic love of science and sense of purpose, she set up major new programs, and in recognition of her achievements was promoted to the position of Professor of Nutrition and Associate Professor of Psychiatry. Over the years, her work ranging from infants to the elderly has brought her a strong international reputation, and nearly one hundred research publications in leading scientific journals including the *New England Journal of Medicine, JAMA,* and *The Lancet.*

Meanwhile, she and her husband started a family. The birth of their daughter in 1993, she tells me, was a turning point that made her think beyond the frontiers of science. As she described it, it was as if a light had been switched on. One day she was primarily a scientist who studied nutrition from birth to old age. The next day she was a scientist and mother with a mission to help other parents and pediatricians to feed children in the best possible way.

Enter Melvin Heyman, M.D., a renowned pediatric gastroenterologist and researcher from the University of California at San Francisco, who spent a sabbatical year in Dr. Roberts' laboratory. Dr. Heyman's professional specialties, which include pediatric nutrition and gastroenterology, seemed to provide a perfect complement to her own, as did his love of children and his family of three young boys.

They decided to write a book together. A book that would share with other parents groundbreaking new research into nutrient and food needs for long-term health and development as well as short-term growth. A book that would also give parents simple but effective psychological strategies for ensuring that children learn to *enjoy* these healthy foods, based on understanding the instinctive way children think and behave about food. In the process of refining these themes, Dr. Roberts and Dr. Heyman have created a new guide to childhood nutrition that should revolutionize the way parents approach feeding their families—and help bring about a healthier and brighter future for all children.

I am proud to introduce their book and the talented scientists who produced it.

Irwin H. Rosenberg, M.D.
Dean, School of Nutrition
Tufts University

PART ONE

The Power of Food in Your Child's Life

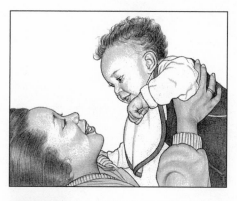

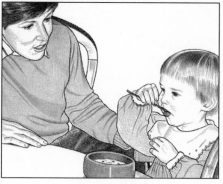

CHAPTER I

—⊹—

Metabolic Programming

What It Is, and What It Can Do for Your Child

With her baby due in three weeks, a mother-to-be visited her local supermarket to buy some diapers and check out the baby food aisle. What an excitement—and a shock—it was. Those rows of jars, packets, and cans made impending motherhood seem so real! But she had thought she was ready to feed her baby, and here was a whole world of new decisions to make. She wouldn't be using formula at first, but which of the sixteen kinds (some costing three times as much as others) would be right for later? And would she need any of these other items? The pear juice in tiny bottles looked delicious, but wasn't her niece's tummy pain traced to an allergy to baby juice? Should fluoridated spring water go on the shopping list? And those jars of nutrient-packed spinach—could she really get her baby to like something she hated? Should she even try?

This book began in that moment six years ago, when I* was that excited and puzzled mother-to-be. As a nutrition researcher, I have spent twenty years studying the importance of healthy food at all stages of life. But it was only when I became a mother that I realized how much parents needed the information we were discovering. Studies from my own laboratory and others around the world had taught me that, contrary to the advice in the parenting books in my house, the foods my daughter would eat during the first months and years of life would have long-lasting—and in some cases permanent—effects. I knew that nutrition was not the whole story, of course. But it would make an important difference in virtually

---

* Susan Roberts speaks in the first person as the principal writer of this book, with extensive and invaluable input from Melvin Heyman, and in literary collaboration with Lisa Tracy.

3

everything, from her mental and physical development to her vitality, personality, and health from childhood through old age. The way I behaved about her food would be critical, too, preventing difficult eating behavior in the short term and lifelong struggles with disorders such as obesity and anorexia. With this valuable knowledge as my guide, I began helping my daughter learn to enjoy the foods best for her development and health, a rewarding and joyful task that continues with her entry into kindergarten.

My first insight into the power of childhood food came some years ago when I worked with a research team in a village in West Africa. At first I was surprised to see no children who looked malnourished: They all seemed fine—and were extremely well behaved! It was only after I started studying them that I realized they were permanently stunted due to a lack of good food. Their quiet behavior stemmed not from superior discipline techniques (as I had first supposed) but from inadequate nutrition that left them without the vitality and exuberance of well-nourished children. Even worse, their lack of normal exploratory behavior was preventing them from learning all the things that children need to learn if they are not to be left behind in a fast-paced world.

Later, when my research moved to Cambridge University in England and subsequently to Tufts University in Boston, I realized that my observations in Africa were only the tip of the iceberg. Research from my laboratory and others was showing that even in affluent countries such as the United States, good childhood nutrition is not what many pediatricians and concerned parents currently think it is. Yet it can make the difference of a lifetime, conferring long-term, even permanent advantages in mental and physical development and health.

While my experience on three continents was teaching me about the importance of childhood nutrition, my partner in this book, pediatric gastroenterologist Dr. Melvin Heyman, was having similar revelations in his nutrition clinic at the University of California at San Francisco. Mel had also observed that poor childhood nutrition was not confined to families struggling to make ends meet. Affluent, well-educated families were also vulnerable, even to problems such as the nutritional stunting I had seen in Africa. This was obviously not for lack of money or even for lack of concern, but sometimes because the families were eating extremely low-fat, whole-food diets that were healthy for the parents but contained the wrong nutrients to allow for normal childhood growth.

Raising our own children and spending time with other families, we also saw that knowing *what* to feed your child is not enough. *How* children are fed is as important as what goes on the table—because food counts only if it's eaten! Children can often seem difficult when it comes to food, but there are actually good reasons why they think and behave the way they do—reasons grounded in the normal psychology and biological programming of childhood. By learning how to work with, rather than against, our children's natural instincts, we can reduce feeding conflicts while at the same time teaching a lifelong enjoyment of healthy foods.

Combining our insight into childhood psychology with the latest research on childhood nutrition, we saw we could point the way to a whole new approach to feeding children—one that would make parents' lives easier while ensuring that their children reach their full potential in development and health. This book was born out of our desire to share that knowledge with other parents and health professionals, and to give every child the benefits that an enjoyment of healthy foods can bring.

METABOLIC PROGRAMMING:
THE POWER OF CHILDHOOD FEEDING

Behind the big eyes that scan your face and the tiny hand that grasps your finger, an event known as *metabolic programming* is unfolding in your child. Metabolic programming is the new term being used to describe the fact that foods eaten in childhood can have lasting effects on the way your child's body grows and functions.

How do foods consumed early in life exert effects beyond the short time they are physically present in your child's body? Scientists believe that metabolic programming happens in part because growth and cell division in many parts of the body occur only in childhood. During this time individual cells are sensitive to the availability of nutrients—in other words, the body's basic building materials.

We now know that each organ, tissue, and nerve cell within the body develops in its own unique window of time, in response to a complex set of biological signals arising from the body's DNA. The nutrients physically present at this crucial time for cell division and growth help determine which cell types become predominant within each tissue. The same nutrients also influence how large or small each cell within the different body components ultimately becomes, and how efficiently and well it functions

SIX MYTHS ABOUT FEEDING CHILDREN

MYTH: *Left to his own devices, your child will select a nutritionally balanced diet.*

REALITY: Parents need to help their children learn to enjoy foods that promote long-term development and health.

MYTH: *What is healthy for you is healthy for your child.*

REALITY: Children are not small adults when it comes to food. Although they can eat many of the same foods you do, the proportion needs to be quite different to ensure that their very different nutritional needs are adequately met. Higher needs for fat and lower needs for fiber are just two of the many ways your child's nutritional requirements differ from yours.

MYTH: *Colic can't be treated by changing what your baby eats.*

REALITY: As many as 25 percent of colic cases can be improved or even cured by changing a baby's diet. This is true even for breast-fed babies, when it is the mother who makes the dietary changes.

MYTH: *Children need many more calories, pound for pound, than adults.*

REALITY: Children do need more calories than adults when their small size is taken into account, but actual caloric needs are much less than the current RDAs—which have recently been described as "a prescription for overfeeding."

MYTH: *If you delay weaning onto solid foods, you will prevent your child from becoming overweight.*

REALITY: Late weaning can actually compound a tendency to gain too much weight.

MYTH: *Vitamin supplements are not needed by children gaining weight normally.*

REALITY: Weight and height are only two indicators of healthy growth. More than *50 percent* of American children under the age of three years do not get the recommended amounts of several essential nutrients without a daily multivitamin/mineral supplement.

in the future. And because organ and tissue functions determine such essential body processes as hormone production and enzyme activity, alterations in normal development can have far-reaching effects. Once the cells' period of sensitivity to growth signals has passed, the function of each individual cell is largely fixed. In other words, it has been metabolically programmed by the food your baby, toddler, or preschooler was eating during that cell's growth spurt.

You can think of metabolic programming as being somewhat like the set of signals that controls the switches on a railroad track. Sitting in a train in New York or San Francisco, you could go to many places. What determines which direction your train actually takes depends on the signals that set the switches on the track. If they're set right, you'll reach your destination. But if they are set wrong, especially near the start of your journey, you may end up in the wrong place or have to make a real effort to get back on the right track.

Like those signals, metabolic programming gives your child's body directions for his future. We now know that first foods can have permanent effects on growth, strength, the immune system, and intelligence—with long-term consequences for many other aspects of health and even personality. Through metabolic programming, our children's whole lives are influenced by what they eat in their early years.

We also know, of course, that metabolic programming doesn't tell the whole story, and that genetic makeup and family circumstances are tremendously important, too. Understanding metabolic programming and using it to advantage certainly doesn't guarantee that our children will grow up to be athletes, opera singers, or doctors, or that they'll live to be 122. What it does enable us to do is help them realize their own best potential in development and health.

Is working with your child's metabolic programming something you have to start right from day one, or forfeit its benefits? In most cases, the answer is an emphatic no. Raising a healthy child involves trial and error for all parents—ourselves included—and we have time to make mistakes and recover from them. Health benefits, in particular, are cumulative, and the child who starts to eat well only when he is five will still be much healthier in the long run than the one who doesn't begin until his teen or adult years.

At the same time, certain ages present a special window of opportunity for specific metabolic programming. Height, for example, is metabolically programmed primarily during the first five years of life. When it comes to intellectual development and IQ, your child's brain is growing especially fast during the first year, and this is when food can make the difference of a lifetime. For the immune system, a major window of opportunity is during the first few *months.*

Although metabolic programming affects virtually all aspects of our children's lives, there are five major areas where you can expect food to have an especially big impact.

1. PROMOTING HEALTHY WEIGHT GAIN AND PREVENTING OBESITY

More people are overweight in the United States now than at any previous time in history: well over half of all adults, and now about 15 percent of preschoolers—double the number twenty years ago. At the same time, research is showing a link between excess weight gain in childhood and remaining overweight throughout adult life. Helping your child avoid becoming overweight is a good example of how you can influence metabolic programming to prevent future problems. Fortunately, new strategies suggested by the latest research make this easier than ever before.

But while we want to help our children avoid excess weight gain, it is also important to prevent inadequate weight gain. This form of malnutrition in childhood—often termed "failure to thrive"—surprisingly does not occur only in families below the poverty level. About 15 percent of American children seen by pediatricians for poor weight gain suffer from *accidental* malnutrition. Often this is simply due to a misunderstanding on the part of affluent, health-conscious parents about what foods constitute a healthy diet for a baby or child. Paradoxically, children who gain *too little weight* in early childhood are at greater risk of becoming overweight adults. This seems to be because the caloric deficit metabolically programs their bodies to be more efficient in storing calories.

2. AVOIDING ALLERGIES

Protecting your baby's immune system by avoiding high-risk foods during the vulnerable first twelve months of life is a simple step that pays big dividends. Most childhood food allergies arise when the immature infant digestive system allows partially digested food proteins to get into the bloodstream. These protein particles in turn activate the immature immune system, programming it to overreact in the future to foods and non-foods such as pollen or dust. An overactivated immune system may also destroy some insulin-producing cells in the pancreas, leading to an increased risk of childhood diabetes.

Allergies often run in families and may not be totally preventable. But with what we now know about the role of nutrition, a lot can be done to minimize the risks. Breast-feeding, the use of a new generation of hypoallergenic formulas, and a modified program for introducing solid foods are just three of the ways parents can help lower the risk of allergies by at least 50 percent in a susceptible son or daughter.

3. OPTIMIZING BONE STRENGTH AND HEIGHT

"Drink your milk so you'll grow up tall" was the standard advice for many decades, but recent research has shown that calcium actually doesn't influence height: Height is largely in the genes. And the nutrients that influence it the most are calories and zinc, not calcium!

Calcium is, of course, vitally important for bone and tooth strength. Less than 50 percent of American children consume as much as they need. The metabolic signals for absorption of calcium begin at birth and continue through adolescence. Once we become adults, bone and tooth strength is largely fixed, and the best we can hope for is to hold on to what we developed as children. For a lifetime of strong bones, and for preventing eventual osteoporosis and tooth loss, your baby needs an adequate calcium intake now and throughout childhood.

4. BOOSTING INTELLIGENCE

During the first three years of life, and especially during the period from birth to age one, your child's brain is developing rapidly and can be influenced to a remarkable extent by what he eats. The mineral iron is essential for optimal brain development and future intelligence. Iron is a vital component of the red blood cells that transport oxygen to the brain. It also has additional diverse roles around the body, including helping control synthesis of the myelin sheath that surrounds brain cells and is essential for normal brain activity. Even a briefly inadequate supply of iron, as when mild anemia develops, has been shown to have permanent effects on IQ, motor development, attention span, and behavior. Yet according to a recent survey, a shocking one in seven American children is clinically iron-deficient.

Another critical nutrient for brain power is fat, because the brain is 60 percent fat by weight. For your new baby's brain cells to grow, divide, and develop into the billions of interconnected cells he will need in the future, he needs to consume about 50 percent of his calories as fat—about twice the amount that is healthy for you. One of the reasons that breast milk is widely accepted as the best food for young babies is that it supplies exactly the right amount and kinds of fat for optimal growth of the brain and nervous system.

This crucial connection is especially clear in research on premature infants. Children who as preemies were fed their mothers' milk for *just the first three weeks of life* showed an eight-point advantage in IQ scores in tests at age seven over those who had been fed formula. New research is showing that babies born at term may receive comparable benefits. A recent study of teenagers born at the normal time and breast-fed for even a few weeks showed higher IQ, better school grades, and only half the risk of leaving school early compared to teenagers fed formula after birth. This finding was true not only in a straight comparison of the two groups, but also after statistically adjusting the results for such factors as maternal smoking and family income.

5. PREVENTING CHILDHOOD CANCERS

This is a difficult topic for parents even to think about. Yet one recent study reported that children who eat a low-risk diet—one with plenty of fruits and vegetables and few high-nitrite foods—have only one-seventh to one-tenth the incidence of brain cancer and one-third the incidence of leukemia seen in other children.

Cancers start when the DNA in a single cell gets irreparably damaged and causes uncontrolled cell division and growth. And although DNA damage is caused by a number of environmental factors, of which food is only one, it is possible to substantially reduce our children's risk of cancer by controlling the types of foods they eat.

One way to help is to minimize children's consumption of nitrite-containing foods including hot dogs, ham, bacon, and sausages. The body can convert harmless nitrites into potent carcinogens called nitrosamines and nitrosamides, which increase the risk of DNA damage.

Ensuring that children get plenty of the antioxidant vitamins A, C, and

E is another way to help. These vitamins, found in fruits and vegetables—and, in the case of vitamin E, nuts, seeds, and oils—literally soak up the dangerous free radicals (products of normal metabolism) that attack DNA. It's important not to rely on supplements alone for antioxidants, because plant-based foods also contain thousands of other substances called phytochemicals, many of which have anticancer properties.

HOW YOU FEED YOUR CHILD IS JUST AS IMPORTANT AS *WHAT* YOU FEED

Feeding your child healthy foods doesn't have to be the daunting task it is often made out to be. In fact, much of the conventional wisdom on how to get the right foods into children is positively counterproductive. Your child is equipped with an incredible set of innate instincts and behaviors that can become your best helpers in the feeding process. Your newborn's instinct to suck, and his instinct to put everything in his mouth at about six months, when he begins to need solid food, are just two examples of how your child starts life ready to help with the important job of getting himself fed.

This is not to say that your child's instincts will automatically make him eat the right foods no matter what. Far from it! We have to channel our children's instincts, particularly when it comes to the foods we want them to enjoy in the future. This is necessary because we live in a world surrounded by a vast array of highly refined commercial foods for which evolution didn't prepare us. It's also necessary because medical and technological advances now allow us to live far longer than the forty-year life expectancy of our ancestors. Almost any food will allow us to survive for forty years. But for double that life span, a much better diet is needed.

To teach our children to enjoy healthy foods, we need to understand why they think and behave about food the way they do. Why do they instinctively avoid foods they know we want them to like? Why at age two are they cautious about vegetables, and how can we work around this innate behavior? Why do they pick up the bad habits of their peers from about age three on, and how can we prevent this? Once you understand why children think about food the way they do, you can use "smart strategies" to actually mold your child's food preferences and eating habits. These strategies work because they tap into the way children instinctively learn. You and your child become collaborators in healthy eating.

PROGRAMMING YOUR CHILD'S FUTURE FOOD PREFERENCES

Eating is one of life's great pleasures. When you introduce your child to healthy foods in the right ways, she learns to actually enjoy the foods that are best for her development and long-term good health.

Why should the foods your child enjoys now determine her future preferences? One reason lies in the way childhood memories are formed. Up to the age of about two and a half or three years, children do not form conscious memories, but instead are busy using their daily experiences to create the instinctive emotions and likes and dislikes that will become intuitive feelings in the future. So if your young child learns to enjoy vegetables for dinner every night and fresh fruit for dessert, she incorporates these healthy foods into her developing subconscious blueprint for what a proper meal should be. Not only does it taste good to her, it feels right, too. It nourishes her soul while feeding her small but growing body.

Many of us have unhealthy internal blueprints for what foods make us feel whole and content, and they dominate our lives more than we would like. When we crave the pies our mother made for us or overindulge in chocolate and cookies when we are stressed, we are living through the subconscious feelings about foods that were built up during our early years.

Your child doesn't have to develop these associations. With your help she need never learn to crave the items you want her to avoid. Instead, she'll have the kind of blueprint that makes her enjoy eating the foods that put her on the right track for a long and healthy life.

HOW THIS BOOK CAN HELP

Our book is designed in four parts to help you make the best possible feeding team with your child. In Part One you'll learn how science is redefining our knowledge of childhood food and feeding: the what, how, and why of nourishing your son or daughter. We urge you to read Part One even if you sometimes skip the theory section of books, because it has information you will find nowhere else. If you are pregnant or recently had your baby, you may want to read Part Two next, which will walk you through the essentials of breast milk and formula, and what to do if your baby was born early. If your child is older, Part Three will take you through all the food transitions from four months to six years and will explain how to prevent and treat common food-related problems as they arise. Part Four is devoted to concerns such as feeding a sick child, food-related allergies, weight gain, hyperactivity, and sleeping disorders.

Have confidence that you can do a great job. Your baby comes equipped not only to survive but to thrive with your help. The master plan for this seemingly enormous task is unfolding in every cell of her body. You're her guide and caregiver, and you too can learn everything you need to know. Our role is simply to help you do it in the best and easiest way possible.

CHAPTER 2

---◇---

Inside Your Child's Head

Why Children Eat the Way They Do—
Starting from Day One

*Jane has three girls between twelve months and ten years. The baby will eat
anything and has the glow and vitality that a healthy diet provides, but the
older two eat ice cream twice a day and get about 50 percent of their calories from this one food.*

*Four-year-old Mason will usually eat most things his mother cooks, but
only under the table, with his food passed down in bite-size servings.*

*Six-year-old Robert is picky to the last degree. At home, his mother gives him
whatever he will eat at that meal, and then cooks a proper meal for the rest of
the family. When Robert goes on play dates, he takes emergency rations from
home in case he gets hungry and there is nothing there he is prepared to eat.*

Why is it that so many infants eat anything, but then become fussy,
difficult eaters as they get older? The problem is so widespread as
to be considered normal. Almost everyone knows older children who
refuse vegetables and fruit, are too picky, don't eat enough or eat too
much, or want to snack instead of eating meals at regular times. Even families who appear to manage well are often cooking two dinners instead of
one, or dining nightly on pasta or pizza.

One thing Mel and I have learned from our work over the last twenty
years is that behavior problems over food are easier to prevent than to
cure. But you need to start early. If your baby is between one day and two
years old, there are surprisingly simple things you can do *now* to get feeding on the right track. If your child is older, the same techniques will also

help eliminate established difficulties, although you'll need some patience and persistence.

With your help, your child can learn to:

- Like healthy foods, and not prefer less healthy ones
- Self-regulate—or be in control of—his own caloric intake to maintain a healthy weight
- Be an adventurous eater who enjoys a wide range of foods
- Be a contented eater, comfortable with family meals and family favorites
- Eat an age-appropriate balance of meals and snacks

This chapter goes inside your child's head to explain why he thinks and behaves about food the way he does. You will then be ready to use the "smart strategies" detailed in Parts Two and Three to prevent common problems or fix them as they surface at each developmental age.

WHO NEEDS SMART STRATEGIES?

You've probably been told—as I was when I was pregnant—that infants left to their own devices will select an adequate diet. My well-meaning informant added that research studies had shown it. As it happens, that research was done seven decades ago, when much of the highly processed food of today didn't exist. Choices were fewer, to say the least. And while it is true that healthy children instinctively eat to satisfy their bodies' needs, there are two qualifiers:

- Nature has been bypassed by technology. We're not living in a world where healthy choices are the only choices. Your child is going to encounter potato chips, candy, ice cream, and fast foods, all containing the calories and other nutrients that his body recognizes as food. But his body doesn't automatically distinguish between a deep-fried potato chip with calories and little else, and a vitamin-packed stir-fry with vegetables, oil, and perhaps some chicken. That part is up to you.

- As we mentioned in Chapter 1, until quite recently in human history, the average man or woman lived to about forty years of age. Just about any food will keep us alive that long. What our bodies aren't equipped to do is automatically prefer the foods that will give us the best start in life and then *keep us healthy for eighty or a hundred years.* But those healthy preferences can be learned.

There's another theory you've probably heard: All parents have to do is provide healthy food at each meal, and children will eat that food if nothing else is available. Providing healthy food is certainly important but will not by itself create good eating habits. The army of parents who've tried the eat-it-or-leave-it approach and failed is testimony to the futility of the inevitable food stand-offs. It's just too hard to be tough all the time. When your nine-month-old wants only milk and refuses solid food, you're not going to let him go hungry. When your two-year-old says she isn't hungry for dinner and then asks for ice cream, you may not feel good about leaving her crying over a plate of carrots.

In any case, these scenarios miss the real point. What you really want is for your children to *like* healthy foods. Being starved into submission doesn't accomplish that and will often have the opposite effect. Leaving it all to chance is no better. To help your child rise above the tide of bad food influences and actually *enjoy* the healthy foods you want him to eat, you need to use strategies—smart strategies based on understanding why your child thinks and behaves about food the way he does.

BUILDING ON YOUR CHILD'S INSTINCTS

Eight powerful instincts related to food and feeding surface at different times between birth and three years of age. Working with these instincts from your child's earliest days will make her introduction to the world of healthful food both simple and enjoyable. No single instinct will be effective for every feeding issue, of course, or will even work on every day of the week! But that's okay. You have eight at your disposal, and when one doesn't help, another will.

1. YOUR CHILD'S BODY HAS A SAY, TOO. FROM THEIR FIRST DAYS OF LIFE, CHILDREN INSTINCTIVELY SEEK CONTROL OVER THEIR OWN LIVES

Imagine that a friend is spoon-feeding you. She gives you a huge spoonful of strange food, and before you have even swallowed it, she is trying to push another huge spoonful into your mouth. When you start to refuse, she attempts to push the spoon between your closed lips. You're revolted by the spoon and the food. Next mealtime, you decide you'd rather just skip it and stay hungry. Sounds grotesque? Many infants are fed in just this way.

Our bodies are certainly fallible when it comes to food—which is why you need to shape your child's tastes. But in some respects, our children's bodies know exactly what they need from the earliest days. The most striking example is appetite. Strong metabolic signals from the brain ensure that a healthy child will never willingly go short of calories. Her body knows precisely how much it needs to eat to gain weight properly.

Trying to fight these metabolic signals by overencouraging a baby to take solid food when she isn't hungry, or by refusing to feed her when she is ravenous (perhaps because it isn't dinnertime yet), is wrong for three reasons. First, it teaches her to ignore the very signals she will need in the future to prevent overeating and obesity. Second, even infants seem instinctively to want to control what goes into their mouths. If we ignore these powerful feelings, we risk losing the fight and setting up more battles for the future. Finally, being forced to eat things she doesn't want is a scary experience for a child. The likely result is that she'll develop aversions to precisely the foods you want her to like, and will become generally conservative about trying new foods in the future.

Between twenty-one months and two years this instinct becomes even more apparent: Your child wants to be assertive and do it herself. Why does this happen? Nobody knows for sure, but it is probably linked to our human drive for independence and achievement. Although it may be hard to believe now, the child who drives you crazy by refusing to eat the things you most want her to like may rise to future greatness through the same behavior—channeled into, say, art, cooking, or politics.

Whatever the reason, two-year-olds feel compelled to defy their parents, and will do it with any tools they can find. If you let them know there are battles to be fought and won over food, they will be delighted to engage you! And while it is true that your child definitely needs to find something to defy you about, there are much easier and less harmful opportunities than tantrums over what is for lunch or whether candy is okay at the dinner table.

What you can do: Right from day one, accept a division of control, and learn age-appropriate feeding skills. You, as an adult, are the only one who can make an informed choice about what foods are good to eat in general, and what particular foods are right for each meal and snack. Your child is the one with the biological signals that determine hunger, fullness, and whether a particular food looks and smells appealing. One key to growing a healthy eater, then, is to focus on getting healthy foods on the table that she can reasonably be expected to enjoy, and then—most important—letting your child feel in control of *how much* of those foods she eats.

As you get to know your infant, you will recognize that crying, fist chewing, and looking irritable are signs it ought to be lunchtime by now. Your older baby signals that she wants to continue eating by leaning forward, watching her bowl, and even opening her mouth for more when she has swallowed the last mouthful. As she starts to get full she will take smaller amounts off the spoon and will swallow more slowly. Finally she refuses to open her mouth, turns her head away, or lets the last spoonful dribble back out. Let her have the last say and you'll both be happier.

For a child of two to five years, loud demands for high-calorie snacks, irritability, or lethargy are all signs that the gas tank is low. When provided with food, she will start eating at a great rate, and her humor will usually improve as the food disappears. Conversely, some days she may not be hungry when a meal is ready, and picks at the pasta she usually likes. Maybe she is coming down with something, or perhaps she simply ate a larger afternoon snack than normal. Whatever the reason, give her a chance to change her mind while you eat your dinner, but don't insist she clean her plate or try to get her to eat "just a tiny piece" of chicken. Micromanaging can prompt future food refusals and fussiness at any age.

2. ONE-YEAR-OLDS ARE PROGRAMMED TO PUT EVERYTHING IN THEIR MOUTHS

Thirteen-month-old Darryl is busy eating while his mom and dad are clearing up from a New Year's Day brunch and chatting. Says his mother, "Darryl must have tried every single food on the table—I had no idea we would have such an adventurous eater. I'm not like that, and neither are you!"

Your newborn's sucking reflex gets him started on the milk he needs for early growth. A few months later he develops another important instinct that can be one of your best allies when it comes to food, although you may not have thought about it this way.

This instinct makes your little angel want to put *everything* in his mouth from about six months until about age two. Toys, coins, dirt . . . anything lying around is fair game. It may make you frazzled or irritable on occasion, but this determination to put everything in his mouth is most likely evolution at work, guaranteeing that he is able to make the essential transition to adult food.

What you can do: Exploit this special window of opportunity to introduce foods you want your child to like. Between twelve months, when your child can eat virtually any food you do, and twenty-one months to two years, when conservative instincts start to surface, your child can learn to enjoy almost any new food you offer. By the time he is two, he will have a repertoire of one hundred to two hundred healthy foods that he has learned to recognize, eat, and enjoy. It may be years before he is this adventurous and experimental again.

3. YOUR CHILD HAS A POWERFUL INSTINCT FOR VARIETY

Thirteen-month-old Aaron seems fussy. If he eats carrots today, he probably won't eat them tomorrow. Natalie, age five, eats lightly at mealtime and then demands huge snacks. What their frazzled parents don't realize is that these two different but common problems both stem from basically healthy impulses.

Most children older than about eight months instinctively seek variety unless discouraged by bad food experiences. They push their parents to provide variety by refusing to eat what they ate two days ago. This is a common source of irritation, but doesn't need to be if you understand what it's about.

You can think of this behavior as nature's way of making sure that your child's high needs for essential micronutrients are met. Almost any menu can supply enough calories and protein, but only a varied diet with a rotating supply of different vegetables, fruits, and protein sources can supply the right balance of vitamins, minerals, and phytochemicals needed for lifelong health.

If you watch your child's eating patterns, you'll find that fruits and vegetables are often consumed for interest after he's gotten his calories from denser foods containing more calories per ounce. Be patient. Don't assume that just because he ate the hamburger and potatoes first (foods denser in calories), he won't try the string beans. Given enough time at each meal, and a low-key atmosphere, most small children will regularly graze through a good proportion of the variety on the table.

What you can do: Make an ally of your child's variety instinct to mini-mize fussiness. Many food refusals are caused by boredom, and demands for less healthy foods may really be a plea for something different. So offer your child a varied and interesting selection of the foods you want him to like, and a very limited variety of the things you want to deemphasize. A different vegetable or two with dinner every night of the week encourages vegetables to disappear, while keeping only one brand of plain cookies in the house keeps an excessive cookie habit from forming.

A general rule of thumb: Plain staples such as milk, bread, and cereal, which are eaten for hunger and thirst, can be offered every day, but variety foods such as fruits, vegetables, entrees, and lunch dishes are better offered only every three to fourteen days. This doesn't mean that you can serve chicken or carrots only once a week. A little inventiveness makes a big difference. Tomatoes can be raw or cooked, potatoes baked or mashed, apples sliced or as applesauce, chicken as fingers or in a stir-fry. Change the appearance, taste, or texture and you have variety. Even something as simple as cutting toast into soft inner parts and crispy crusts will provide interest to a curious toddler.

Making sure that your children over one year have enough time at the table to get to the variety of foods is important, too. If your toddler never voluntarily stays still, a rule requiring that everyone sit at the table until the adults have finished their main course may be what you need.

The variety instinct also helps you balance meals and snacks. Most children are good at keeping their daily caloric intake constant. If they eat more at meals, they'll snack less. If you want your child to eat more dinner so that she doesn't need a snack before bed, try adding an extra food or two to the table. Research shows that, given variety, diners of all ages will amazingly manage to eat more. Conversely, keep snacks a moderate size by offering only one drink and one food—perhaps just a few crackers, some fruit, a small container of yogurt, or one kind of cookie—and see an excessive snacking habit drift back into balance. Of course, this principle can also work against us. Rich desserts provide variety without high-quality nutrients. And because they are so different from the rest of the foods typically offered at dinner, they appeal to the variety instinct more than, say, two kinds of lettuce in the salad.

What if your child doesn't seem to want any variety? Some children do get stuck in a rut, wanting the same few foods day in and day out. This conservatism is usually a temporary change between two and three years, but it can become entrenched if the child feels he is being forced into changing. As explained below and in Part Three, there are several good ways to help your child back to a more normal pattern of food without any battles or coercive dining.

Your child's variety instinct may also disappear when life becomes un-settling—for example, following the birth of a sibling, or when the family moves or there are marital problems. Under these circumstances, many children try to re-create some sense of security by insisting on eating the same thing every day. If this happens to your child, be understanding and loving but don't fall into the trap of giving in because you feel guilty. Hot dogs every day for dinner for a year after the birth of your second child or bologna sandwiches every day for six months after moving will do nobody a favor. Offer alternative ways to make life seem more settled while you nip developing food jags in the bud. All it will take is nicely making the problem food unavailable for two or three days every week while providing alternatives that you can reasonably expect your child will enjoy.

4. TWO-YEAR-OLDS ARE CAUTIOUS DINERS WITH A DEEP SUSPICION OF THE UNFAMILIAR (THE RULE OF FIFTEEN)

Two-year-old Anna will not eat green vegetables. Her mother has tried them all without success. When Anna is presented with a new vegetable to try, she peers at it, maybe she sniffs it—and then leaves it untouched on the plate. What should her mother do?

Counterbalancing the variety instinct and tremendous adventurousness of a nine- to twenty-one-month-old is an equally powerful and instinctive cautiousness that starts to show itself later, around two years. It can drive you crazy if you don't know why it's happening—and it may even make you give up on trying to introduce your child to foods you love and know are healthy choices.

But imagine yourself at age two in the long-ago past, when humans were hunter-gatherers. You are now able to move around independently, and perhaps you are encouraged to do so because your mother has a new baby on the way. While a small amount of something poisonous would probably not kill you, a whole meal might. A tendency to have a small taste of something several times before making a whole meal of it would enable you to find out which wild foods were good to eat while also minimizing the chance of fatal poisoning. Put in the context of our human ancestors, the cautiousness of a two-year-old makes perfect sense.

What you can do: Use the rule of fifteen and low-key persistence to introduce new foods. Working with this instinct means being patient—really patient—and offering a child who is two years or older a particular food *up to fifteen times* until it is accepted. Research has shown that it really does take this much repetition for many foods to be accepted as good to eat! Yes, there is some potential here for food waste, but kid portions are small, and if you eat it yourself, or freeze it for another meal, it needn't be a problem.

Don't try to offer the food in question at every meal. Let it go for three to fourteen days, then offer it again. It may be rejected again—and again—and *it is very important* that you treat it as no big deal. By all means say, "Okay, I'll eat it." But don't use bribery, threats, or active encouragement. At some point your child will suddenly, miraculously accept it, perhaps even eating a whole portion of it with gusto, without ever realizing that you wanted him to do so.

5. YOUR CHILD LEARNS BY COMPARISON: FOOD LIKES AND DISLIKES EXTEND TO FOODS THAT ARE SIMILAR

Monica loves green beans, and recently learned to love snow peas too! Is it a coincidence, or because they are similar?

Psychologists have shown that children, like adults, learn by comparing new experiences to their internal blueprint of familiar ones, and this is as true for foods as for other things in life. Appearance, taste, and texture are all things your baby or child notices when you give her a new food, and she compares them to her memories of foods she already knows. Thus she recognizes that roast chicken is similar to grilled chicken, but realizes immediately that spinach is very different. If she likes one food and you give her another that's similar, she's likely to enjoy the new food, too. By exploiting similarities, you increase your child's repertoire of healthy foods. This is an especially handy strategy for conservative two- and three-year-olds, but can be used with equal success for babies and older kids.

What you can do: Build a "bridge of familiarity" to speed acceptance of new foods. If your son already likes oranges, it won't take fifteen tries before he accepts tangerines. Toast with peanut butter and jelly is similar to toast with peanut butter and banana, which is similar to fruit salad with banana. Mashed sweet potatoes resemble mashed potatoes and cooked carrots. By moving from one food to a similar one, you can make introducing new foods much simpler.

You can also build a bridge of familiarity to rescue a difficult food for which there seems no hope. My daughter at eighteen months didn't like roast chicken, but I was unwilling to give up on such a family favorite. When the rule of fifteen didn't appear to be working, I switched to two other chicken dishes—nuggets and chicken with barbecue sauce. Success. At this point she suddenly decided to like all chicken dishes. Now my husband and I celebrate our victory each time we cut into a dinner of roast chicken—enjoyed by all!

6. YOUR CHILD LEARNS BY IMITATION. LONG BEFORE THEY CAN UNDERSTAND COMPLEX EXPLANATIONS, CHILDREN ARE COPYING OUR BEHAVIOR

Three-year-old Julia tries on her mother's dresses. She also watches what her mother eats. "I love milk," says Julia, "and water." "I love them, too," says her mother. This low-key encouragement tells Julia that she is making choices that are approved of, and are what her role model chooses for herself.

Children start mimicking their parents soon after birth, and they become startlingly precise observers of your likes and dislikes. Once your child reaches three years, she is also strongly influenced by her small friends. Learning by imitation is part of the social instinct we all share and is a good strategy—as the success of the human race demonstrates. It can work against you, but you can also use it to advantage.

What you can do: Be a good food model, and keep undesirable outside influences outside. When your nine-month-old sees you enjoying squash, she wants to do the same. The same is true for your two-and-a-half-year-old, although she is instinctively more conservative and may need to watch you a few more times before trying it.

What you don't eat at home is as important as what you do. When you keep candy out of the house, your child will never learn to crave it, even if you love it and eat it when you are at work. The day your five-year-old refuses the one food that is your major weakness, you will know that being a good role model has really paid off.

What you say and how you behave about food is also important. Kids learn to love virtually anything that they see their parents enjoy, from ants in some parts of Africa to raw fish in Japan and snails in France. It puts cauliflower in perspective!

When your child begins to emulate her peers, between three and four years, you can harness this powerful force for the good. The tomatoes and carrots she refused at home may well become favorites after she sees a friend eating them with enthusiasm, so try offering those items for a play-date snack or for lunch when the friend comes to visit.

Soaking up good influences and avoiding bad ones is not always possible, of course, and some patience will be needed when your preschooler learns to lick the frosting off birthday cupcakes after watching a small friend do the same thing. As she becomes more aware of the world around her, she may also try requesting unhealthy foods she's seen in commercials on TV.

If you take the position that it is okay for your child to try different things, and at the same time *keep outside influences outside,* you can keep a frosting habit in its rightful place—which is at other people's birthday parties. Or you can hold out successfully against chips at home because they are only eaten during a weekly trip to the pool. When you do this, you establish the important principle that home food is different from outside food. Children are remarkably place-specific in their food requests, which makes maintaining a healthy home menu much easier than it might sound.

7. CHILDREN INSTINCTIVELY RESIST PERSUASION AND ACTIVE ENCOURAGEMENT

Three-year-old Sarah was snacking happily on carrots in the kitchen. She paused to pick up her doll, and her baby-sitter immediately offered her another carrot, praising her for being such a good girl, eating something that was so good for her health. One minute later Sarah had quietly put down the carrot. She didn't eat another for more than two months.

Groucho Marx once remarked that he wouldn't want to be a member of a club that would have him as a member. Audiences laugh at that line because we all recognize the universal truth about human behavior—one that's been known to psychologists for decades. It's an aspect of the "discounting principle," where we instinctively think, "How great can this really be if they're selling it so hard?"

Even tiny kids respond this way. As much as they want to imitate what and how we eat, they'll learn to reject the very same foods if we actively encourage them—or use incentives or demands. Preferences for less-healthy foods are actually reinforced by pressure to eat healthy ones, coupled with the absence of pressure to eat the less-healthy ones. When was the last time you heard a parent urge a child to eat that last piece of chocolate, or finish up the candy?

What you can do: Don't use overt persuasion. Do offer food opportunities. Starting on day one, avoid trying to breast-feed or bottle-feed your baby when he is clearly not hungry. For a baby starting solid foods, giving food opportunities means offering spoonfuls without playing "airplanes" to get them into his mouth if he looks uninterested.

At twelve to eighteen months you can start verbalizing the opportunity, asking, "Would you like to try some salad?" If a particular opportunity is rejected, be relaxed about it: He'll be pleased to have similar opportunities later if he feels free to sometimes say no. Just don't actively encourage him ("What a good boy you are, finishing your salad—here, have some more") or resort to bribery or threats. Telling your child "You can have ice cream only if you finish your spinach" sends the clear message that dessert is nice and spinach is an unpleasant chore. Yes, the spinach may get eaten at this meal if the threat or bribe is strong enough, but over time he will come to hate it.

By the time your child is three or four you can also use a kind of reverse psychology derived from the discounting principle to encourage him to try things. Say you've given your three-year-old an omelet and peas and by the end of the meal the peas are still rolling around his plate. Tell him, "I'm glad you haven't eaten your peas, because I want them. Give them here!" Almost no preschooler can resist a challenge like this, and you may see the peas disappear in short order. Of course, you have to be prepared to follow through and eat them if he doesn't. Use this trick only occasionally, or it will lose its effectiveness.

If you are feeling bold, you can even try using the discounting principle to discourage foods you don't want your child to eat. One father we know inadvertently used it to put his daughter off ice cream—something few people would think possible. They were on a family vacation and he took her for a nostalgic trip to an ice cream parlor that had been a favorite of his twenty years ago. Arriving after a big dinner, he told her enthusiastically about the wonderful ice cream they were about to have. After only a few spoonfuls she said she'd had enough, and his disappointment showed: "Are you sure? It's so good. Have some more. Here, try some of mine." Next night the same thing happened—and excursions for ice cream have not been requested since.

8. CHILDREN ARE DRAWN TO FOODS THEY HELP GROW OR HARVEST

With fall in full swing, I bought an acorn squash. It was green, ridged, and heavy, and not very appetizing to look at. My daughter showed no curiosity about the squash, and I realized it had a slim chance of being welcomed at dinner. So I cut the squash in half and asked her if she would like to hear the story of how the squash grew. By the time I had moved from seeds to plants to flowers to squash, she was demanding seeds and raw squash to eat right then and there. It got eaten for dinner, too.

From the time they can walk and talk well, many children seem to like nothing better than helping grow things. They are thrilled to plant a seed, thrilled to see that it has come up, and thrilled to pick the crop when it is ready to eat. In fact, the concentration with which they zoom in on agricultural activities looks like instinctive behavior straight from our long-ago ancestors, who survived by hunting and gathering.

What you can do: Tap your child's hunter-gatherer instincts. From the time your child is about two years old, use her interest in growing things as a way to introduce her to foods she otherwise might not eat, especially vegetables. Gardening and even talking about items while shopping together at the supermarket are also valuable ways to make otherwise unglamorous foods interesting.

SMART STRATEGIES IN BRIEF

1. *Accept a division of control.* You control the foods, your child controls the amounts.

2. *Use your window of opportunity.* Between twelve and twenty-one months your child will learn to enjoy virtually any new food you offer.

3. *Exploit the variety principle.* You can help shape your child's appetite and preferences by the number and kinds of foods you offer.

4. *Understand the rule of fifteen.* Cautious two-year-olds may need to be offered a new food up to fifteen times before it is accepted.

5. *Use bridges of familiarity.* Introduce foods by moving smoothly from established favorites to similar but new items.

6. *Teach by example and keep outside influences outside.* Your child learns by imitating you.

7. *Forget persuasion.* Your child will learn to dislike any foods you push on her. Focus instead on offering food opportunities.

8. *Understand your hunter-gatherer.* Growing and gathering—or even shopping for—foods encourages consumption.

A FINAL WORD: FOOD IS ONE EXPRESSION— BUT NOT THE ONLY EXPRESSION—OF LOVE

Grace, a woman overweight all her life, was comforted with food instead of love from the earliest age. She never succeeds in dieting because whenever she starts she feels so deprived that she turns to the very comfort—food— that made her overweight in the first place.

Certainly you show your love for your child by feeding him, from his first helpless days onward. He rightly feels loved when you feed him. And food in itself is a powerful source of pleasure and satisfaction. What it should not be is a *substitute* for love, comfort, physical contact, affection, play, and all your child's other needs. Breast-feeding a fretful baby who is not hungry or giving a toddler a lollipop as a treat after dinner are just two of many ways we may inadvertently teach our children to eat when they don't need to. If this happens repeatedly, then our children learn to turn to food—instead of to us—when they need to feel comforted, loved, or joyful. Then they may be at increased risk for obesity, eating disorders, and a host of emotional problems.

At the other extreme, families who don't eat together, who rarely sit down to a well-cooked and relaxed meal, or who bolt their food and rush from the table are sending a message that food is merely for stemming hunger and for nothing else. Apart from the fact that it is terribly hard to get children to eat vegetables and fruits when they eat in this way, they also miss out on the emotional connection to food that we all instinctively need. Enjoyable meals eaten with family and friends do satisfy our souls. And if we don't get this soul nourishment, we may end up eating more calories than we need to get the satisfaction we instinctively crave.

So our final smart strategy is to keep food and life in balance. Later in the book we'll talk more about how to make mealtimes and snack times enjoyable—and about how to avoid using food as a substitute for comfort, love, or attention. Learning how to read your baby's emotional needs actually goes hand in hand with learning to feed him. Sometimes he needs a cuddle or a story; sometimes he needs a snack. Recognizing the difference is a skill you can learn to help your growing child keep food in a healthy perspective.

CHAPTER 3

⸻ ✦ ⸻

The Key Eight Nutrients

A mother tells me that her lively eighteen-month-old boy craves "bad" foods. When I sympathize and inquire what these bad foods are, I find that the child wants foods containing large amounts of fat—in cream cheese, peanut butter, and so on—so much that he desperately tries to eat them straight from the tub or jar! This goes against all the nutritional principles that his mother has ever learned. On questioning her further, I learn that household meals are low in fat. No butter or oil is used at the table. Very little is used in cooking. Salads are made with no-fat dressing, and desserts aren't ever on the menu. The family also consumes a good amount of fiber and no red meat. Their diet is, in fact, exactly what is considered healthy for most adults.

Their little boy, however, is nutritionally deprived. Children have very different nutritional needs than adults. What this child is doing, then, is craving the very foods that give him the fat he is lacking from his regular diet and which his growing body and developing brain critically need.

During most well-baby visits, your doctor will measure your child's weight, height, and head circumference, and maybe ask about whether he is eating basic foods—breast milk or formula at first, and later pasta, bread, or cereals. If the answer is yes, and growth is normal, you will probably be told everything is fine. Good doctors provide this important reassurance because they know that relaxed, confident grown-ups make the best parents.

There is, however, increasing recognition that the traditional ways of assessing a child's development just don't go far enough. There are so many aspects of health and development that are influenced by what your child eats but can't be seen with a scale and tape measure. As your baby gains in pounds and inches, her brain is developing in subtle ways that determine

THE KEY EIGHT

BASIC NUTRIENTS

1. Fat
2. Fiber
3. Calories

MINERALS

4. Iron
5. Calcium
6. Zinc

VITAMINS

7. Folate and related B
   vitamins
8. The antioxidants:
   vitamins A, C, and E

future IQ, motor development, and even personality. Her immune system is maturing and will influence her susceptibility to infections, diabetes, and cancer. Not only are her bones and muscles growing longer, but their eventual strength is being determined. All these essential developmental processes and more need nutrients—the right ones in the right amounts.

For this reason, knowing that your child is eating a healthy balance of nutrients is as important as knowing what her weight is. Fortunately, there are only eight major nutrients or nutrient groups that you really need to focus on when it comes to giving your children the best start. That's because:

- In most cases, these eight nutrients are the ones that have the biggest impact on metabolic programming.

- Some are in short supply in today's society. This is true even in the most affluent households.

- If your child is getting enough of the key eight, most likely she is getting enough of all the other essential nutrients, because the same foods that supply the eight also tend to supply the others.

You may be surprised not to find protein on the list of essentials. Protein is essential for growth and development, of course, but if your child's needs for the key eight are being met on a daily basis with foods including at least 16 ounces of milk or formula, and regular servings of bread and cereals, you can be confident he will also be getting at least 130 percent of the Recommended Dietary Allowance for protein for his age. Similarly, if he is getting the recommended amount for iron, zinc, and the antioxidant vitamins, he will likely also be getting enough magnesium, potassium, and trace minerals.

Keep in mind that we *won't* be asking you to keep every RDA (Recommended Dietary Allowance) or the new DRIs (Dietary Reference Intakes, used where available) in your head, or to calculate how many milligrams of selenium or molybdenum your child ate today. As busy parents ourselves, we know that *portion goals* for basic foods are much more useful when it comes to keeping a child's intake on track, and these will be used in the remainder of the book.

FAT, FIBER, AND CALORIES

FAT

Fat Recommendations (in percentage of calories in daily diet)

Under 6 months	50%
6–12 months	40%
1–2 years	35%
2–3 years	30–35%
3–6 years	30%
Adult	Less than 30%

This is the recommendation most likely to startle new parents. A newborn's requirement for 50 percent of calories from dietary fat is in distinct contrast to adult nutritional needs. Most adults are told to consume only 20 to 30 percent of their calories in the form of fats. In the widely recommended USDA Food Guide Pyramid, fat provides only about 18 percent of calories. But most nutrition experts agree that a low-fat diet of this kind is *harmful* for infants and young children.

Dietary fats provide the concentrated calories that are essential for normal infant growth during infancy and up to age three. They also provide fatty acids, the building blocks needed for critical metabolic programming of brain growth and development. The many kinds of fatty acids in each fat determine the fat's unique properties, such as being liquid or solid at room temperature.

Fat and Brain Development
Babies' brains undergo astounding growth in the first year of life. The brain is 60 percent fat by weight, and most brain tissue is formed after birth. A newborn starts out with only 30 percent of the number of brain cells he'll possess as an adult, and yet he has fully 90 percent by 12 months of age and 95 percent by 18 months—a fact that emphasizes the particular importance of early fat consumption. Simultaneously, another critical

process called myelination is taking place, in which new brain cells, and other nerve cells throughout the body, are coated with a fatty myelin sheath. This allows the transmission of essential electrical and chemical messages between different parts of the brain and body.

It is this combination of an increase in brain cell number, growth in brain cell size, and myelination, fueled by dietary fat, that leads to the developmental stages that parents are so delighted to witness. Being able to consciously grasp objects of interest at five months, having hands and eyes that work together to make self-feeding possible, and crawling soon afterward are just a few of the many skills that proud parents watch for in the first year of life. Brain growth continues up until about age three, when an essentially adult brain emerges from the whirlwind of developmental stages.

Does it matter where the necessary fat comes from? Most certainly yes. Breast milk is a critically important food for babies because it contains not only the right amount of fat, but also the right kinds. In particular, it supplies the essential fatty acids linoleic acid and alpha-linolenic acid, which are the primary building blocks for new brain growth and myelination. Apart from breast milk, the only good sources of linoleic acid are formula, vegetable oils, nuts, seeds, and foods made with these ingredients. This is one of the reasons why whole cow's milk is not recommended during the first year of life: It contains only a *fifth* of the linoleic acid of equivalent amounts of breast milk or formula. Breast milk also contains many other fatty acids (more than 160 in all) whose functions are still uncertain but which may well be identified by future research as important in brain development.

After your baby is one year old, there are easy ways to ensure that he continues to get the essential fatty acids he needs in foods that are healthy for the whole family. Cooking not with butter and margarine but with vegetable oils such as canola, which contain essential fatty acids, is one easy way. Keeping several vegetable oils in your kitchen is good because each contains different valuable fatty acids. Whole milk and other whole-milk dairy products are also valuable after one year because they contain alpha-linolenic acid, even if they are low in linoleic acid.

Foods containing trans fatty acids, such as margarine and shortening and baked goods made with them, should be avoided for babies under twelve months of age. Trans fatty acids (which are produced when liquid vegetable oils are partially hydrogenated to form solid margarine and shortening) are bad news for babies because they inhibit the interconversion of fatty acids essential for normal brain growth and so theoretically may impair or delay essential developmental processes.

Different Ages, Different Needs

Jimmy's pediatrician referred him to the gastroenterology clinic when he was just three years old, to see why his height and weight had fallen steadily from the 50th centile at birth to their current position on the 5th centile. The problem was eventually tracked to his diet. The combination of a very low-fat, high-fiber diet (the whole family was careful because Jimmy's dad had high cholesterol) and Jimmy's fussy eating habits was keeping Jimmy from getting the calories and essential nutrients he needed for normal growth and development.

Although your child's total fat needs decrease as he gets older, as brain development nears completion and the rate of growth slows down, it is important to make sure that he continues to get enough fat to fuel remaining growth and development.

A decrease in fat intake happens naturally as solid foods are introduced. Baby cereals and fruit and vegetable purees, the foods infants try first, are so low in fat that they cause the overall dietary fat percentage to drop. By about one year, after the transition is made to a diet of 16 to 24 ounces of whole milk and a modest amount of solid food, most babies will appropriately be eating a diet that provides about 35 to 40 percent of calories as fat. This amount can continue until about two years. At two years, you can switch from whole milk to 2 percent milk, and restrict eggs to three per week. These two changes alone will bring the fat content of your child's diet down to the 30 to 35 percent that is best for this age. By three years of age, changing to 1 percent milk or skim milk will reduce your child's fat intake to a level that can stay with him throughout his childhood.

If the family diet is very low in fat, can the extra fat needed by children be supplied with butter, margarine, ice cream, and cake? No, because even after eighteen months, when brain development is less of an issue, these foods contain large amounts of saturated fat or trans fatty acids without the benefit of valuable nutrients (such as calcium in milk and cheese). The fatty arterial plaques that accumulate when saturated fat is consumed in excess, eventually culminating in adult-onset heart disease, have been found in children as young as eight and undoubtedly start developing at a much earlier age. Trans fatty acids are thought to have a similar (and perhaps stronger) effect on arteries and so should be consumed only in moderate amounts.

You can prevent cumulative artery damage from starting by preparing family meals that are generally low in saturated fat and trans fatty acids, and using smart strategies to ensure that your child learns to enjoy eating them while not especially enjoying unhealthier options. Milk with the right amount of fat for your child's developmental age, combined with home-cooked meals containing lean meats, poultry, eggs, modest amounts of cheese, oils such as canola, corn, or olive, and spreads such as hummus and peanut butter (the kind without added "partially hydrogenated vegetable oils") will give your child the good fats in a healthy amount and plenty of other essential nutrients, without an excess of saturated fat or trans fatty acids. This plan, with a substitution of skim milk for whole or low-fat milk, is also healthy for you. Parents certainly don't have to compromise their own health to feed their child the best diet.

FIBER

Fiber Recommendations

Under 1 year	no recommendation
1–3 years	5–8 g
4–6 years	9–11 g
Adult	25–30 g

Many parents who have tried, without success, to get their child to eat whole-wheat bread are surprised to learn that children actually don't need large amounts of fiber—and their child is being constructively selective, rather than picky, in the foods she chooses or rejects. Fiber, also called roughage, helps digestive function and prevents constipation by providing the bulk needed to keep waste moving down the gastrointestinal tract. The bulk also helps prevent overeating. In addition, fiber is thought to reduce the risk of colon cancer and adult-onset diabetes.

Most people assume that fiber is indigestible. This is actually not the case. Although the human gastrointestinal tract does not possess enzymes to break fiber down into digestible subunits (as it does for carbohydrates, fats, and proteins), we do possess intestinal bacteria that do the job for us. In adults, about 75 percent of dietary fiber gets fermented into fatty acids by a complex colony of more than four hundred types of bacteria living in the lower intestine. Only undigested fiber and waste products are excreted. The fatty acids are taken up by the body to be used for energy. This energy probably contributes to the satiating effects of fiber, along with the increased sense of fullness that fiber gives. However, fiber is considered to contain no calories, because the calories provided by the fermented fatty acids are about equal to the fat calories that fiber traps in the intestine, making it unavailable for digestion.

Fiber is good for adults for all these reasons, but it has notable drawbacks for children. Newborns actually don't need any fiber at all. We know this because breast milk—the most perfect food for babies—contains no fiber and yet doesn't cause constipation! If newborns were given highly fibrous foods, either they would suffer from gastrointestinal distress or the foods would simply pass through unfermented. Babies gradually acquire their intestinal bacteria during the first two years of life, and until that time they lack the stable balance of the right kinds of bacteria that they need for full fiber processing. This is part of the explanation for why you may see undigested kernels of corn pass right through into your toddler's diaper. It may also explain why she is more susceptible to food-borne bacterial contamination: She lacks the buffering effects of friendly bacteria in the gut. In large amounts, and if coupled with a low-fat diet, fiber may also keep children from consuming the calories they need for activity and growth. It can also capture important micronutrients such as iron, zinc, and calcium in the intestine, reducing the amounts that are absorbed.

For these reasons, fiber recommendations for infants and young children are considerably lower than for adults. The equation most experts use to calculate a healthy fiber intake for children is *years* + 5 *grams* per day. So a three-year-old needs 8 grams daily and a five-year-old needs 5+5 = 10 grams. The daily fiber recommendation for adults, in contrast, is much higher, at 25 to 30 grams.

Making sure that your child has enough fiber is actually quite simple. For children over two years of age, ³/₄ to 1¹/₂ cups of mixed fruits and vegetables per day will make a good start in providing what is needed in a form she will enjoy. High-fiber whole-grain breads and cereals should certainly be introduced for additional fiber, enjoyment, variety, and to shape future food preferences. However, they are not needed in large amounts to make up a daily fiber requirement before age four or five years, provided that your child eats fresh fruits and vegetables (which are also important for other nutrients) in the recommended amounts.

So don't be dismayed if your two-year-old rejects the high-fiber whole-wheat bread you like for lunch in favor of squishy store-bought white. She may just be avoiding foods that her body doesn't need now, or that actively reduce her ability to eat enough calories. You'll have more success getting her to like whole wheat if you start by offering bread made from a mixture of white and whole-wheat flours, or even serving white-bread sandwiches on a regular basis and small portions of whole wheat as a "special treat" toasted with honey. You may find she grows to love your bread this way.

You can also try offering higher-fiber foods regularly, but if you do this, make sure that each individual item is not low in calories (for example, avoid the cereals containing *mostly* bran) so that your child doesn't go hungry in the process. By the time she reaches about age three and her body is ready for higher-fiber items, you may be surprised to see how easily she takes to exclusive use of items she previously rejected.

Constipation is one of the few reasons that you may need to be particularly conscious of fiber. Ways to increase fiber intake in a susceptible child are described in Part Three, along with nonfiber treatments that can often be effective when fiber intake is already adequate.

CALORIES

Greg's mother worried that her son wasn't eating enough. At thirteen months, he was showing good growth but taking very little solid food on top of his four 8-ounce bottles of milk a day. When his mom wrote out a list showing a typical day's food for her son, it did appear to be much less than recommended in most parenting books. Only when we told her that the old estimates of calorie needs are inaccurate and far too high did she stop worrying, reduce his milk a little, and concentrate on the important job for this age of introducing small portions of a wide range of adult foods.

In our experience, parents of young children tend to be more concerned about calories than any other nutrient. Sometimes they worry that their child is eating too many, but more typically, like Greg's mother, they worry about him not eating enough.

Calories are actually a measure of energy and are found in all foods, especially those with a high proportion of carbohydrates or fat. They are essential for daily activity, for healthy growth, and for maintaining normal metabolic functions in the body. However, one of the important recent discoveries in nutrition research is that most infants and children up to at least age three grow normally, and avoid obesity, on approximately 15 percent fewer calories than experts used to recommend.

This new information on calorie needs comes from new research methods. Calorie requirements used to be calculated from records of what infants ate. But as every parent can well imagine, distinguishing between exactly how much gets eaten and how much is left on the floor, the plate, or the high chair is a problem. Researchers can now measure the calories that are used metabolically by infants and children instead of having to rely on individually kept food records.

Typical Calorie Needs of Infants and Children

	OLD RECOMMENDATION	WHAT CHILDREN ACTUALLY NEED (AVERAGE)	(RANGE)
3 mos.	640 calories	550	400–700
1 year	1,050	850	550–1,100
2 years	1,250	1,050	700–1,400
3 years	1,500	1,250	850–1,650
6 years	1,800	1,550	1,000–2,050

This new knowledge goes a long way to explain the discrepancy that has worried so many parents and grandparents. Judged by the old calorie and meal estimates, their children did seem to be eating like birds. We now know that the calorie standards were the problem. Many children simply do not need that much food, and trying to make them eat it is a prescription for behavior problems and possible overeating.

Suppose your one-year-old usually has about a pint (16 ounces) of milk a day, one slice of bread with peanut butter, ¼ cup of cereal, and ¾ cup total of fruits and vegetables. If you compare this to meal plans in most parenting books, it will look like a pitifully small amount. But if you know that it is within the new definition of the normal range, you can relax— and you can more easily avoid the pitfall of overencouragement and the resulting problems of fussy eating and resistance.

Your child's individual calorie needs depend on his size, activity level, and temperament (calm versus excitable); there will also be substantial daily variations. Growth spurts can make your child seem constantly hungry for a few days, while hot weather or a minor illness may turn a big eater into one who picks at everything.

THREE ESSENTIAL MINERALS: IRON, CALCIUM, AND ZINC

Recent diet surveys have reported that more than 50 percent of children in the United States consume inadequate amounts of one or more of these three crucial minerals. This is one of the major public health problems of our time. Virtually all children are at risk, both affluent and poor alike. Surprising? The reason is that these minerals can be hard to get in adequate amounts without knowledge of the best food sources plus some smart strategies for making sure those foods get consumed. And they really matter. Even mild shortages of these essential three can have serious long-term consequences.

IRON

Alex, eighteen months, is brought to his pediatrician for a checkup. Although he is growing normally, he seems pale, and a blood test reveals severe anemia. The problem, it turns out, can be traced to milk. Alex loves drinking milk and has been drinking five or six bottles a day, with very little solid food, since he was switched to whole cow's milk at one year. A multivitamin/mineral supplement, combined with a decrease in milk intake and an increase in solid foods, resolves Alex's problem in a short while. But his parents are left wishing they had been told more about iron before their son got to the point of anemia.

Iron RDAs

Under 1 year	6–10 mg
1–3 years	10 mg
4–6 years	10 mg
Adult	10–15 mg

All minerals are important for your child's healthy growth, but iron is perhaps the most important of all. Iron is needed by children in quite large amounts relative to body size. It is used in many of the body's enzyme systems and is an essential part of hemoglobin, the protein in red blood cells that transports life-sustaining oxygen around the body. It is also essential for the myelination of delicate nerve cells within the brain and throughout the body during the first two years of life. Without adequate iron levels throughout early childhood, the brain may not get enough iron to ensure normal growth of critical areas. As documented in several recent studies, persistent iron deficiency can cause permanent damage to mental and motor functions, resulting in a measurably decreased IQ throughout childhood (4 IQ points in one study), lower scores on general developmental tests, poor attention span, and aberrant social behavior.

Although many common foods are fortified with iron, including baby cereals, iron deficiency is common in the United States. Surveys suggest that about one in seven of all young children has anemia—the clinical result of iron deficiency. Why is this? Partly, we think, it is because many parents aren't aware of how important iron is, and thus don't monitor their child's intake of this nutrient.

Until they are about six months old, breast-fed babies don't need much iron. They are born with substantial stores in their liver, provided by the mother during pregnancy, and breast milk can supply the necessary balance. Even though breast milk contains very little iron, it is in a form that is taken up by the body very efficiently. Babies fed formula also do fine provided the formula is fortified. Although more iron is excreted when formula is consumed (because iron in formula is poorly absorbed), fortified formulas contain extra iron to make up the difference. However, when infants are switched at one year from formula containing iron to whole cow's milk, which contains virtually no iron, they need a really good dietary iron source or a multivitamin/mineral supplement in order to meet their daily iron needs.

This is where the trouble often begins. Many pediatricians do not recommend multivitamin/mineral supplements, even though they are valuable at this age. And many parents come to rely more heavily on milk than is truly healthy. Children like Alex need to be restricted to between 16 and 24 ounces of milk daily so they can consume other foods that give them an overall better balance of nutrients.

There is another reason why iron deficiency happens in nutrition-conscious families today. Two of the best natural food sources of iron are red meat and eggs, which many of us are eating less of than in years gone by. Fortunately, you don't have to feed your child red meat and eggs every day to prevent iron deficiency, because fortified foods or a supplement will do the job just as well. But bear in mind that children often seem to like the foods that supply the nutrients they critically need. So keep an open mind about all the options on our iron-rich list, even sardines and spinach!

GOOD SOURCES OF IRON

- Lean beef
- Lamb
- Eggs
- Sardines
- Fortified cereals
- Fortified baby cereals
- Spinach and other dark green leafy vegetables
- Wheat germ
- Fortified breads
- Egg noodles
- Beans
- Peas
- Dried apricots

In addition to keeping high-iron foods on your shopping list, you can plan menus to maximize the usefulness of the iron your child eats. Once she gets to one or two years and no longer needs milk with every meal, separate dairy and high-iron foods into different meals, and offer your child fruit or fruit juice whenever high-iron foods are on the menu.

The reason for this is that not all the iron a child eats is absorbed. In fact, the dietary recommendation of 10 mg is made with the expectation that only about 10 percent will actually be available to the body. Vitamin C in fruits aids iron absorption by keeping the iron soluble. Milk and dairy products, on the other hand, have been shown to decrease iron absorption by as much as 30 to 50 percent.

If, like most families, you tend to eat meat at dinner but rarely with breakfast or snacks, you'll get your best return on your iron investment if you give your child milk or yogurt with breakfast and snacks, but not with dinner. Lunch can go either way, depending on what is on the menu. You don't have to be fanatical about this separation, especially since not all studies confirm the results reported above. If your child wants a piece of cheese with today's egg-salad sandwich, go ahead and let her enjoy it. But by making a general schedule that provides for some separation, you potentially give her a health boost.

It's interesting to note that Jewish scholars in the third and fourth centuries made strict dietary laws dictating the separation of milk and meat, which many religious Jews continue to honor when they keep kosher. Whatever the origin of the dietary law, the weight of scientific evidence suggests that the separation was an excellent idea.

CAUTION: IRON EXCESS IS DANGEROUS

With iron, as with so many good things, it's important to know that too much is as harmful as too little. It is almost impossible to get too much iron from regular foods, even fortified ones. Supplements, however, are a different story. Children's multivitamins containing iron are considered safe, and indeed recommended. But supplements containing only iron *should never be given to children* unless prescribed by their pediatrician for a specific problem. You should also keep any supplements that contain iron out of children's reach. Accidental ingestion of iron supplements is the leading cause of poisoning in young children in the United States.

CALCIUM

Emily, age four, won't drink much milk. Her mother says she spends all day trying to get an ounce consumed here and there, and adds skim milk powder to many of her recipes. Even so, Emily only consumes the equivalent of about 8 ounces of milk daily. With Emily's body at its peak for absorbing calcium from now through late adolescence, Emily's parents can focus on diversifying their food sources of calcium and using some smart strategies to make sure they are consumed and enjoyed.

Calcium DRIs

Under 1 year	270 mg
1–3 years	500 mg
4–6 years	800 mg
Adult	800–1,200 mg

Calcium is familiar for its role in making strong bones and teeth. But what many people don't realize is that the essential calcium deposits in bones and teeth occur almost *entirely* during childhood and adolescence. After that time, calcium is gradually lost. A child who doesn't get enough calcium may suffer no ill effects for forty years, but then may be diagnosed with osteoporosis or suffer tooth loss, and treatment is extremely difficult.

I myself was made uncomfortably aware of this fact when I was twenty-five. A researcher friend offered to test me with her new machine for measuring bone density, and I found to my horror that my bones were far on the weak side of normal. Looking back, it was clear that not drinking milk as a child was a precipitating factor. I had disliked whole milk (the only kind kept in our house) so much that I even got my mother to write a note to school saying that I never had to drink it. In retrospect, it would have been better if my mother had tried different milk products to find one that I liked, rather than pushing me to drink whole milk and then giving in when I refused. Now I like skim milk, cheese, and yogurt but still don't care for the whole milk I developed such an aversion to nearly forty years ago.

The body's use of calcium is a perfect example of metabolic programming. It is part of a vital growth process that we cannot see in our babies and children but which can have a huge impact on their later health. Current expert opinion is that children over one year of age need at least 500 mg of cal-

GOOD SOURCES OF CALCIUM

- Milk
- Yogurt
- Calcium-fortified juice
- Cheese
- Frozen yogurt
- Canned sardines
- Broccoli, kale, and other dark green vegetables
- Tofu

cium daily, and up to as much as 800 mg to grow the best bones and teeth, which is about the same amount that their mothers and fathers also need.

Providing your child with the recommended daily amount is generally not difficult. Just 12 ounces of milk daily will provide your one-year-old with most of the calcium she needs, and 16 to 24 ounces will also ensure other important nutrients such as protein. There are also other rich sources of calcium that children enjoy, including yogurt and cheese. If for some reason your child won't eat dairy foods, you can also use some fortified juice to help make up the difference, but be sure your child also gets enough protein and vitamin D, which dairy products supply but orange juice doesn't. Using a calcium supplement is also an option, as described in Chapter 11 (pages 202–203).

If you want to give your child's bones a further boost, there are two things you can do. First, encourage her to be physically active. Calcium deposition in bones is determined not only by how much calcium is eaten, but also by weight-bearing activity, such as walking, running, jumping, or dancing. The pressure these activities put on bones sends a local signal to the bone cells to pull in additional calcium from the bloodstream, and in this way causes a valuable increase in bone strength. The other thing you can do is make sure your child eats the recommended amounts of fruits and vegetables and avoids very salty foods. The combination of plentiful potassium from produce and avoidance of excess sodium promotes additional calcium availability for bone strengthening.

ZINC

Zinc RDAs

Under 1 year	5 mg
1–3 years	10 mg
4–6 years	10 mg
Adult	12–19 mg

Many scientists believe that zinc deficiency may be one of the most common hidden health problems in children today because, unlike iron deficiency, zinc is not something pediatricians routinely test for. Things that can't readily be measured in a doctor's office are all too easily put on the back burner.

Why is zinc so important? Zinc has had a lot of press lately for its purported ability to strengthen the immune system and help prevent or reduce the severity of the common cold. But where this otherwise relatively little-known mineral really stars is in the many enzyme processes that speed up or slow down metabolism. Zinc is an essential partner to more than two hundred of these enzymes. It is especially responsible for controlling the cell division, growth, and protein synthesis that occur only during childhood. Too little zinc will stop a child from growing. If the deficiency persists, it will cause permanent stunting.

Zinc deficiency does not have to be very severe for growth impairment to be seen. Intakes of 6 to 7 mg per day, instead of the RDA of 10 mg for young children, have been linked to deficiency signs. Low intakes are common not only in poor communities but also among children in affluent families.

Why is zinc often low in children's diets? For a start, there is no single good source of zinc that parents can give their child every day—and children's multivitamin/mineral supplements for age two and under don't even contain zinc. Even the best food sources for zinc supply only about 10 percent of the daily allowance when a child-size portion is eaten. Two of the best sources are red meat and egg yolks, which many nutrition-conscious families are limiting. This, plus the fact that many common kid foods (including fruits and vegetables and many refined grain foods) contain virtually no zinc, means that some careful zinc accounting needs to be done to meet your child's needs by food alone.

You might think it is strange that humans have evolved to need a nutrient that is difficult to get in adequate amounts. In fact, nutritional historians estimate that Paleolithic hunter-gatherers consumed about four times as much zinc as the RDA, with red meat being a major source (and making up a third of the total weight of consumed food!). All that red meat may have been fine for them, but not for us. With their average lifespan of only forty, they died before they acquired the late-life degenerative diseases that excessive red meat fosters.

Breast milk and formula contain zinc, so infants under six months

BEST SOURCES OF ZINC

- Lean beef
- Lamb
- Turkey
- Dark chicken meat
- Egg yolk
- Yogurt
- Milk
- Hard cheese
- Peanut butter
- Fortified cereals
- Whole-wheat bread
- Beans
- Yellow wax beans
- Peas

manage well without any additional help. After six months, the zinc content of breast milk decreases, and weaning foods or supplemental formula are needed to provide additional necessary zinc to breast-fed babies. After twelve months, zinc intake falls off in the switch from breast milk or formula to cow's milk, and a varied diet coupled with a multivitamin/mineral supplement is the best way to prevent a slowing of height gain resulting from subclinical zinc deficiency.

As with other nutrients, too much zinc is harmful—in particular, it prevents essential copper from being absorbed from the diet and so encourages a different micronutrient deficiency. Supplements other than the daily multivitamin/mineral kind should never be given to children unless prescribed by a pediatrician.

FOLATE AND B VITAMINS (B$_6$ AND B$_{12}$)

B Vitamin DRIs

	FOLATE	B$_6$	B$_{12}$
Under 1 year	65–80 mcg	0.1–0.3 mg	0.4–0.5 mcg
1–3 years	150 mcg	0.5 mg	0.9 mcg
4–6 years	200 mcg	0.6 mg	1.2 mcg
Adult	400–600 mcg	1.3–2.0 mg	2.4–2.8 mcg

As recently as the late 1970s, the B vitamins were considered pretty ho-hum even among students and teachers of nutrition. If you didn't have enough, we learned, you showed classic deficiencies such as beriberi, but this happened only in Third World countries.

Since then, however, it has been discovered that the B vitamins—particularly folate (also called folic acid), but also B$_6$ (pyridoxine) and vitamin

B_{12} (cobalamin)—prevent the buildup in the body of a harmful chemical known as homocysteine. Homocysteine has been linked to heart disease and strokes because of its suspected role in increasing arterial plaque, and to colon cancer for reasons as yet unknown. In effect, folate and other B vitamins are now thought to help prevent heart disease and colon cancer. Especially if you have a family history of these problems, now is the best time for both your child and you to start eating for lifelong prevention.

Folate has other important functions, too. As you were probably told when you were expecting your baby, it prevents neural tube defects if taken before conception and during very early pregnancy. Folate also plays a role in the myelination of brain cells in the first months of life, making it another powerful promoter of good development.

Folate and the other B vitamins are not hard to find. They're natural components of lots of different foods that are probably already part of your diet. In addition, flour manufactured in the United States and all products made with it, including bread and pasta, are now fortified with folate. This vitamin complex is at the heart of a good diet, and, as the gatekeeper of the foods in your family's house, you can do a lot to make sure the B vitamins are on the table in abundance.

One valuable source of folate that you may not be aware of is Marmite, a vegetarian yeast-based spread that is delicious, even though it doesn't look it! Long popular with children in England and Canada

GOOD SOURCES OF FOLATE

- Spinach
- Beans
- Bread
- Oranges and orange juice
- Marmite
- Broccoli
- Dark green lettuce

GOOD SOURCES OF B_6

- Eggs
- Milk
- Oatmeal
- Bananas
- Avocados
- Chicken
- Beef
- Fish
- Wheat germ
- Prunes

GOOD SOURCES OF B_{12}

- Milk
- Peanut butter
- Beef
- Chicken
- Fish
- Eggs
- Cheese

(it was a childhood favorite of mine), it is increasingly found in U.S. supermarkets and health food stores. This vitamin-packed product contains more than 30 percent of the children's daily requirement for folate in just ¼ teaspoon (the perfect amount for a small slice of fresh bread).

ANTIOXIDANTS: VITAMINS A, C, AND E

Five-year-old Johnny won't eat any vegetables except potatoes. His mother worries, but his grandmother insists that everything will be fine. "His father never ate anything green the whole time he lived at home," she says, "and he's certainly okay now. No child ever starved himself, and you don't need to fuss about Johnny!"

RDAs for Vitamins A, C, and E

	VITAMIN A	VITAMIN C	VITAMIN E
Under 1 year	375 mcg RE[1]	30–35 mg	3–4 mg
1–3 years	400 mcg RE[1]	40 mg	6 mg
4–6 years	500 mcg RE[1]	45 mg	7 mg
Adult	800–1,300 mcg RE[1]	60–95 mg	8–12 mg

[1] RE, retinol equivalents, the measurement used for vitamin A.

Contrary to the advice of well-meaning friends and relatives, we now know that the aging process starts very early in life, and many scientists believe it begins in our DNA, the vital component of every cell that carries the genetic code and directs what proteins and hormones are to be synthesized and how much of them. When there is DNA damage, one effect is susceptibility to a range of cancers. Research suggests the antioxidants actually prevent damage to the DNA, in particular damage from molecules known as free radicals. Because free-radical damage to DNA starts early in life and is cumulative over time, we can decrease our children's risk of cancer by promoting adequate consumption of foods containing these vitamins starting at four to six months, when solids are first introduced.

You probably know where to find vitamins C and A (or its dietary precursor, beta carotene): in fruits and vegetables. Unfortunately, knowledge and consumption are not the same thing—few families eat enough of these important health boosters. The average American family eats only *half* the recommended daily servings of fruit and vegetables, and the majority of these servings come from only three foods—potatoes, iceberg lettuce, and canned tomatoes (none of which are high on the list when it comes to vitamin-packed produce).

As outlined in Chapter 2, psychological strategies can help ensure that this valuable group gets consumed and enjoyed, including exploiting the variety principle (more choices today + different choices tomorrow = more eaten) and giving your child the *opportunity* to eat them rather than using active encouragement, bribes, or threats. As long as you are casual about these great health-boosters and cook the delicious fresh sort rather than less-enticing frozen or canned options, you will probably be surprised at how easily he takes to them. By using vitamin E–rich oils such as canola, corn, olive, and sunflower in your cooking, your child also gets the benefit of that antioxidant as well.

Foods containing antioxidant vitamins can also help to protect against potentially carcinogenic nitrosamines and nitrosamides—which can be made in the body from the otherwise harmless nitrites added to hot dogs, ham, and other cured meat products. Say you visit friends who are making hot dogs for dinner. One option is to refuse them for your child and ask for something else, but another option is to relax and let him have one, since you know he eats them only rarely and enjoys plenty of vitamin-packed fruit. Approaches like this, based on the science of how nutrients and food chemicals in-

GOOD SOURCES OF VITAMIN A AND BETA CAROTENE

- Sweet potatoes
- Broccoli
- Carrots
- Spinach
- Squash
- Cantaloupe
- Dried apricots
- Milk
- Eggs
- Cheese

GOOD SOURCES OF VITAMIN C

- Kiwi fruit
- Oranges and orange juice
- Sweet peppers
- Cantaloupe
- Broccoli
- Strawberries
- Tomatoes

GOOD SOURCES OF VITAMIN E

- Milk
- Canola, corn, and sunflower oils
- Nuts and seeds
- Avocados
- Peas
- Wheat germ

teract, can help you to maintain a high-nutrient child without worrying about every bite that he eats.

WHAT ABOUT SUPPLEMENTS?

It's important for children to obtain most of their essential nutrients from foods, rather than relying on supplements. Even "complete" children's vitamin and mineral supplements lack some of the essential known nutrients. In addition, while the classic vitamins have been known for decades, there are many other substances in foods that have important effects on health.

Already more than *four thousand* of these *phytochemicals* have been identified, and many are believed to have a protective role against the diseases associated with aging, particularly heart disease and cancer. Phytochemicals are present in fruits and vegetables and whole-grain cereals—yet another reason to help your child enjoy these all-around health-givers.

Bioflavonoids are one class of phytochemicals that recently made headlines. They're abundant in red grape skins—and as such are now suspected to be part of the answer to the question that had long intrigued researchers: Is there a connection between red wine and the low incidence of heart disease among the French? We now think it's in the skins!

We're definitely not suggesting wine for your child. But red grapes will provide the same protection, and so will other bioflavonoid-rich foods such as onions, broccoli, berries, cherries, apples, and string beans. Phytochemicals are just one example of why unadulterated nature is still the best primary source of nutrients for your child and yourself.

This said, we also recommend daily supplements (though not megavitamins) for infants and children up to at least three years, because they can provide insurance against a shortfall in any of the key nutrients—especially for such hard-to-get nutrients as zinc and iron. Details of supplements for each age group are given in Part Three.

A WORD ABOUT WATER

We didn't count water among the "key eight" nutrients because many people don't look on it as a nutrient (even though technically it is considered to be one), and because sensitive thirst mechanisms usually ensure that healthy babies and children never willingly go short of fluid.

Nevertheless, water is among one of the most important substances your child gets from her food. Fifty to 70 percent of a typical child's body is water, and virtually all metabolic processes occur in the watery body fluids. Water is also needed to replace that which is lost continuously through the skin and from the lungs, and is the vehicle used to transport essential oxygen (via the blood) around the body and to excrete waste and toxic substances in urine and stools. For all these reasons, a regular intake of water is essential.

When babies are first born they usually get all the water they need from breast milk or formula. In fact, one of the ways new parents can be reassured that feeding is going well is by keeping track of how many wet diapers are generated daily! Later on, after solids become regulars on the menu, additional fluids are necessary because solid foods contain less water than milk. Many parents slip into the habit at this time of giving their child milk, juice, diluted juice, or even soda whenever a drink is needed. This is definitely something that should be avoided. Milk, and to a lesser extent juice (though not soda), do have a valuable place in your child's diet, but both contain lots of calories and in excess amounts can lead to unnecessary weight gain.

So what should you do? Sometimes your child will be hungry and thirsty, and milk and juice in amounts healthy for her age fix both problems. But at other regular times during the day, your child will be thirsty but not hungry. Water is then the right beverage because it fixes the thirst without giving unnecessary calories. Faucet water (straight from the tap if it has low lead, or filtered if necessary) and bottled water are both good. Be reassured—you absolutely don't have to feel guilty about giving your child something so plain. Children who have been brought up with regular drinks of water love it for the pure feeling of refreshment it brings, and will often request it over calorie-laden or sweet alternatives.

MAKING A MEAL OUT OF NUTRIENT RECOMMENDATIONS

At the beginning of this chapter we told you that understanding individual nutrients is helpful in keeping your child's food on the right track— but that you didn't need to keep all the nutrient recomendations in your head in order to feed your child well. And this is true! Part Two takes you through feeding during the first months of life, when all your child's nutritional needs are supplied by breast milk or formula. At the start of Part Three, Chapter 8 gives portion goals for different food groups that will supply the right balance of essential nutrients between six months and six years. Armed with this information, and the details about individual foods in later age-group chapters, you will know everything necessary to give your child the best start.

PART TWO

⸺ ◈ ⸺

Your Baby Arrives

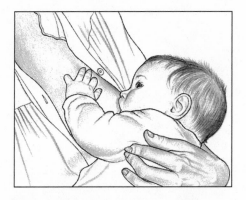

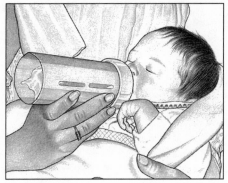

CHAPTER 4

————— ✦ —————

Food for Thought

Preparing to Feed Your New Baby

Three weeks before her due date, Laura was still confused about how she should feed her new baby. She wanted to try nursing, but she was planning to return to work and agreed with her husband and mother that formula would probably be easier. With her doctor's strong support, however, Laura threw caution to the winds and gave nursing a try. To the delight of the whole family she found it easy and practical, and is now the mother of a baby who has received all the important benefits that breast-feeding provides.

All experts agree that breast-feeding is the best option for most newborns.[1] Breast milk has the perfect composition, with nutrients, hormones to stimulate growth and regulate metabolism, and antibodies for immunity your baby can get in no other way. Breast-feeding also creates a bond with your infant that many nursing mothers find is an experience of a lifetime.

So why would anyone choose formula, which is never a perfect match for breast milk, the food that nature designed especially for human babies? In some cases it's because no one has explained all the advantages of breast-feeding for the whole family. So we'll start there.

- Breast-fed babies are measurably smarter and have better visual development and fine motor coordination than babies fed formula—probably because of the unique kinds of fats that breast milk contains.

---

[1] Exceptions are: babies whose mothers have tested positive for HIV (because this virus can be transmitted to the baby through mother's milk) and babies with the rare disease galactosemia.

Astonishing though it may seem, you can expect to give your baby a permanent IQ advantage when you breast-feed for even a few weeks, as well as better scores in math and general achievement tests during her school years.

- Breast-fed babies are healthier. They have fewer colds and ear infections than babies fed formula, because breast milk contains the mother's own antibodies, which confer immunity in the vulnerable early months when a baby's own immune system is maturing. In consequence, studies show that nursing moms actually take less time off work than moms using formula. As we pointed out in Chapter 1, breast-fed babies also have fewer allergies than babies fed formula. This is because breast-milk proteins do not activate the delicate newborn immune system, whereas formula increases the risk of allergies up until at least four months of age.

- Breast-fed babies bond naturally and easily with their mothers. New research suggests that the smell of breast milk is what infants instinctively use to identify their mother in the days following birth.

- Breast-fed babies are easier to care for. In addition to being sick less often, they are more contented generally, go to sleep more quickly, and rarely become constipated. They even have sweeter-smelling diapers compared to formula-fed infants.

- Breast-feeding is more convenient. You don't have to worry about buying formula, carrying it with you, or keeping it sterile when you go out. And you don't have to make and warm up bottles in the middle of the night!

- Breast-feeding is less expensive. By the time your baby is five months old you will have saved between $300 and $800 if you nurse rather than use formula.

- If your baby is born prematurely, breast-feeding is even more valuable because, in addition to all the other benefits of nursing, it helps prevent the life-threatening diseases that preemies are especially susceptible to in the first weeks of life. We have devoted the whole of Chapter 7 to helping you get nursing off to a good start if you deliver early.

BREAST MILK AND FORMULA—
WHAT'S THE DIFFERENCE?

Formula is just a food. Breast milk is much more. Here are some of the powerful substances in breast milk that your baby needs but is unable to make for herself for several months after birth—and even up to two years in some cases.

Digestive factors	At least three *digestive factors* ensure that milk fats are easily broken down so they can be absorbed during the early months when the digestive system is immature. Several breast-milk proteins also aid absorption of other nutrients, such as iron. Breast milk not only supplies essential nutrients but provides the means to digest them, too.
Protective factors	*Antibacterial molecules* prevent intestinal diseases by inhibiting bacterial growth in the intestine, directly killing bacteria such as *streptococci,* and encouraging growth of the friendly microorganisms that inhibit overgrowth of bad bacteria.
	Antiviral and antiparasitic molecules kill viruses and common parasites such as giardia.
	Antibodies and white blood cells protect the infant against diseases the mother has experienced in the past, and also help strengthen resistance against new diseases.
	Anti-inflammatory agents help protect the delicate intestine against damage by milk components.
Hormones	At least ten *hormones* help regulate growth and maturation of the intestine and other body tissues.

• Last—but certainly not least—breast-feeding is healthier for the mom. Nursing mothers have the edge in losing extra weight gained during pregnancy. The hormone oxytocin—produced by the mom when babies nurse—also helps contract the uterus back to its former size, which in turn reduces your abdomen. Perhaps most important, some research suggests that breast-feeding decreases the risk of breast cancer before age fifty by as much as 30 percent.

Some parents have heard the advantages of breast-feeding but hesitate for other reasons—perhaps nobody in their family ever nursed and it seems difficult, or, like Laura, the mother needs to return to work quickly and doesn't want to be "tied down." In other families, it's the husband who doesn't want his partner nursing, for fear of being excluded or because it just doesn't seem "nice." Grandmothers from a generation where formula was the rule can also be a problem, particularly if they withhold the emotional support that nursing mothers find invaluable.

These common concerns often disappear when parents have a chance to think and talk about the options. Breast-feeding is really not the difficult skill it is sometimes made out to be. If it were, none of us would be here today, because the survival of generations of our ancestors depended on it. Breast-feeding is also no more time-consuming than using formula. Once it's established, it's actually more convenient, and it can be fitted into a working mother's schedule quite easily, as we'll show you in Chapter 5. And although breast-feeding is a mother's job, there are plenty of other important tasks to go around. Dads are indispensable for cuddling, playing, walks, a share of diapering, baths, and bedtimes—and for giving bottles of expressed breast milk, and later introducing solid foods. When both parents see themselves as part of a team, breast-feeding clearly becomes only one of the many important tasks that are shared.

So if you are still undecided about how to feed your newborn, we urge you to give breast-feeding a try. Talk it over with your doctor if you need additional input. Even if you are able to breast-feed only for a limited time, just a few weeks of nursing will give your baby important developmental advantages. You can then switch over to formula or a mix of breast-feeding and formula, and your baby will be all the healthier for the breast milk she did get. Chapter 5 tells you how to get started on a rewarding nursing experience for everyone in the family.

If, after careful consideration, you are sure that breast-feeding is not for you, Chapter 6 explains new options in commercial infant formulas.

Manufacturers have come a long way from the early years of mass-marketed formulas. Even though formulas are still far from identical to breast milk, they're a much better alternative than they were in the past.

HARNESS INSTINCTS—YOUR NEWBORN'S AND YOURS—FOR A TROUBLE-FREE START

Whichever choice you make, getting started on feeding is easier than you might think if you are expecting your first child. Contrary to his appearance, your newborn is far from being a helpless little bundle. He has already developed a swallowing reflex, which he practiced in utero by taking in up to a pint a day of the amniotic fluid that surrounded him. Another powerful set of reflexes helps him find a nipple (whether breast or bottle), take it in his mouth, and suck. And, astonishing as it may seem, if you didn't need the delivery drugs that make newborns drowsy, he may even be able to wriggle up your abdomen to find your breast within an hour or two of delivery!

Another thing your newborn knows is exactly how much milk he needs and how to get it when he wants it. He'll let you know—he's frantic, angry, inconsolable, crying wildly, or chewing on his fists. This perfectly normal behavior taps your newly activated parental instincts; you figure out the problem and rush the food to his hungry mouth. Soon you have a contented baby, ready for a nap or some entertainment. He no longer wants food, any kind of food. In contrast to his earlier eagerness, he's now indifferent to breast or bottle.

This repeated pattern of hunger, eating, and contentment is one of your first glimpses of the incredibly strong life force in your child. He's instinctively determined to live, thrive, and ultimately grow up.

PARENTS HAVE INSTINCTS, TOO

Let's take one step back. It takes two to make a good feeding team, and just as your child starts life with all the skills he needs to eat, so you too have feeding instincts ready to surface when your baby is born. We are not the purely rational, cerebral creatures that many of us like to think we are, and in fact have biological instincts ready to help us with many major life transitions, including becoming new parents. Acting on these instincts gives you the best possible start with your new baby.

One important instinct mothers have is an instinct to nurse. New mothers who put their babies to the breast soon after delivery, and continue to feed frequently, may never realize how strong this instinct is. But mothers who have to leave their babies, or mothers who start on formula, are very much aware of *not* feeding. For a start, the physical and emotional discomfort can be considerable. Some women also report vivid dreams and waking fantasies of nursing. We believe that evolution has created this discomfort for a reason: to ensure that mothers everywhere—whether they're in the midst of their family or alone on a desert island—think about nursing.

One thing this instinct gives you is a second chance to start nursing. Studies have shown that women who don't nurse for the first week after birth can go on to produce enough milk for twins. You shouldn't deliberately take this risk, but if you start on formula and discover some days later that you are longing to nurse, you can be successful.

Both parents share the instinct to care for their newborn and to meet his every need. Feeding, of course, is a major part of caring for a new baby. And when your child cries for food, it is astonishing how those wails affect you! They may make you feel tender and nurturing, or frantic and irritable, but the end result is the same: They are impossible to ignore. And however tired you are, they ensure that your baby gets all the food he needs in short order.

A FINAL WORD: HAVE CONFIDENCE IN YOURSELF

When your baby is born, if she is your first, you may feel as if everyone around you knows more than you about how to look after her. Try to relax and have confidence in yourself. Although family, friends, and even strangers may give you advice, you and your baby have a special bond that will help you work out everything you need to know and do. Growing a baby takes nine long months, and feeling like a parent just a few days longer!

CHAPTER 5

---◆---

Breast-feeding Made Easy

Mary was twelve weeks pregnant when she learned that she was carrying twins. They were born early, weighing less than 4 pounds each, but she was able to breast-feed them both successfully for many months. Jane also succeeded under seemingly difficult circumstances—she nursed her baby for one year although she had the same inverted nipples that had caused her own mother to give up. Mary and Jane illustrate an important point, which is that nursing is a natural female skill, not the difficult task it is sometimes made out to be, and one that all mothers can accomplish with flair.

In the West African village where I researched breast-feeding in the late 1970s, all mothers nursed their babies. There were no failures and no exceptions. Difficult deliveries did not interfere with lactation, nor did inexperience or even quite serious health problems. One of my village friends had only one functional breast, yet she managed to produce as much milk as everyone else—we knew this because we were measuring breast milk as part of our research study. Another woman in our village had twins and produced twice as much milk as the other nursing mothers.

If these women sound like breast-feeding superwomen, think again. Two simple things helped them succeed. The first was confidence. They *knew* that they could nurse because they had seen other mothers manage just fine. The second was the good advice and support that ensure an easy start.

Confidence, good advice, and support are all you need, too, for this most natural of womanly abilities. In this chapter we are going to walk you through the essentials. A lactation counselor or nurse from your hospital will also be helpful during the first days. Breast-feeding is instinctive, but in a world where you're not surrounded by your "village," an experienced advisor can make all the difference when it comes to a trouble-free beginning. If your hospital doesn't have a counselor on staff, the International

BRIEFLY: WHAT TO EXPECT, AND WHY

Colostrum: During the late stages of pregnancy and for the first two to five days after birth, breasts make small amounts of a thickish fluid called *colostrum*. In addition to containing essential nutrients, colostrum contains antibodies and special proteins that protect infants from disease in the first vulnerable days outside the womb.

Breast milk: Two to five days after birth, breasts start to make real, or *mature*, breast milk. Breast milk changes during a feed, starting as watery *fore milk*, and gradually becoming fattier *hind milk* toward the end. Babies need both kinds of milk—fore milk to provide protein and satisfy thirst, and the richer hind milk to give them the energy and fat they need for brain growth, neurological development, and tissue synthesis. On average, fully 50 percent of breast-milk calories come from fat, which would be too much for an adult but is just the right amount for a baby's development and growth.

Milk production: Mature breast-milk production starts suddenly, over a period of a few hours, when the circulating concentration of the pregnancy hormone *progesterone* decreases enough to allow the lactation hormone *prolactin* to become active. This is often referred to as your milk *coming*

Lactation Consultants Association can refer you to a private consultant in your area (919–787–5181), or La Leche League can put you in touch with a trained local volunteer (847–519–7730; www.lalecheleague.org). Many insurance companies now pay for lactation assistance, so getting help doesn't have to be expensive. If you want to do some additional reading, you may also wish to consult some of the books we list at the end of the chapter.

GETTING STARTED

Nursing is truly a wonderful experience for both babies and their mothers—but not necessarily in the first few days. It typically takes a week to ten days for you to become a comfortable nursing pair.

in. Prolactin is produced in the days after birth whether or not the mother plans to breast-feed, and it continues to be produced when your baby *suckles,* or *nurses.* After your milk has come in, the *law of supply and demand* determines how much milk you produce. You supply as much as your baby demands!

Let-down: After a baby latches on to the nipple at the start of a feed, it usually takes about a minute or two of nursing before milk starts to flow. In addition to maintaining production of prolactin, the baby's sucking activates the mother's *let-down reflex.* A neurological loop from the breast to the brain sends a signal to release the hormone oxytocin, which then causes contractions inside the alveolar cells of the breast that make milk. These contractions squeeze milk from the cells into the breast ducts that lead to the nipple, making it easily accessible to your baby.

Weaning: Weaning is the process of gradually introducing your baby to solid foods until eventually you give up nursing. You certainly don't need to stop nursing when you start feeding solid foods. A period of several months to a year when you continue to breast-feed while offering solids is best for both you and your baby.

For the first two to five days after your baby is born and while he is just beginning to get used to the world around him, your breasts produce colostrum rather than actual milk. Despite the fact that it's produced in tiny amounts—from a mere teaspoon up to a tablespoon per feeding—it contains large amounts of essential antibodies and growth factors. It also coats your baby's gastrointestinal tract to prevent the absorption of harmful substances. The antibodies, in particular, are essential because they provide your baby with immunity against common diseases until his own immune system is up and running. It's important that your baby get the benefit of colostrum, so don't be dismayed by the small amount of nutrition it seems to provide.

Many mothers worry during the time before their "real" milk comes in. They worry about whether their infant is going hungry. They worry about whether their milk will eventually come in. These fears are needless.

Nursing *should* start slowly—it's what is best for your baby and best for you. And your milk *will* come in; it virtually always happens, and you will certainly know when it does. You also get second and third chances if you get off to a rocky start.

You may ask, why is it good for nursing to start slowly? Nobody knows the answer for sure, but we have a theory: Aside from the special protective properties of colostrum, the wait itself seems to be valuable. Your body has invested nine months in this baby, and evolution has worked out that a respite between birth and full lactation gives both of you the best start. Your baby has time to practice real-life sucking and swallowing before there is too much milk to make it complicated. Meanwhile, you have time to recover from giving birth, and your nipples can get used to nursing before your baby gets serious about needing milk. During this adjustment time, your baby will use the surplus nutrients and water present in his body at birth. That is why babies lose a small amount of weight in the week after birth before they start gaining again.

You may have heard that you should nurse immediately after birth, and worry if for some reason this is not possible. In fact, some studies have found that mothers who put their babies to the breast immediately after birth have an overall easier start, and are able to nurse for more months. On the other hand, a study of mothers who had pre-mature babies showed that mothers who didn't nurse their babies for several days after birth were just as successful two months later as mothers who fed within twenty-four hours of delivery. On balance, if your baby is ready and you are able, we suggest you go ahead and feed right away. On the other hand, if you had a tough delivery and both of you want to take a nap first, that's fine, too. Just try to get as much nursing practice as you can before your insurance policy says it's time to leave the hospital, because many of the helping hands on your ward will have enough experience to make sure your positioning and technique are right.

THE IMPORTANCE OF POSITIONING

Getting your baby correctly positioned at the breast is the single most important thing you can do to ensure getting off to a good start. Surprising? Many people think so. The value of positioning was not understood when our mothers gave birth, and this lack of knowledge contributed to many of the breast-feeding problems that women in those days experienced. Now, however, we know that good positioning coupled with your baby's

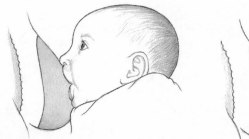
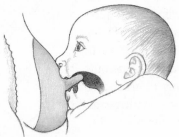

A correctly positioned baby. Babies do not suck on the nipple during feedings. The nipple should be well back in your baby's mouth to allow milk to flow.

instinctive reflexes will make nursing feel easy and natural when you've both had a bit of practice.

What's essential is that your baby must not suck on just the nipple. The nipple merely *guides* your baby to the right place on the breast, and it needs to be well back in her mouth during sucking, with at least some of the areola (and perhaps all, especially the portion below the nipple, depending on your breast configuration) inside her mouth. This ensures that your baby's mouth is in the right position to squeeze the milk ducts behind the areola, activating the flow of milk. With proper positioning, women with flat or inverted nipples—who used to be told they'd have problems—can nurse as well as other women.

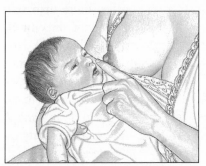

Touch one side of your baby's face with your finger or nipple.

You and your baby may be comfortable in any of several positions. Most mothers start with the classic "cradle" position, but you can vary positions if you want, as soon as you feel comfortable doing so. Some lactation experts believe that rotating positions helps prevent breast infections, while others think it doesn't matter. We recommend that you at least try each one until it feels familiar, and then your own and your baby's preference can be your guide. However you hold your baby, be gentle, support her head, and make sure that her nose is not blocked by your breast (especially if you have large breasts). You can use a finger to keep the breast clear of her face, being careful to press gently so as not to block a milk duct inside. Alternate the breast you use first at each feed, to keep milk production equal on both sides.

At the start of a feeding, make sure that your baby is awake and alert. Cradle her in your arms (with a pillow underneath for support if you like) and, with your breast in your free hand, touch *one* side of her face near her mouth (she'll get confused if you touch both sides). This acti-

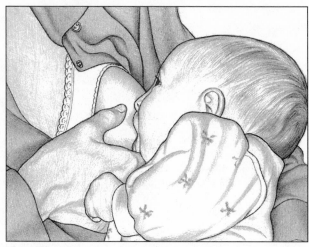

Your baby will move toward the touch and open her mouth. Move her to your nipple to start nursing.

vates her rooting reflex. She opens her mouth and turns toward the breast. You quickly move her so that when she puts her mouth on the breast, her lips cover most of the areola, activating her sucking reflex. *Voilà!* Your baby is latched on.

Your baby's bottom lip should be well under your nipple, so that you can feel her tongue under your breast, not over it. If you feel more than very

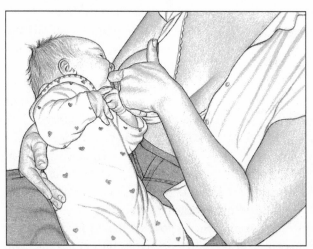

If you feel any discomfort, or want to stop a feed for some reason, break the suction gently with your finger before taking your baby off the breast.

minor discomfort, gently break the suction with your finger and reposition your baby. *Pain is not normal;* it's a sign that you need to start again.

If this all feels tremendously awkward—as if three or four hands would help—don't worry. It will feel like second nature in a surprisingly short time.

COMMON NURSING POSITIONS

In the "cradle" position, you cradle your baby's head in the crook of your arm with her body resting across your stomach and facing yours, tummy to tummy. To move her around, simply shift the crook of your arm and use your other hand tucked under her body.

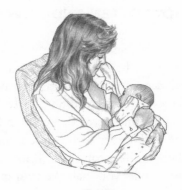

Cradle

The "football" position is particu-

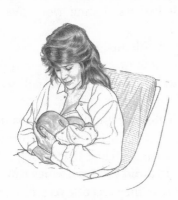

Football

larly good for feeding very small babies, and also works nicely with twins. Hold your baby facing you with her legs and body tucked under your arm on the side you are nursing. That same arm supports her back,

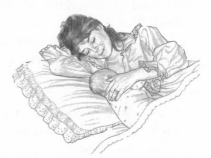

Horizontal

and your hand cradles her head; you can easily move her to where you want her to be. You can make this position more comfortable using a pillow or two to support your arm and the baby.

Mothers also like the "horizontal position," which lets you lie down while nursing. Turn onto the side you want to nurse on, and cuddle your baby up close so that she is lying on her side facing you. Move her up or down until she is level with your breast, with your upper-most arm curled behind her for support and guidance. Once you have her latched on to the breast, you can slide your lower arm under the pillow that your head will be resting on. This is a great position for resting and feeding at the same time.

HOW OFTEN AND HOW LONG?

New mothers always want to know, "How often and how long?" Your baby will be happiest, and you will get off to the best start, if you nurse on demand as much as possible—which means whenever your baby seems to need a feeding. She'll let you know by crying or chewing her fists and looking agitated. Nurse on the first breast until she stops sucking or the milk seems to be gone (which may be five to fifteen minutes), and then on the second breast until she stops sucking. There is no rule about time, so let your baby be your guide. If a feeding is what she wants, you'll see the contentment nursing gives her. Although it varies from infant to infant, newborn babies typically want to nurse about eight to twelve times per twenty-four hours, with individual feedings lasting from five to twenty minutes.

If your baby is fussy more than every two hours, don't automatically assume she is hungry. It can be easy to slip into the mistaken habit of fixing every problem with a breast-feeding when what she may actually want is a cuddle, or entertainment, or some nonnutritive sucking. Most small babies need lots of sucking, and it doesn't always have to be accompanied by food. Both moms and dads can offer a little finger, clean and turned soft side up with a blunt, short nail, and enjoy feeling that strong little suck as she practices her "technique." Try to avoid pacifiers, which can increase the risk of nursing problems because they teach a very different kind of sucking.

If your baby does not demand to be fed at least every four hours, she may simply be sleepy. Drugs given to you during delivery are transferred to your baby through the placenta, and (depending on the drug) can make your baby sleepy and disoriented during the first two days—and sleepy, disoriented babies don't suck well! Be patient and tell your doctor, who will want her monitored carefully and may suggest that you wake her every four hours and encourage her to nurse. This extra monitoring is important to prevent dehydration, but you don't need to worry about being able to establish nursing eventually—remember that nature allows you extra time for just such adjustments.

Whatever your baby's need for nursing right now, don't assume it is a pattern for the future. Nursing changes when your milk comes in and then changes again as you and your baby settle into a routine after about three weeks. Although we don't recommend scheduled feeds, most babies develop their own routine after a while, which smoothes the way for easier days and—in time—the return of unbroken nights of sleep.

In the first three to five days, there is one important don't: Don't give your baby water or formula unless your doctor says it is medically necessary. Water is not usually needed at this time, and in large amounts may upset the delicate balance of water and sodium in your baby's body, leading to a dangerous condition known as *water intoxication* (causing a reduced level of consciousness, and even seizures). This remains true until about two months, when babies' kidneys are more mature and better able to control water and sodium excretion. Sometimes water is necessary, for example if your newborn is very yellow or when the weather is extremely hot, but don't give it unless your pediatrician says you should. Formula can sometimes seem tempting before lactation is completely established, or if you have been exhausted by the delivery. But it makes getting started with nursing harder, and increases the risk that you will give up nursing prematurely. In any case, it isn't needed except in very unusual cases.

FROM THREE DAYS TO FOUR WEEKS

Before her milk came in, Silvia wondered how she would know it had happened and whether it would be enough for her new baby. But when it happened, there was no mistaking it. Silvia's experience is typical. Milk is produced by all new mothers, even those who do not plan to nurse and those who did not nurse during the first days after delivery.

One of the amazing things about babies is the way nature has arranged for all their needs to be met. Just at the time your baby starts to get genuinely hungry, you start to produce the milk he needs. On both sides, nature has created joy to encourage you to nurse, and some discomfort as penalty for not nursing, as if to make sure that it *will* happen. Your baby has an urgent need to suck for some time every day; he now has the discomforts of hunger and thirst, as well. Pretty soon he learns that nursing fulfills his need for sucking, stops the hunger and thirst, and provides a glow of contentment. Meanwhile, your breasts are uncomfortable if you don't nurse. His cries when he is hungry or needs to suck tug at your heart like nothing else, and his contentment during nursing, once established, will make your heart soar.

Your "real" milk, coming in at two to five days, is thin and white or

STAYING COMFORTABLE

Healthy nipples. Making sure your baby latches on correctly helps you avoid sore nipples and infections. If you're uncomfortable or he hasn't taken a good mouthful of the areola, break the suction gently with your finger and start again. Spread a little breast milk around the nipple after nursing and let your breasts dry before closing your bra afterward. Your breast milk's fat lubricates, and the protective factors may also help prevent infections.

Clothing. Nursing bras with flaps that open up in front can make your life a lot easier. You can also buy nursing clothes that make it simple to feed your baby in public, although regular clothes work well if they open in front or pull up from the waist. Drape a towel or baby blanket over your shoulder for privacy.

Leaking. Some women leak milk from the other breast when they feed, or they leak between feeds. This is completely normal and easy to deal with. Simply wear breast pads tucked inside your bra—the cotton ones are most comfortable, but disposables are fine, too (look for the kind without a plastic lining, to prevent breast infections). Carry spares when you go out, so that you can replace damp ones after you nurse.

Catching messes. Buy some cotton diapers (the kind that are not pre-folded) and keep one handy at all times for catching spit-up before it gets on your clothes.

bluish, and contains all the nutrients your baby needs for growth in the next four to six months. At first your breasts will feel as hard as footballs and it will seem as if you're producing a huge amount. But the actual volume is less than it seems. Later, after the normal engorgement of the first few days has subsided, you'll produce more, even though your breasts will feel softer and more comfortable.

You may now become very aware of the let-down reflex that starts soon after your baby begins to suck (or even before, when you hear him crying for milk). It comes as a mild or strong feeling of relief from pressure, warmth, or tingling in the breast. It can also be accompanied by quite strong uterine contractions (good for getting your waistline back), although some women feel very little. You may also notice your baby

ESSENTIAL BURPING SKILLS

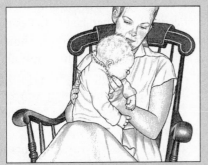

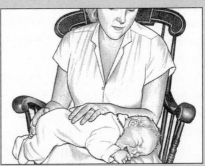

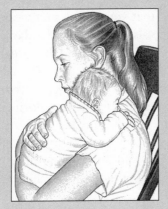

Some, but not all, babies swallow air when they nurse and need to be given the chance to let it come up without bringing too much milk with it. Burping is the solution. At the end of the feed (and in the middle of the feed, if necessary) hold your baby gently in a sitting position, or lean him over your shoulder, and gently stroke and pat his back for three or four minutes. Some mothers also find that laying their baby tummy down across their knees works well.

changes the pattern of his sucking after let-down. Rapid, strong sucks change to bursts of sucks, with rests in between, as he settles in to feed on the full milk flow.

ON-DEMAND OR SCHEDULED NURSING?

Feeding your baby at fixed three- or four-hour intervals, known as "scheduled feeding," was widely recommended in the past. However, it has now been almost completely superseded by "on-demand" feeding. This simply means feeding your baby when he is hungry, and not pushing him to eat when he is reluctant. Scheduled feeding often discouraged nursing by putting mothers and babies at odds. In addition, it sent the harmful message that eating is not connected with hunger. In contrast, on-demand feeding encourages the instinctive caloric regulation that will be one of your baby's best lifelong protections against obesity and eating disorders.

Almost as soon as your milk comes in, your baby starts working on increasing your supply to keep up with his needs. To do that, he has to be able to feed as much as he wants. This might mean once every two or three hours for ten to twenty minutes, but can occasionally be as often as thirty minutes out of every hour. This may sound like a lot, and during a growth spurt it can seem like a lot, too, but don't panic. The frequency and length of feeds will decrease as he gets older. Most babies also develop their own "routine" by three to six weeks, so life will soon take on a more orderly pace.

In the meantime, if your baby at two to three weeks naturally wants to feed at two- to three-hour intervals during the day and wakes up once or twice during the night, you can feel pleased that you have it pretty easy. Even if he feeds at two- to three-hour intervals for most of the day or night, and wants to nurse more in the afternoon or evening, this is perfectly normal, even common.

Some "nibblers," however, like to take a little bit of milk now, a bit more in an hour's time, and so on all through the day. A few pauses during a feeding are normal, but extended breaks of several minutes, or even a quick nap, are not. Apart from the inconvenience, regular short feeds are not a good idea because your baby needs the calorie-rich hind milk to grow properly. To get it, he should nurse for at least five to fifteen minutes on the first breast during most feeds.

Nibblers who are otherwise healthy can be helped toward a better pattern of feeding. If your baby starts to fall asleep after a few sucks, nudge him gently, stroke his hair, and maybe start to undress him or sit him up, and he'll start to suck again. Keep doing this until you feel he has had a good feed. If he won't take a full feeding, he simply may not be hungry. Give him a clean finger to suck on, or a cuddle or a stroll or some playtime, and make sure he is good and ready next time. A combination of encouraging full feedings and discouraging short ones will get most babies on board within a few days. Babies who never seem to take a good feed at any time of the day should be seen by a pediatrician.

Be aware that growth spurts, illness, or vaccinations can disrupt whatever pattern seems to be emerging, raising or lowering feeding demands dramatically. It can be disconcerting, but growth spurts typically last just a few days—and recovery from illness will be heralded by the return of a hearty appetite.

EXPRESSING

Expressing can be helpful after about three weeks if you find yourself short of milk in the afternoon, or need to go out and want to leave a supply of breast milk for your baby.

If expressing is going to be a routine, look into renting a large electric pump from your hospital or a local lactation consultant, or contact a company directly (Medela, 1-800-TELL-YOU; Ameda-Egnell, 1-800-323-4060). If you can't find a large pump to rent, the small electric pumps that are for sale in most baby-supply stores do work, even if not quite as well. There are also small hand pumps for sale, some of which work fine for some women, while others (especially the "bicycle horn" type) don't. If you don't like using one type of pump, try another. You may also find that manual expression works for you. It is certainly good for emergencies, but most women find it slow and difficult for large volumes.

If you can, try expressing from one breast while feeding your baby with the other. It is easier and will provide a larger supply of expressed milk, since the let-down reflex works for the other breast, too. This is especially useful if there are feeds during the day when you have more milk than your baby needs. If you pump milk when you are away from your baby, find a quiet, relaxing room where you won't be disturbed. Take a few minutes to rest first and get in the right frame of mind. Having a picture of your baby to look at will help with your let-down reflex, or you can even consider making a tape of him crying. Expect to wait one to five minutes after starting to pump before the milk starts to flow. Expressing should not be painful. If it is, reposition your breast and/or turn down the pressure until it feels comfortable.

Collect expressed milk in sterilized bottles or plastic storage bags, available from your hospital or a nursing consultant. Store in the refrigerator for up to twenty-four hours or in the freezer for up to three months. If you express milk at work, use an insulated bag and ice pack to transport it home.

Clean your collection and storage containers well after every use, by washing with hot soapy water and then boiling in clean water on the stovetop for five minutes, or by rinsing well and then washing in a dishwasher with a heated drying cycle. Nipples and nipple rings should also be sterilized in boiling water for five minutes.

Make sure the expressed milk is body temperature when you feed it (but not hotter—be careful to check this before feeding), and cuddle your baby close in a nursing position. Feeding with a bottle is usually easier than with a spoon or cup, but you need to wait until your baby is three to four weeks old before you start using a bottle, to prevent the "nipple confusion" that can reduce his ability to nurse well. See Chapter 7 for information on heating milk and making bottle feeding a good experience for you and your baby.

ONE BREAST OR TWO AT EACH FEEDING?

You may have been told that you have to nurse with both breasts every time you feed your baby. Actually, this is not true. Research has shown that nursing with one breast at each feeding sometimes works just as well. If you offer one breast at each feeding, alternate every time and nurse for as long as your baby wants to. If you go with nursing on both sides each time, your baby should nurse until he stops sucking or for five to fifteen minutes on the first side, then switch to the other side for as long as he wants (alternating the breast you start with each time). Many mothers go with a combination of the two techniques depending on how hungry their baby seems and how much milk they have.

IS YOUR BABY GETTING ENOUGH MILK?

This is the question that new mothers often worry about most. Fortunately, there are several good ways to tell if your baby is getting enough to eat.

- Has he returned to his birth weight by two weeks of age?
- Does he become content soon after starting a feed?
- Is he content immediately after you have finished feeding him?
- Can he last at least two hours between some feeds on most days?
- Does he usually have six or more wet diapers every day?

If your answer is yes to all of these, you can feel reassured that all is well. You really don't need to weigh your baby before and after feeds (which some new mothers try) to be confident that everything is fine. If the answer to some of the questions is no, it may mean one of two things. Your milk supply might be a little short right now, even if it is usually adequate. Or maybe your baby is having a growth spurt at the moment and is especially hungry.

The first growth spurt usually occurs at two to three weeks. Just when mothers think they have gotten the hang of nursing, it suddenly seems that their milk supply can't keep up with a rapidly escalating demand. The solution is to take your baby's hunger as a cue to nurse more than usual, and make yourself an extra snack or two and a drink, and perhaps have an afternoon nap. Within two or three days your milk supply and your baby's demand should be back in balance again. If it isn't, talk to your pediatrician, and ask yourself these troubleshooting questions:

- How often and how long are you feeding your baby? You may need to keep track by jotting it down for a day. If it's less often than every two and a half hours, with a total of less than two hours per day, try giving longer and more frequent feeds to build your supply.

- Are you trying to lose weight? If you are, stop now and plan to start when your baby is older. Dieting and nursing are poor partners during the first two months after birth.

- Are you getting enough sleep and rest? An afternoon nap can work wonders for both your peace of mind and your milk production.

- Do you have plenty of milk in the morning but seem to run out by midafternoon? This common pattern (reported by nine out of ten nursing mothers in a recent study) can be remedied by nursing more in the afternoon, or by expressing milk in the morning (perhaps expressing from one breast and nursing with the other at the first morning feeding) and saving it for the afternoon. Expressing increases your milk supply (the law of supply and demand again), and gives you extra to feed by bottle or cup if you need it later.

- Is your last feeding of the day a complete one? Make sure you allow your baby to take a full feed from both breasts to provide the proper stimulus for good overnight production.

- You don't, by the way, have to increase your fluid intake provided that you are already drinking the equivalent of eight 8-ounce glasses per day. Excess fluid intake doesn't increase milk production.

NUTRITION AND YOUR MILK SUPPLY

Breast milk contains high concentrations of many nutrients, which must be supplied by your diet if they are not to be taken from your body's valuable reserves. You need more calories than you did before or during pregnancy, and these calories need to be nutrient-dense.

Recommended Nutrient Intakes for Nursing Mothers

DAILY NUTRIENTS	BEFORE PREGNANCY	DURING NURSING	PERCENT CHANGE
Calories	2,200	2,700	+25%
Protein (g)	50	65	+30%
Vitamin A (mcg)	800	1,300	+63%
Vitamin D (mcg)	5	5	0%
Vitamin E (mg)	8	12	+50%
Vitamin C (mg)	60	95	+58%
Thiamin (mg)	1.1	1.5	+36%
Riboflavin (mg)	1.1	1.6	+45%
Niacin (mg)	14	17	+21%
Vitamin B_6 (mg)	1.3	2.0	+54%
Folate (mcg)	400	500	+20%
Vitamin B_{12} (mcg)	2.4	2.8	+17%
Calcium (mg)	1,000	1,000	0%
Iron (mg)	15	15	0%
Zinc (mg)	12	19	+58%

Many of the nutrients you eat go directly into breast milk. Your fat consumption is particularly important. There are many different fats in breast milk, and the nursing mother's diet determines the balance her baby receives. For the best milk fat, your diet should emphasize a variety of monounsaturates and polyunsaturates, making sure to include some of the good sources of essential fatty acids (canola, soy, sunflower, and saf-flower oils, plus cow's milk). Try to keep your intake of saturated fat from red meat modest for general health. Also try to avoid frequent servings of trans fatty acids (in solid margarine, shortening, and many commercial baked goods and peanut butters), which can also get into your milk and may interfere with the synthesis of special fatty acids necessary for normal brain development in your baby.

Food flavors also get into milk. If you eat garlic for dinner, your baby will have garlic-flavored milk for breakfast! But this is not bad at all—quite the contrary. These first tastes introduce your baby to a spectrum of subtle but distinct flavors. Studies have shown that babies usually like these early flavor experiences—including garlic—and that they go on to be much more receptive to a diverse range of solid foods than babies who have been fed a uniform diet of formula.

CAUTION: PCBs AND OTHER HAZARDS

Unfortunately, harmful substances can also get into your milk. Besides medications of all kinds, widely accepted drugs such as caffeine, nicotine, and alcohol enter breast milk. They should all be avoided. Ask your obstetrician or pediatrician about any prescriptions or over-the-counter medicines you might want to use.

In some areas tap water contains high amounts of lead, which is known to have permanent harmful effects on IQ. Check the lead count of your home water supply, and consider switching to bottled water with a listed low lead count if necessary.

Some industrial pollutants are also a concern because they get into breast milk and have the potential to cause permanent neurological damage—particularly mercury and polychlorinated biphenyls (PCBs). The FDA has issued an advisory to nursing mothers recommending that they eat wild game fish (for example, swordfish, tuna, and shark) only once per month or less. These fish may contain high levels of mercury because they are at the top of the food chain, where toxic chemicals and heavy metals accumulate. Some species of lake fish (for example, walleye, trout, and bass) are also considered unsafe because of lingering high levels of water contamination, and many states recommend restricting consumption to once per month or less and then to only smaller fish (less than 9 inches long). Inshore sea fish such as bluefish, bass, catfish, and crabs can also be cause for concern, again because of water contamination. The safest bet is probably to contact your state fish advisory board for information on fish safety in your area.

SO WHAT *SHOULD* YOU EAT, AND HOW MUCH OF IT?

- *Eat a varied diet with a normal (30 percent) fat content.* This means eating daily helpings of whole grains, fresh fruit and vegetables, low-fat dairy products, and some lean meat, poultry, or fish. For fish, concentrate on low-pollution deep ocean varieties such as cod and pollock. Use vegetable oils, rather than butter, margarine, or solid shortening, in cooking. Good nutrition also means going outside on fine days: Your skin needs sunlight to make vitamin D for your baby.

● *Take a daily multivitamin/mineral supplement* (50–150 percent of RDAs, not more).

● *Don't try to lose weight before two months postpartum.* Between two months and six months you may safely lose up to 1 pound per week. More than this and you risk reducing your milk supply. If your baby seems hungrier than usual, nurse more to boost your supply, or be prepared to back off and diet more slowly. When you are ready to give up nursing, dieting to lose 2 pounds per week may possibly make weaning easier, by decreasing your milk supply.

● *Be aware that your baby may not tolerate some foods in your diet.* In some women, small food particles are absorbed undigested into the bloodstream and pass into the breast milk. These particles can occasionally cause colic and food allergies. As we've noted, variety in Mom's diet is a plus for most babies, but some are sensitive to certain foods—among them cow's milk, soy products, chocolate, onions and garlic, and cruciferous vegetables (including cabbage, broccoli, and cauliflower). If you think your baby is at risk for allergies or appears to be developing colic, check Chapter 16 for ways to identify offending foods. Very spicy foods are something to be wary of, too—causing diaper rash in rare cases.

● *Stay away from processed foods with additives.* These include nitrites in hot dogs, sausages, and ham; coloring agents; artificial sweeteners, and MSG. All of these chemicals can get into breast milk and may cause metabolic reactions in your baby. Also avoid caffeine—which, among other things, will keep your baby awake when you want to sleep. Herb teas are generally off-limits, too, since they can contain chemically active components whose effects haven't been well documented.

● *Drink eight cups of water or other fluids every day.* You don't need to force yourself to drink more, but eight cups is important for your milk supply—and for your own good health. You will probably get thirsty and want at least this amount in any case.

FROM FOUR WEEKS ON

By the time your baby is one month old, you will have mostly gotten over your delivery and weathered your milk coming in. Some babies have already settled into a comfortable routine by four weeks. Others, especially those with colic, will take a bit more time but nevertheless you and your baby *will* get to a contented, happy stage.

WHAT SHOULD YOUR BABY'S GROWTH LOOK LIKE?

Many parents of breast-fed babies worry that their baby is gaining too much weight in the first few months. Let us reassure you: This is perfectly normal. The growth charts that most pediatricians use are based on data from the 1950s, when the majority of babies were formula-fed. Breast-fed babies have a quite different pattern of growth—in particular, they gain weight faster during the first three months of life and then slow down until between twelve and eighteen months. If you aren't aware of this pattern, you may also worry later that your baby is not eating enough. Check Appendix 2 (pages 319–322) for the World Health Organization's new weight and length charts that are designed especially for breast-fed babies.

HOW LONG CAN YOU EXCLUSIVELY NURSE?

By four to six weeks, your baby will have worked your milk supply up almost to its maximum. So how will you continue to satisfy her? In fact, while her body weight is increasing, her growth is slowing down. The net result is that her milk requirements won't change much for the next few months. On average, babies have almost constant calorie needs between the ages of one month and four to six months. This means that when you have successfully reached one month, there is no biological reason why you can't nurse exclusively for several more, as long as you continue to nurse regularly. Some mothers can even increase their supply beyond six months. However, exclusive nursing is not usually a good plan after this time, because breast milk no longer satisfies essential nutrient requirements. In addition, the introduction of solid food by six months is valuable because it gives your baby's facial muscles the exercise they need for speech in a few months.

WHAT ABOUT SUPPLEMENTAL BOTTLES?

If your baby needs a feed when you can't nurse her, you will find that it's easier to give expressed breast milk or formula with a baby bottle than with a spoon or cup. Chapter 6 gives details of different formula options. Be aware, however, that it is good to avoid giving multiple daily bottles of formula unless you intend to move to a mixed breast-feeding/formula regimen—otherwise you may find that your baby decides to stop nursing before you want to.

HOW CAN YOU HANDLE SEPARATIONS?

Many women are unable to spend all their time with their newborn babies. Even if you don't have a job that takes you away from home, you may have other commitments. Separations while nursing are certainly possible, but they need to be managed carefully.

The basic problem is that separations tend to reduce your milk supply. When you are away from your infant, you get overfull breasts. This sends a nerve signal to your brain to make less milk. You can deal with this by expressing your milk and following other suggestions for keeping your supply up. Or you can accept that regular separations will decrease your milk supply, and supplement with formula. In this case, your baby will still be better off than if you simply switched over to an exclusive diet of formula.

Occasional separations, when you're away from your baby for half a day, are easy to manage. You can leave expressed milk behind and take a hand pump to relieve the pressure in your breasts—or you may learn from experience that you'll be fine until you get home, at which point you can feed your baby immediately and catch up with an extra feeding or two in the next few hours.

The regular daily separation of working mothers takes more effort.

- Nurse fully before you go to work, when you get home, and at least once at night if possible.

- Nurse more frequently over weekends.

- Leave expressed milk or formula for the hours you are gone.

- Keep a pump at work and use it once or twice during the day. With proper refrigeration you can take that milk home; otherwise it should be discarded. Some companies are now providing private rooms with pumps for nursing women. If yours is not one of them, you may wish to ask your supervisor or Human Resources department to see if it is possible.

- Let your baby sleep in your bedroom to make nighttime nursing easier. You can even consider sleeping with your infant so that she can nurse more frequently and so keep your supply high. If you do this, make sure that your baby can't fall out of bed and that there is enough room so that you or your husband won't roll over on her.

Separations of several days are difficult but possible. Some mothers, faced with a sudden family crisis, illness, or important business trip, choose to give up nursing (using firm bras, breast pads, and analgesics to help with the discomfort). The better solution if you can manage it is to take along a breast pump and try to pump as often as you would normally nurse. Your milk supply will dwindle but, provided you continue to express milk, you should be able to work your supply back up with extra feedings once you are able to nurse again. This is not as amazing as it might sound. During most of human history, lactation was so essential to babies' survival that evolution has equipped us to keep it going as long as there is any demand at all.

NURSING IN PUBLIC

In the best world, nursing would be fully accepted by everyone, and you would simply nurse your baby when and where you needed to. Until this utopia arrives in the United States, nursing blouses, a cloth draped over your shoulder, or an awareness of the location of the nearest dressing room for more privacy, will give you the freedom to nurse outside your home.

CAN YOU EXERCISE AND NURSE?

By all means! Studies have shown that women who exercise five times a week starting six weeks after delivery are just as able to supply all their babies' milk needs as mothers who don't exercise. Any kind of exercise will be good for you now, ranging from a brisk walk to an aerobics class or workout with weights.

You don't, incidentally, have to worry that the lactic acid produced by your muscles during exercise will get into your breast milk and stop your baby from wanting to nurse. Recent research has documented that the vast majority of babies like breast milk just as much after their mothers' exercise. If your baby is one of the very few who doesn't, nurse before you exercise and keep a spare bottle of expressed milk in the freezer. Feeding beforehand is a good idea anyway, because full breasts can make some exercises uncomfortable.

SHOULD YOU GIVE YOUR BABY MULTIVITAMINS OR FLUORIDE?

Breast milk has the perfect balance of nutrients for most babies until four to six months. Multivitamins and fluoride are not usually considered necessary when a baby is breast-fed up to this time. One exception: Babies whose mothers don't drink vitamin D–fortified milk and who either live in northern latitudes or can't spend regular time outside (so their skin can make vitamin D) need a supplement prescribed by their pediatrician. In addition, babies born prematurely need special supplements, as described in Chapter 7.

WHEN SHOULD YOU INTRODUCE SOLID FOOD?

Most babies start to need extra calories at some point between four and six months. This milestone is also the point at which breast milk no longer supplies your baby's total requirements for essential micronutrients such as zinc, iron, and vitamin C. You don't, of course, need to give up nursing just because you are starting solids. We'll discuss how to combine the two, and the signs that tell you when your baby is ready for solids, in Chapter 9.

WHEN TO STOP NURSING: IT DEPENDS

The American Academy of Pediatrics recommends nursing throughout the first year. This is certainly good if you can manage it. If you can't, or if your baby decides to wean herself earlier, remember that she will still have benefited from most of the advantages of breast-feeding.

The easiest way to stop nursing is simply to gradually reduce the time spent feeding. Let your baby be your guide. Most babies decide to completely wean themselves from the breast between nine and fourteen months, refusing to nurse even though they are hungry for solid food or formula in a bottle or cup, though a few happily go on until two or even three years.

If you want to be the one who makes the decision, cut out one feeding every few days, replacing it with formula (before four months) or formula and solid foods (after four months). Start with the lunchtime feeding, when your baby is feeling lively and independent, then move to other daytime meals. The last feeds to stop should be the first one in the morning and the last one at night, feedings for which there is the greatest emotional need. Weaning as gradually as possible is easiest on your baby and on you. Your milk supply will decrease naturally, preventing the physical discomfort of stopping suddenly.

COMMON PROBLEMS AND FREQUENTLY ASKED QUESTIONS

Leah is expecting her first child. She would like to breast-feed but has inverted nipples and fears that this will make it too hard for her baby to suck properly.

About one in five women has inverted nipples. This does not have to interfere with breast-feeding. Babies don't suck on the nipple; they use it as a guide to get the areola into their mouths. The critical factor is correct positioning rather than nipple shape. Getting off to a good start, however, can take two to three weeks, rather than the usual seven to ten days. Leah does not need to "prepare" her breasts during pregnancy, even though this advice is still sometimes given. She can use breast shields between feedings, and apply a minute of suction from a breast pump before feeds during the first few weeks. However, she should not wear breast shields while she is feeding, because this reduces a baby's milk intake by about 50 percent. Breast shields, also called breast shells or breast cups, are plastic domes with a center hole for the nipple, and can be purchased in most baby stores.

Jennifer has small breasts and fears that she won't be able to produce enough milk for her baby, due in eight weeks.

Fortunately, Jennifer's concerns are groundless. Studies have shown that breast size is unrelated to milk production. There is no reason why Jennifer cannot produce as much milk as larger women.

Suzanne has sore nipples. Her baby is four days old, and she is worried that her nipples are going to get worse and that this will cause her to give up nursing.

Nipples *can* feel a bit tender in the first days after you deliver, but they should not bleed or crack. If they do, the problem needs to be fixed quickly with the help of a midwife or lactation consultant, who will probably check first on positioning. It can help to rub a little breast milk on the nipples and allow them to dry thoroughly before closing the flaps of the nursing bra. Other things to try: Avoid soap (warm water is all the washing that is needed), make sure to break the suction with your finger before taking the baby off the breast, and start feeds on the less sore side until the irritation subsides. Creams and lotions, tea bags, and other topical remedies (other than breast milk, which has antiseptic properties) have not been shown to work.

One week after giving birth, Rose is ready to give up. Her breasts are uncomfortably full, her baby is finding it hard to latch on, and she can't imagine going on like this for the next several months.

Rose is experiencing something that quite a few women go through for a few days after their milk comes in—mild engorgement. Once the law of supply and demand starts working properly, the engorgement will disappear and her baby will find it much easier to latch on. In the meantime, Rose should wear a nursing bra with good support and hand-express a teaspoon or two of milk before she starts feeding so that it is easier for her baby to latch on.

Christine has plenty of milk for her ten-day-old baby, Thomas, but he finds it very hard to start feeding. As soon as Christine feels her let-down reflex working, Thomas starts to pull away or cough.

Some women have a powerful let-down reflex, and the strong jet of milk can make it hard to suck. Christine should try expressing an ounce of milk before she feeds Thomas, to make it easier for him. The surplus can be frozen for a rainy day. In a very short time Thomas will be bigger and stronger and will cope without any help.

Ann has been nursing well for two weeks, but she has suddenly developed a pain in one breast, a fever, and some swelling and redness. She wants to keep nursing and is worried that if she goes to her doctor, she will be told to stop.

Breast pain, with or without fever and swelling, is not a normal part of breast-feeding. It should be thoroughly investigated when it happens. Most likely Ann has a breast infection that can be cleared up with antibiotics, and she should see her doctor immediately. She should not stop feeding; her milk is fine (the antibiotic will get into her milk, but only baby-safe varieties are prescribed for nursing mothers). In fact, feeding is vital for keeping breast ducts open and helping to clear the infection. She should make sure to change breasts and positions so that milk from all areas of the breast gets removed.

Rachel is five weeks old and has recently taken to crying inconsolably for several hours in the late afternoon. She cannot be comforted and appears to be in pain.

Rachel should be taken to her pediatrician to make sure she has not developed an infection, allergy, or other problem. More likely, however, the diagnosis will be colic, a condition of unknown origin that affects about one in four babies age two to sixteen weeks. Ways to relieve colic are described in Chapter 16.

James is five weeks old, and his mother is worried about her milk. James' stools are very watery. Is something she is eating giving him diarrhea?

Watery stools are normal—not just common—in breast-fed babies. However, stools that are much more watery than the baby's usual pattern are cause for concern, though they are rarely connected to the mother's diet. If the change persists for more than a day or two, his parents should contact their pediatrician. In the meantime, James' mom should continue to nurse, because this will give her baby the fluid that he needs to replace what is being lost. If she is feeding expressed milk, she should take care to keep her pump and containers sterile.

Barbara has nursed well and enjoyed it for seven weeks, but now her infant seems to be constantly hungry and unsatisfied. Does this mean she should give up nursing or supplement with formula?

Fear of an inadequate milk supply is the major reason that women stop nursing. It is unlikely that Barbara has reached a point where she is physically unable to satisfy her infant, because milk requirements are more or less stable from about six weeks until four to six months. More likely she has started to cut corners (decreasing nursing time or cutting her calorie or fluid intake, and perhaps trying to rush around as well) and her milk has actually decreased.

The first things Barbara should do are to increase nursing time to two or two and a half hours a day and make sure she is drinking enough and eating at least 2,500 calories daily (enough to avoid weight loss greater than ½ pound a week). Making time to relax and trying to get enough sleep are also important. If she has plenty of milk during the morning but seems to run short later in the day, Barbara can express milk early and feed it late. This will also increase her milk supply.

Jason is four months old. He continues to be satisfied with nursing as his only food source, but he is not gaining much weight. Is it time for Jason to start solid food?

Usually babies who have been exclusively breast-fed should start to have some additional food between four and six months. However, if Jason has fed well up to now and shows no signs of being hungry, there is no particular reason to start offering him solid food right now rather than when he is six months old. It may be that, like most breast-fed babies, he gained a lot of weight early on and is now taking a break. His parents should make sure they are using the new breast-feeding growth curves (pages 319–322) to compare him to, and that he is continuing to gain some weight, even if not very much. If he has grown poorly all along and his mom and dad are a normal size, he should be evaluated by his pediatrician for growth failure.

Alison tells the pediatrician that her breast-fed three-week-old has not had a bowel movement for five days. Little Jeremy is fine and not crying, but she is worried nevertheless. The doctor suggests a suppository, but it produces no results. After another week she is frantic—at which point Jeremy has a perfectly normal bowel movement, with no crying or straining or any of the other signs of constipation.

The moral of this story is that a few breast-fed babies simply don't have much in the way of bowel movements. Constipation (hard, difficult bowel movements) is rarely seen in normal breast-fed babies. Infrequency (unlike in adults) doesn't mean constipation; rather, it is evidence that the milk is being very efficiently used.

Joey's mother took him to a pediatrician at two weeks because she became concerned that his skin was yellow. She was told the problem was breast-milk jaundice and that she should stop nursing until the problem was resolved.

Breast-milk jaundice affects 5 to 10 percent of all newborns. Although the cause is not fully understood, it is thought to happen when a mother's breast milk contains unknown substances that stop a newborn's liver from eliminating bilirubin (a waste product of hemoglobin) from the bloodstream. A switch to formula is sometimes required if the bilirubin level is very high. However, this does not mean that nursing has to stop. Joey's mother can express milk and throw it out during the three to five days it takes for the problem to resolve. If for some reason Joey is not better within a week, another trip to his pediatrician will be needed.

Additional Reading

The Complete Book of Breastfeeding. Marvin Eiger and Sally Wendkos Olds. Bantam, revised edition, 1999.

The Womanly Art of Breastfeeding. La Leche League International. Penguin, 1997.

Breastfeeding Your Baby. Sheila Kitzinger. Knopf, 1998.

CHAPTER 6

———————— ✧ ————————

New Options in Formula Feeding

When Robin was eight months pregnant, she went to check out formulas in her supermarket. What a shock! She discovered an enormous section devoted to different brands and types, each with different medical claims. In the end, she picked the one she had seen leaflets for in her obstetrician's office. But she wondered whether another one might be healthier or safer for her baby.

Irene nursed her baby during maternity leave from work, but at three months was finding it too difficult to express breast milk at work and needed a backup of formula. When she went shopping for formula, she wondered whether she should buy a standard formula, a soy product, or one of the many other types she could see.

Today's infant formulas range from the traditional or *standard* formulas that have been on the market for a number of years to the much newer *hydrolysate* and *elemental* varieties. This proliferation has given parents the important power of choice, but with this choice has come some potential confusion. How do you decide which one is best for *your* baby?

In some ways all these types of formulas differ remarkably little—for example, they all contain the known essential nutrients in approximately the right amounts, and all provide a safe alternative to breast milk when the mother doesn't nurse. In other areas the formulas differ quite a lot, particularly in their ability to treat and potentially prevent allergies and intolerances. On the face of it, the hypoallergenic formulas would seem to win hands down. However, this is not necessarily the case. At the frontiers of baby-formula research there are a number of important unresolved questions about what the optimal formula should contain, and it is in this gray area that we have to balance the tried-and-tested older kinds against the newer generation.

Take, for example, the hydrolysates, the group of formulas whose proteins have been broken down into very fine particles to reduce the risk of allergies. Can we be sure that the proteins they contain are really as good as those in standard formulas when it comes to promoting growth and development? The consensus from multiple short-term studies is yes, but there are not enough data from long-term research trials for a really comprehensive answer yet. Just as when treating chronic diseases with new drugs, you have to balance the improvements in the newer products against the known value of the tried and proven.

SIX FORMULA TYPES: WHICH IS BEST FOR YOUR BABY?

The following questions can help you narrow down your choice.

1. *Was your baby born at term without any particular problems?* If so, and if you have no strong family history of allergies or childhood diabetes, then a standard "with iron" formula is good to start with. You can stay with this formula until one year or move to a follow-up formula at six to nine months.

2. *Do you have a strong family history of allergies?* If so, consider using a hydrolysate formula until one year.

3. *Do you suspect that your baby has colic or is intolerant to a standard formula because you see symptoms of gastric discomfort, distention, persistent vomiting, diarrhea, or nasal or upper airway congestion?* If so, you may want to consider changing to a hydrolysate formula in consultation with your pediatrician. First, however, we suggest you read more about colic, food intolerances, and allergies in Chapter 16.

Once you have chosen the formula group that is right for you, the next question is: Which one in the group should you pick?

FORMULAS AT A GLANCE

FORMULA TYPES	USES	BRANDS
Standard	This is the cow's-milk-based formula type designed for infants who have no special problems. Most babies fall into this category.	Good Start with iron[1] Enfamil with iron[2] Enfamil low iron[2] (*not recommended*) Similac with iron[3] Similac low iron[3] (*not recommended*)
Hydrolysate	Hydrolysates are a type of cow's-milk-based formulas with proteins broken down into small pieces in order to minimize allergic reactions.	Alimentum[3] Nutramigen[2] Pregestimil[2]
Elemental	Elemental formulas are composed of essential nutrients broken down into very basic components to minimize digestive problems and allergic reactions.	Neocate[4]
Lactose-free	Lactose-free milk-based formulas are designed for infants with lactose intolerance but no other milk-related allergy problems.	Lactofree[2]
Follow-up	Follow-up formulas are alternatives to standard formula for infants older than six months. Some are milk-based and some are soy-based.	Enfamil Next Step Soy[2] Follow-Up with iron[1] Follow-Up soy with iron[1]

FORMULAS AT A GLANCE (CON'T)		
FORMULA TYPES	**USES**	**BRANDS**
Soy	Soy formulas, which contain soy protein and a carbohydrate-like corn syrup or sucrose instead of milk sugar, are suitable for infants in strict vegetarian families and possibly infants with milk protein allergy or lactose intolerance.	Alsoy[1] Isomil[3] ProSoBee[2]

Manufacturers: [1]Carnation, [2]Mead Johnson, [3]Ross, [4]SHS North America

STANDARD FORMULAS

There are three good and widely available options in this group—Enfamil with iron, Similac with iron, and Good Start. They all contain a good balance of nutrients, and in addition have recently been supplemented with nucleotides (which may possibly improve disease resistance and so make them similar to breast milk in this respect, though this is not yet proven).

We do not recommend any of the supermarket house brands because their composition is sometimes very different from the major brands that have undergone extensive testing. We also do not recommend any low-iron formulas because they increase the risk of anemia and resulting impaired development. This is because iron is poorly absorbed from formulas, necessitating an increased amount to prevent problems. For this reason, the American Academy of Pediatrics has issued a warning against using low-iron formulas. The main reason they were sometimes recommended in the past was an unsubstantiated belief that iron in formula causes constipation or gastrointestinal irritation, and that a low-iron formula would prevent it. Some formula-fed babies do experience constipation, and there are effective ways to deal with it (see page 98). A low-iron diet isn't one of them.

Of the standard formulas, Enfamil and Similac most closely resemble the formulas of old and so are probably the most "tried and true" of the three, with very little difference between them. The third standard formula, Good Start, was originally marketed as a kind of hydrolysate because its proteins are broken down into small pieces during the manufacturing process. Some research studies have suggested that Good Start does offer protection against allergies, but recently documented cases of allergic reactions to its whey-protein base (which it uses instead of the less-allergenic casein-protein base of the other hydrolysates) have resulted in withdrawal of its hypoallergenic status.

If you want to use a standard formula but have mild allergies in your family and want the potential (though not proven) benefits of a mildly hypoallergenic brand, Good Start may be a good choice, especially considering that it is much cheaper than the casein-based hydrolysates.

One of the frontiers of formula research today concerns fatty acid composition. Fatty acids (there are many different kinds) are the main component of fat. They're important because the brain is 60 percent fatty acids by weight, and the *type* of fat our infants eat may affect their actual brain structure. Research controversies continue to swirl around whether the fatty acid composition of current formulas is good enough to allow optimal brain development. Following is a summary of what is known to date.

The two chief essential fatty acids that infants need (those their bodies can't make from other fatty acids) are linoleic acid and alpha-linolenic acid, and both are present in breast milk and formula. These two fatty acids are used to synthesize new brain tissue, and they are also used to make two other fatty acids—arachidonic acid and decosahexaenoic acid (DHA), which in turn are also used for brain growth. Therein lies the controversy: Some research studies, but not all, have suggested that newborns can't synthesize enough arachidonic acid and DHA and so need to get these fatty acids from the milk they drink. Breast milk contains both, and many others besides, but formulas sold in the United States don't—yet. Added to this is the fact that some studies (but again, not all) have reported poorer visual development in formula-fed babies. Furthermore, one recent study showed better problem-solving ability at ten months in babies whose formulas had been supplemented with just 1 to 1.5 grams per day of DHA compared to babies fed with standard formula. As a result, questions have been raised about whether formulas should be modified to contain arachidonic acid and DHA, or some other of the many different fatty acids contained in breast milk. No commercial formulas in the United States currently do, but some may in the future if the consensus of scientific evidence becomes more conclusive than it is now.

HYDROLYSATE FORMULAS

The name *hydrolysate* refers to the fact that the proteins in these formulas are hydrolyzed, or enzymatically broken down into submicroscopic pieces, with the result that they are much less likely to induce allergic reactions than the whole proteins in standard formulas.

A rare option until recently, hydrolysates are becoming increasingly popular despite their greater price (about three times that of standard formula) and poor taste, as their reputation grows for alleviating colic and symptoms of milk intolerance. Families with a history of allergies may also be attracted to hydrolysates. However, more research is needed before hydrolysates can be strongly recommended for routine use (as opposed to treatment for specific intolerances and severe family histories).

Hydrolysates or elementals are also necessary for babies who develop problems with their gastrointestinal tract, and babies who have undergone surgery or severe infections causing intestinal damage. Among the three currently on the market, Pregestimil and Alimentum have more easily digested fats (medium-chain triglycerides), making them the most suitable for babies who have a particular problem with fat absorption.

ELEMENTAL FORMULAS

Most elemental formulas are designed for infants and children with impaired intestinal function that makes complete absorption of normal foods impossible. They are also given to babies who have severe symptoms of milk protein allergy that do not resolve with a hydrolysate. While most elemental formulas are for children over one year, one (Neocate) is specifically designed for infants. Neocate is even more expensive than the hydrolysates, but because each nutrient is supplied in its most basic form, it is theoretically without any allergy risk at all. This said, elemental formulas should be used only in consultation with your baby's pediatrician because they are relatively new to the market and have not undergone all the long-term testing of standard formulas.

SOY AND LACTOSE-FREE FORMULAS

Soy-based formulas were once widely recommended for babies with milk allergies but have been largely superseded by hydrolysates for treating medical problems. We now consider them primarily as an option for families who want to start their children on a strict vegetarian diet and for infants with the rare disease galactosemia (who are unable to digest lactose). Soy formulas were originally designed with cow's-milk intolerance in mind, but several recent studies have suggested that quite a number of infants who cannot tolerate cow's milk are also intolerant of soy-protein formula. So although soy formulas are worth considering if your child appears to have a milk protein allergy, you may find you need to move to a hydrolysate if there is no improvement. In addition some, but not all, research studies have suggested that soy formulas may have other drawbacks, including less-than-optimal calcium availability.

We don't recommend routine use of lactose-free formulas for young babies, except those with galactosemia. Lactose-free formulas are marketed for infants who are "lactose-intolerant," but true lactose intolerance generally occurs only after the age of three to four years, when a formula is no longer needed. The hydrolysates appear to be a better way of addressing the needs of families in which allergies might be a problem.

FOLLOW-UP FORMULAS

Follow-up formulas are designed with a slightly different balance of nutrients and are suitable for older babies. If your baby is growing well with a standard or soy formula, you can consider switching to a follow-up brand at six to nine months and staying with it until one year. But in fact, the formula you used up to six months will be fine until your child is one year old, at which point formula will no longer be necessary and you can switch directly to cow's milk.

Among the follow-up formulas designed for six months and older, the main difference is that one is milk-based (Follow-Up) and one is soy-based (Follow-Up soy). If you started with a milk-based standard formula, continuing with either the same formula or a milk-based follow-up is your best bet. If you found that a soy formula worked best for you in the first six months, continue with it or with a soy follow-up. Next-Step products (Enfamil) are designed for children one to three years, when formulas are not usually needed.

YOUR BABY'S FIRST FEEDINGS

If, like most families today, you have your baby in a hospital or birthing center, you will get advice from one of the nursing staff about when to give your baby her first feeding. Probably about two to four hours after your baby is born, or as soon as she is awake and lively, your nurse will suggest a feed. If you have decided on a formula, you can bring a supply with you. Otherwise the hospital staff will supply whatever brand they are using. Hospitals often rotate through the different brands of formula on a monthly basis so as not to favor one manufacturer over another. For this reason, don't be surprised if your baby is given a different product from the one your neighbor received six months ago.

Giving your baby a bottle is a great opportunity to cuddle up, so relax and soak up the experience. Cradle your baby in one arm in a semi-upright position, with your free hand in reach of the bottle. Touch your baby on *one* side of her face with the nipple of the bottle (she'll get confused if you touch both). This activates her rooting reflex. She then opens her mouth and turns toward the nipple. You quickly and gently slide it into her mouth so that most of it is inside. By doing this, you activate her sucking reflex. If she doesn't start sucking straightaway, or tries and starts spluttering, take the nipple out and gently try again in a few minutes. It may not go totally smoothly the first time or two, but most babies learn pretty quickly and it will soon seem like second nature.

When she has had 2 ounces (which is all she will probably want for now), or her sucking stops, or she drops off to sleep, you can gently remove the bottle. If she is still awake, it's time to see if you can get up any burps. Babies on formula usually swallow air when they suck and need a chance to let it come up without bringing too much milk with it. The number of burps will depend on your baby, ranging from none to several with each feed!

The best way to burp your baby is to prop her on your knee or lean her over your shoulder and gently stroke and pat her back for three or four minutes (see page 69). For the first few days, when she is taking only a little milk, you can do it just at the end of each feed. When her milk intake increases to 4 or more ounces per feed, some gentle burping halfway through may be called for as well. Babies who swallow a lot of air or who tend to spit up a lot may need to be burped more often, sometimes as frequently as every ½ to 1 ounce of milk.

The type of nipple you use in feeding your baby can help diminish the amount of air she'll swallow. Some babies manage fine with the first nipple you try; others need to try several before finding one they can suck easily. Nursing counselors often recommend one such as the Gerber Nuk or the Playtex Nurser to allow a good, vigorous sucking experience without too much air getting swallowed in the process.

By the second or third day after birth you will be able to see that your baby has become a much more experienced feeder and that her sucking is actually not continuous but occurs in bursts with little rests in between. You will also see her vigorous, rapid sucking at the beginning of a feeding when she is hungry, and the weaker, slower sucking toward the end as she gets full and contented. And while you are enjoying watching her feed, you will also see her taking the full measure of you, her universal provider. When you cuddle up with her cradled in your arms, she is at the best distance for her immature eyes to focus, and she will love watching your face to learn about you. Your smiles and loving gestures are all being taken in for her to model herself on in the future.

HOW MUCH FORMULA DOES YOUR BABY NEED?

Every baby needs a different amount of formula, and on-demand feeding is the best way for you to work out what yours needs. Babies fed on demand eat when they are hungry—typically every two to four hours (more frequently at first), and take only as much formula as they want at each feeding. Why is on-demand feeding so important? Mainly because if we force babies to eat when they are not hungry, or to wait when they are starving, we send the very harmful signal that eating is not connected with hunger. Babies need to learn to eat when they are hungry—and not learn to eat when they are not—in order to maintain the intrinsic caloric regulation that will protect them against obesity and related problems in the future.

Feeding your baby on demand means avoiding the temptation to try to get him to take the whole bottle. Just because he usually has, say, 4 ounces at this particular feed doesn't mean he will be hungry for 4 ounces today. Conversely, at some feeds your baby will be hungrier than usual. If he wants more and is still sucking eagerly when he finishes his bottle, give him more. He will be happier with this arrangement—and so will you, knowing that you are meeting his needs and that the two of you are working together as a team.

How do you figure out when to feed? If your baby cries and it is at least two hours since the last feeding, you can offer him a bottle. If he cries more often, try other options first. Perhaps he wants a cuddle, a nap, or entertainment, or quite possibly he wants to suck. If sucking is what he needs—and most small babies need lots of it—a pacifier or your smallest finger turned soft side up, clean and with a blunt, short nail, will probably make him happy. During the first two weeks, if he doesn't wake up and cry for milk every four hours, you should wake him and try a feed after he is alert. Babies who don't wake up to be fed regularly need to be monitored by their pediatrician because of the possible risk of dehydration or malnutrition.

By the time your baby is a month old you can expect him to want feeding about every three to four hours during the day and perhaps one or two times at night. At three months a likely schedule will be five to eight feeds in twenty-four hours, with perhaps one in the middle of the night—unless your baby has gotten the hang of sleeping through, in which case consider yourself lucky!

How much does your baby need to eat at each feeding? Again, everyone is different, and your baby's temperament and activity level will have an effect. During the first few days after birth, he will probably take very little—maybe an ounce or less at each feed—although some babies are hungry and take more from the start. After the first few days, his intake increases over the course of about six weeks. An average-size baby will typically want anything from 20 to 28 ounces per day at six weeks (the equivalent of five to eight feeds of 3 to 4 ounces each), with a range for babies of all sizes of 15 to 30 ounces (roughly 2 to 2½ ounces per pound of body weight). Research on babies growing normally has documented average formula intakes of 29 ounces per day by three months of age (with a range of 21 to 38 ounces), and these amounts or maybe a very little more will suffice up until the age of four to six months, when you can think about adding solid food.

DOES YOUR BABY NEED MULTIVITAMINS OR FLUORIDE?

Multivitamins/mineral supplements are not necessary for bottle-fed babies under one year, because all formulas have the full complement of essential nutrients. Fluoride is not recommended under six months, and details of what to do at that time are given in Chapter 9.

PRACTICAL AND SAFETY ISSUES

- Most formulas can be bought as ready-to-feed liquid, concentrated liquid, or powder. Despite the fact that they look a bit different when made up, they all contain the same nutrients in the same amounts. Powder is the least expensive option and the most work; ready-to-feed is the most expensive and the least work. Many families find that a combination (powder for home use and ready-to-feed for trips) works well.

- If you decide to use powder or concentrate, make sure you follow the manufacturer's advice exactly about how to make up the right strength. Studies have shown that parents of boys (especially dads) have a tendency to make up formula too strong. This is potentially dangerous and should always be avoided, because your baby needs the right amount of water in order to metabolize the formula and remain well hydrated. Be sure also to mix the powder enough to eliminate all the sticky lumps that can block the nipple or get left in the bottom of the bottle (starting with slightly warmed, rather than cold, water will help).

- Be scrupulously careful about cleaning everything you use until one year of age, and throw out leftover milk from partly finished bottles. (The saliva mixed in with the milk contains bacteria that will start to grow in saved milk, increasing the risk of a gastrointestinal upset.) Formula-fed babies are more susceptible to illnesses than breast-fed babies, so cleaning everything thoroughly is important even if it seems like a lot of work. Water needs to be completely contaminant-free (filtered and boiled tap water and distilled water are both fine), and all equipment needs to be cleaned well after each use. One easy way to do this is to rinse baby equipment except nipples and nipple rings by hand and then wash in a dishwasher with a heated drying cycle. Alternatively,

COMMON PROBLEMS AND FREQUENTLY ASKED QUESTIONS

Benjamin is two weeks old, and although he is contented in the morning, he cries without stopping for hours in the evening. His mother and father are frantic because they can't comfort him and don't know what to do.

you can wash well by hand and then put in clean boiling water on the stove-top for five minutes. Nipples and nipple rings should be sterilized in boiling water for five minutes after cleaning to ensure they are completely con-tamination free.

- All newborns should be started on body-temperature formula (98°F), which you can prepare by setting the bottle in a pan of hot (not boiling) water for a couple of minutes. Microwaves are more convenient but heat the formula unevenly. If you decide to use a microwave, mix the formula re-ally well after heating to avoid accidentally burning your baby's mouth. Always test the temperature of a bottle by shaking a drop onto the back of your hand. If it is at body temperature, it should feel tepid, neither hot nor cold. After one to two months you can try moving to more convenient room-temperature or even refrigerator-temperature formula, but be sure you 'don't discourage consumption in the process.

- Nipples with different sizes of holes are sold for infants of different ages. Make sure you use the right size, so that your baby can get the amount of formula she needs.

- Some bottles are better than others at allowing air to flow in as formula flows out (which means that pressure never builds up to collapse the nip-ple and interfere with sucking). Problems with pressure buildup are a com-mon reason why babies sometimes stop sucking in the middle of a feeding. If you suspect this is a problem, gently remove the nipple from your baby's mouth and replace again after the air has rushed in.

- Try disposable bottle liners (sterile bags with special holders) for easy trav-eling and for less sterilization and mess at home. They are usually available where formula is sold.

Benjamin should visit his pediatrician, who will likely diagnose colic. Several approaches can be tried, including using better burping techniques and switching to a hydrolysate formula for two weeks to see if it brings relief. Turn to Chapter 16 for more information on treating colic.

Sam, now one month old, has been fed formula from birth. His problem is that he gets very constipated. Before having a bowel movement, he strains a lot, and sometimes cries.

Constipation is not uncommon in formula-fed babies. Until recently, Sam's parents would have been advised to switch to a low-iron formula. However, this has not been proven to be effective, and low-iron formula increases a baby's risk of becoming iron-deficient. Offering one ounce of water twice a day is probably the best place for Sam's parents to start. If this doesn't work, they can try giving one teaspoon of light Karo syrup two times a day. It softens the stool and can solve the problem in short order.

Angie, at two and a half months, is showing some blood in her stools, which are hard, small, and accompanied by straining and crying. Her mother is in a panic.

Angie's mother is right to be concerned. This is probably a genuine case of constipation that has caused tearing of the tender anal tissue. Angie's mom should talk to her baby's doctor. She may also want to ask about using one teaspoon of Karo syrup two times a day; this is not widely known as a treatment for constipation, but it usually works well within three or four days. Topical ointments (such as A&D) will also provide temporary relief.

Rachel, two months, has had vomiting and diarrhea for two days. Should she be changed to a different formula until she recovers?

Most probably Rachel has a virus rather than the beginning of a food allergy. Research has demonstrated that giving glucose-electrolyte solution, such as Pedialyte, under a pediatrician's direction, is definitely helpful in preventing dehydration during an episode of diarrhea as described in Chapter 13. But as soon as Rachel can tolerate her standard formula she can go back on it. There appears to be no benefit from traditional treatments such as diluting the formula or changing to a lactose-free variety. If Rachel is on a mixed breast-feeding/formula regimen, she can continue to nurse.

Two-month-old Sarah loves to eat but just won't burp. She gulps bottles and then spits up large amounts when it is least expected.

"Spitty" babies are the reason you'll want some cotton diapers, even if you normally use disposables. If Sarah's mom carries one of the non-prefolded kind on her shoulder when Sarah is feeding, it will help. If it's total nutrition she's worried about, she should know that the "spits" probably contain less milk than she thinks. A review of burping positions may also be in order (page 69). But Sarah may also just be one of those "spitty" babies, and provided she continues to grow well, there is nothing to be concerned about. Spit-ups, incidentally, are quite different from projectile vomitting—spits tend to ooze out and are usually not a cause for concern, whereas projectile vomit shoots out over you or the room and is more an indication of a problem.

A trip to the pediatrician is also a good idea in Sarah's case, to check that growth is normal. If it is not, Sarah's parents can talk to their pediatrician about thickening the formula by mixing it with baby rice cereal (one tablespoon per two ounces of formula) for two to three of Sarah's formula feedings every day and enlarging the nipple hole to allow the thicker fluid to flow through. Although solid food before four months increases the risk of allergies, this step (which is usually very effective) may be necessary in cases when so much milk is lost that growth can't be maintained.

Jason—three months old—loves eating so much that he is now on the 95th centile for weight but only the 50th centile for height! His parents are concerned that his eating is out of control.

Although we don't advocate direct steps to influence weight at this young age, there are some simple questions Jason's parents should ask themselves to see if Jason is growing according to his genetic blueprint, or whether there is a problem that can be fixed. First, are they making formula up correctly? If it is too strong, this could be an explanation. Is Jason primarily thirsty? Offering him an ounce or two of water twice daily (though not much more, because it may replace too much milk) may slow his weight gain down immediately. Are they overencouraging him to eat—for example, by ignoring him other than at feeding times? If any one of these factors applies, Jason's feedings can be adjusted to a level that will allow him to "grow into his weight," gaining height until his weight is in proportion.

Baby Caroline is nearly four months old and seems to be fed up with formula. She tries sucking hard and then gives up. Her mother is worried that she is starving herself.

Caroline may simply be coming down with a minor illness, but another likely explanation is that there is a problem with her bottle. Perhaps the nipple holes are blocked and she can't get enough milk out. Perhaps she is ready to move up to the next larger size hole. It may even be that she has not learned how to release the suction on her bottle or Caroline may be sucking so hard she is creating a vacuum (in which case loosening the nipple ring should help). If none of these explanations fits, Caroline should be taken to her pediatrician to search for other reasons for this worrying problem.

> *Vivian, six weeks old, has been on a standard formula since birth and is growing well, but in the last two weeks her parents have started to see bloodstained mucus on the outside of her stool, even though she doesn't have constipation.*

Vivian's symptoms are typical of a baby who has developed an intolerance to the cow's milk protein in her formula, a problem that occurs in about 2 to 5 percent of young babies. She should be taken to her pediatrician, who will probably recommend switching to a hydrolysate formula, which will provide relief in the majority of cases. Symptoms should subside in three to fourteen days. In the unlikely event that they do not, further tests will be needed. If a protein sensitivity is confirmed, an elemental formula will probably be recommended. Information on when Vivian can be reintroduced to cow's milk and milk products is given in Chapter 16.

CHAPTER 7

※

Feeding a Premature Infant

Alice was only thirty-three weeks pregnant when she went into labor. Her twin girls, born by C-section, were tiny—only 3 pounds each—and were rushed to the neonatal intensive-care unit. At first, breast-feeding was the last thing on Alice's mind, and her twins were started on formula by naso-gastric tube. Two days after birth, however, Alice asked for help expressing milk so she could breast-feed them as soon as they were ready. With help and good advice, she was fully nursing her daughters by four weeks after their birth, saying she felt "confident enough to breast-feed until they go to college!"

Few parents think much about the possibility that their baby may be born before the right time. And yet it happens surprisingly often. About one in ten infants in the United States is born prematurely, or before thirty-seven weeks.

If your baby becomes one of this 10 percent, you will have a lot of things to think about in a hurry. Many parents of unexpected preemies are completely unprepared for the sobering reality of a high-tech neonatal intensive-care unit, and it takes a while to come to terms with what is happening. However, whether your baby should be given breast milk is among the most important decisions you will make at this time.

Even if you had decided to use formula, we urge you to reconsider if your baby is born early. At this vulnerable time of life, when essential developmental processes including brain growth are continuing at breathtaking speed, breast milk has the optimal balance of essential nutrients and other factors needed to start life on the right track. Despite the best of intentions, formula manufacturers have been unable to duplicate the many unique benefits and types of protection breast milk provides.

More than any other group of infants, premature babies benefit from being given their own mother's milk. Mothers of premature babies produce a very special milk, with more calories, protein, fat, and special immunological and growth factors compared to normal breast milk. Reductions in bacterial infections, allergies, and potentially fatal diseases of prematurity are all documented advantages for babies whose mothers provide milk during the early weeks. In addition, studies have shown that premature babies fed breast milk during just the first three weeks of life have an *eight-point* increase in IQ by eight years of age compared to premature babies fed formula.

For all these reasons, your decision to breast-feed can really make the difference of a lifetime to your child. The knowledge that you are helping your child in a way that nobody else can, and in a way that will affect his life far into the future, needs to be your incentive in the short term. Once your baby reaches 4 to 6 pounds, you will also start to enjoy the special satisfaction and bonding that breast-feeding mothers with full-term babies experience. But until that wonderful time, your path is a little harder. You will probably start out expressing milk for your baby to be given by tube if he is less than thirty-four weeks or 1,400 grams (about 3 pounds), and gradually switch over to nursing as his weight and strength increase. For larger babies, it may take only a day or two of intravenous or tube feeding before you are able to nurse.

Vitamins and minerals (especially iron) are also particularly important for babies born prematurely. This is because many vitamins and minerals are transferred to your baby during the last four to eight weeks of pregnancy. Without these stores your baby can easily become deficient. Your doctor will prescribe them during hospitalization and for later when you are all home.

GETTING STARTED
BREAST-FEEDING A PREMATURE INFANT

For the best success feeding a premature infant, reach out for advice and support, and let the hospital staff know that you want to take an active role in caring for your baby.

- *Talk with an experienced lactation consultant as soon as possible after delivery.* Unless your neonatal intensive-care unit employs a lactation specialist, and one with whom you feel comfortable, you will need a

IS YOUR BABY SUITABLE FOR KANGAROO CARE?

As we have witnessed time and time again when working in neonatal intensive-care units, being unable to hold your baby is one of the hardest things for many parents of preemies. Fortunately, a new method, called *kangaroo care,* has been developed that makes it possible for you to take your baby out of his incubator for regular periods every day. If your doctor says your baby is suitable (not all are—usually hospitals that use kangaroo care require that the baby weigh at least 3 pounds and be without serious medical problems), a pediatric nurse will show you how to hold him upright on your chest, skin to skin, keeping him warm and comfortable and allowing him to nurse whenever he wants. In a recent study testing whether kangaroo care is safe, premature babies managed to maintain their body temperature, blood oxygen level, and other clinical signs of well-being within normal ranges during four hours per day of kangaroo care. "Back to nature" is not always better, but in this case it seems to be acceptably safe, while at the same time giving back the physical and emotional connections that are so lacking in the modern incubator alternative.

If kangaroo care is not recommended for your situation but you had twins, it may be possible to put them both in the same incubator to boost physical contact. Some sophisticated intensive-care baby units are now starting to do this with good results.

recommendation from your baby's pediatrician or one of the national organizations. (See page 60 for numbers to call.)

- *Use expression to establish and build your milk supply.* Most premature babies under 3 pounds are not able to nurse because they are simply too small and weak. You will need to express milk, and it will be fed by tube as soon as your baby is ready to move from intravenous nutrition to milk. Expression may still be important even if your baby is heavier than 3 pounds and on a milk-only diet, as she may need some of her daily feedings given by tube while she develops the strength to nurse for extended periods.

- *Try to stay in the hospital, close to your baby, if possible.* Some hospitals have "boarding" arrangements.

EXPRESSING MILK

- Your hospital should supply, or you should rent from a lactation consultant, a large electric breast pump. Try to get one that allows you to pump both breasts simultaneously, because this increases your nursing hormone (prolactin) levels and in consequence your milk production. Don't bother with the small portable electric pumps, or hand pumps, at this stage—you need something more effective right now.

- Start expressing within eight hours after birth if at all possible. If this is impossible because of birth difficulties, just start as soon as you can. Research studies have documented nursing successes even in premature twins whose mother did not start expressing until three to five days after birth. Save even tiny amounts of milk—any amount is valuable to your baby now.

- For the highest milk production, try to pump both breasts every three hours around the clock for ten minutes per side. Don't expect to pump much milk in the first two to five days, before your real milk comes in. After that time, the amount of milk you produce will depend on how frequently and how long you pump.

- Very few women can express enough milk for all their babies' needs. However, the developmental advantages of breast milk for premature babies were identified in a study in which mothers provided only about half of their babies' total milk needs on average. So don't feel bad about the milk you can't supply—feel good about the milk you can!

- Talk to your doctor about whether your baby is suitable for kangaroo care—there are some recent data suggesting that it may help moms keep their milk production up.

• *Take part in the decision about how your infant gets fed even before you start nursing.* In the beginning, your infant may need to be fed intravenously, switching over to a nasogastric tube as soon as he can digest breast milk or formula. Once he reaches thirty-four weeks or 1,400 grams, you can expect to start a partial breast-feeding regimen, with the remainder of his milk fed by tube, cup, or bottle, perhaps combined with finger sucking (which is thought to promote growth, perhaps by encouraging production of growth factors). Although some hospitals try to get babies to take formula

- When you get home, do what it takes to give your body the rest it needs to get lactation off on the right track. Accept all offers of help, try not to worry about a messy house and unanswered phone messages, and consider getting someone to do household chores. This can be a tough time, so try to be good to yourself.

- Because premature babies are more susceptible to infection than infants born at term, you need to be very careful to keep your equipment and containers clean, washing your hands before each collection and sterilize your pump according to instructions. Wash your nipples once a day until your baby is able to take all his milk by nursing, using very mild soap or plain water to avoid any drying effect. Expressed milk can be stored in plastic collection bags or bottles and refrigerated for twenty-four hours or kept in a freezer for up to three months. Make sure you date and rotate your frozen supplies so that the oldest containers get used first.

- You may have to express for several weeks or months, depending on how premature your baby is. If you find your supply dwindling after the first month, try eating and drinking more, pumping more, and relaxing more, too. All of these factors, as well as spending as much time with your baby as you can, will help your milk supply. If your supply doesn't improve within four to six days, talk to your doctor about a prescription for metoclopromide, which can increase milk production by raising your prolactin levels. It also gets into your milk supply, and for this reason should be considered only as a last resort.

in a bottle before they start learning how to nurse, many pediatricians feel it is better to start nursing first, to prevent the nipple confusion that can make initiating nursing harder. There is usually no good medical reason for starting bottle feedings first, and the sooner you start nursing, the easier it will be to keep your milk supply up.

- *Be patient when switching over to breast-feeding.* When you do start nursing, be very patient with yourself and your baby. Premature ba-

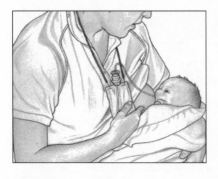

bies often start out with a very weak suck and poor coordination of sucking and swallowing. It may take two weeks or more for your baby to get the hang of it.

Supplemental nursing systems can help you get started on nursing before your baby is able to take a complete feed unaided. These are devices that have a line of fine tubing connected to a reservoir of milk (expressed breast milk or formula). The tube goes into your baby's mouth while he nurses and delivers some milk while he learns to suck at the breast. With this option, you will probably need to pump after nursing him as well, both to provide supplemental milk for the next feed and to fully empty your breasts to keep your milk production high.

Be sure to use a quiet room for nursing during the early weeks, both at the hospital and at home. Many premature babies are easily distracted at first, and may shut down and refuse to nurse if there is too much noise or bright light.

Do be prepared for nursing to take a long time initially. Until your baby grows stronger, he may need to nurse as much as one hour out of every three. Don't panic! This time will pass and you will move on to more normal feeding times quite soon. And whatever other compromises you make, don't skip nighttime feeds. Prolactin levels are higher at night, and feeding then will give your milk supply an extra boost. Don't be afraid to touch and cuddle your baby even when he is too tired to nurse. Some studies suggest that cuddling and touch may improve growth and development, independent of the milk that is consumed.

If you have flat or inverted nipples, don't use a nipple shield during feedings. Nipple shields have been shown to reduce milk production by 50 percent, and they don't make it any easier for babies to latch on. Instead, apply a cold cloth to your breast before the feeding starts to help shape your nipple, and then a little suction from a breast pump to draw it out.

To begin with, the doctors in the neonatal unit will probably ask you to weigh how much breast milk your baby is actually taking, and will supply an electronic scale. Weigh your baby before and after each feed, then add up the total for twenty-four hours. Don't change diapers or clothes during the process or the weights will be inaccurate, and try not to let the weights upset you (even healthy premature babies have day-to-day functuations). Before they reach about 6 pounds, premature babies need a daily total of about 90 grams of milk (3 ounces) per pound of weight. Once your pediatrician knows how much your baby is getting unaided, he or she will be able to tell how much is needed as a supplement.

As you gradually increase the amount of nursing relative to supplemental feeds, you should increasingly encourage on-demand feeding. Be prepared for at least twelve feeds per day in the first week or two. This will seem like a lot, and it is. But it will help your milk supply to increase with your baby's demands and will ensure the best long-term success. Over time you can gradually decrease expression and use of a supplemental nursing system until your baby is able to meet all his requirements by breast alone. At this point, you are a testimony to the success that diligence can bring, and will be able to nurse for as long as you and your baby want.

FORMULA OPTIONS FOR PREMATURE INFANTS

Even mothers who start expressing milk for their premature infants usually find that some formula is necessary, too, until nursing takes off. Expressing can be hard and tedious, and producing the volume that a rapidly growing preemie needs is not something that many women can do. Even if you are one of these unusual few, your hospital will probably still recommend that a breast-milk fortifier be added to your milk while your baby is hospitalized, to give her extra proteins, vitamins, minerals, and electrolytes. Although research on the value of breast-milk fortifiers is at an early stage, the preliminary results suggest that they are beneficial because they increase weight gain with no adverse side effects.

For babies who need formula in addition to breast milk, or who are relying on formula as their sole food source, there are several special formulas that provide a better balance of nutrition for preemies than the regular formulas. These special formulas (which all appear to be similarly effec-

PREMATURE FORMULAS

Standard preemie formulas *(for use in the hospital and up to about 4 to 5 pounds):*
  Enfamil Premature (Mead Johnson)
  Similac Special Care (Ross)

Transitional formulas *(designed for older preemies, up to twelve months, who may still need extra nutrients for catch-up growth):*
  Enfamil 22 (Mead Johnson)
  Similac Neocare (Ross)

Fortifiers *(designed to supplement breast milk when needed):*
  Human Milk Fortifier (Mead Johnson)
  Similac Natural Care (Ross)

tive) are suitable for your baby up to 1.8 to 2.2 kilograms (about 4 to 5 pounds). Once she passes this weight, your pediatrician may switch her to a standard formula, or perhaps to a transitional formula if extra growth is needed.

AFTER YOU LEAVE THE HOSPITAL

Some premature babies need extra physical help for several more months when it comes to feeding, because of weakness and coordination difficulties, and so your special patience, love, and physical contact will continue to be important. Being born early is a major life event, and one that it frequently takes a while to recover from. Keeping up contact with other families you met in the hospital will help provide some of the support you need. Your pediatrician's input will also be important if gastrointestinal, pulmonary, or other disorders persist.

When it comes to feeding milestones, keep in mind how old your baby actually is. Is she four months old because she was born four months ago, or two months old because she came into the world at only thirty-two weeks? Our recommendation is to count her feeding milestones from her full-term due date. So, for example, introduce solid foods at four to six months after the expected time of delivery rather than after she actually arrived. You may even find that delaying the introduction to solids further works better, if your baby doesn't get the hang of swallowing solid food within a week to ten days of first introduction. Don't make the switch from formula to whole cow's milk until twelve months after the expected delivery date. By adjusting for your child's developmental age, you will minimize her risk of allergies and keep her development and health on the best track.

Finally, despite being smaller, many premature and small-for-date babies are often constantly hungry, as if trying to catch up. Our own research studies have documented that premature babies typically eat 200 calories a day more than term babies at nine months of age, despite weighing less. It remains a mystery why this happens, but while scientists work to solve it, your best option is simply to go with the flow. If your baby is constantly hungry, let her eat to satisfaction. Most likely she simply needs more calories. By letting her eat her fill, you will be allowing normal energy regulation to do its job, and ensuring her optimal growth.

———◆———

PART THREE

Food Transitions

Four Months to Six Years

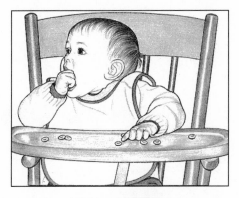

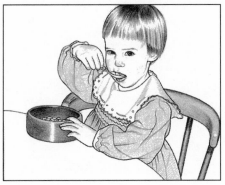

CHAPTER 8

———— ✦ ————

The Family Balancing Act

Alice knows that her two children, six-month-old Sarah and four-year-old Danny, need more fat and less fiber than she does. But how should she give it to them? Would the family diet plus premium ice cream be an easy solution? Or does she need to prepare two separate meals?

Some parents find it easy to feed their newborn but are concerned when the time comes for solid foods. How much, what kind, and how often are just three of many questions at this time. Others negotiate the weaning transition but feel frustrated later, when they want their toddler to like foods he is refusing, or when they have two or more children to feed and providing a healthy diet for everyone seems an impossible balancing act.

These are questions of quality as well as quantity. How much milk should Sarah drink to get all the calcium and protein she needs? Is organic better? Should parents avoid—or seek out—irradiated produce? What extra food safety measures do parents need to employ once there are children in the house?

The good news for busy parents is that making enjoyable meals that are healthy and safe for the whole family doesn't have to be difficult. This chapter answers some general questions parents often raise about feeding their families. Chapters 9 through 12 give age-specific information for four months to six years.

BALANCE FOR THE WHOLE FAMILY

On a day-to-day basis, what we all need are portion and food guidelines that we can keep in our heads. If you and your family eat according to the following plan on most days, you can be confident that everyone in the family is getting the right nutrients in the right amounts.

As you can see from the chart on pages 116 and 117, a healthy diet for your child has more dairy products relative to total calories, fewer high-fiber foods, and a higher density of fat and minerals. This is true for birth through six years, but particularly so during the first two to three years, when metabolic programming is in full swing and brain development, in particular, is still sensitive to what gets eaten.

Six simple strategies will ensure that your whole family eats the balance of nutrients that is right for them.

1. *Vary the balance of different foods for different family members.* Your child (depending on her age) needs about the same amount of milk and other high-calcium dairy products as you do, but only half the fruit and vegetables and *less than half* the grains and cereals (because of her lower calorie needs). Meat and other high-protein foods are not essential if your child eats the recommended amounts of other foods listed and takes a multivitamin/mineral supplement. Amounts can be dictated by preference: up to 1 to 3 ounces daily of meat, poultry, or fish for your child after age one, and up to 6 to 9 ounces for you.

2. *Shop for everyone's fat and fiber needs.* There are at least three food types you can easily keep in the house in two forms—one for grown-ups and one for children.

   - *Milk.* You can drink skim or other low-fat milk, while your baby will start with breast milk or formula, graduate to whole milk at age one, move over to 2 percent at age two, and to 1 percent or skim milk at age three.
   - *Breads.* The adults can get their fiber from whole wheat, rye, pumpernickel, and other whole-grain breads, while your child has lower fiber needs and can be offered white bread as well as adult choices. He will want to try your bread, of course, and gradually increasing amounts will be healthful. But he shouldn't be expected to eat whole grains exclusively unless he actually prefers to.
   - *Cereals.* Breakfast cereals for the family can be stocked in high-fiber varieties for adults (5 grams fiber or more per serving) and moderate-fiber varieties for the kids.

3. *If recipes you like have ingredients that are not suitable for your child, simply leave them out and put them on the table as condiments.* Children under six should have minimal added salt (none at all for babies under six months) and no alcohol. If these are important ingredients in some of your favorite foods, you don't have to give them up. Simply make most entree recipes with half or a quarter of their usual salt, and let those who want to add more (you may find your own salt taste diminishing). If a recipe calls for wine or spirits, add it early and cook very thoroughly so that the taste remains but none of the alcohol. Strong spices such as chili or curry can be cut in half or less and pepper flakes or hot sauce put on the table for grown-ups.

4. *Focus on cooking methods that enhance nutrition for everyone.* Protein, minerals, fiber, and fat-soluble vitamins (A, D, E, and K) are not adversely affected by cooking, but most water-soluble vitamins are lost to a greater or lesser degree, especially when heating is prolonged or when foods are boiled in a lot of water. You can maximize your family's vitamin intake by serving lots of raw salads, and by steaming or microwaving vegetables (rather than boiling them). Stir-frying is also a good way to minimize vitamin losses from vegetables, and is healthy too if you use only a tablespoon or two of oil per family dish. Frozen vegetables and fruits, incidentally, tend to have somewhat less nutrients than fresh ones, contrary to popular belief (though not if you usually leave fresh produce in the refrigerator for weeks before using). Canned vegetables and fruits tend to have far less vitamins than fresh unless the foods have been specifically added back (especially if the foods are packed in syrup or sauce), and of course many are also poor second cousins when it comes to taste and texture.

5. *Unless you have a family medical history that dictates a special diet, you don't need to avoid eggs and red meat entirely.* Most nutritionists recommend eating these foods sparingly. For young children, however, they can be valuable because they are some of the best sources of the essential nutrients iron and zinc, which are needed for growth and development. Your child can, of course, get these minerals from a multivitamin/mineral supplement instead. But some research has suggested that eggs, in particular, are not as unhealthy as they were once thought to be (the old cholesterol measurements were wrong—

FEEDING THE FAMILY

4–12 months	12–21 months	21 months–3 years	3–6 years
Servings:	*Servings:*	*Servings:*	*Servings:*
DAIRY FOODS (FOR CALCIUM, PROTEIN, AND ENERGY)			
Breast milk or formula, 20–38 oz	16–24 oz whole milk, yogurt, or equivalent*	16–24 oz 2% milk	16–24 oz 1% or skim milk
MEAT, POULTRY, FISH, NUTS, LEGUMES, & EGGS (FOR MINERALS AND PROT			
See Chapter 9 on introduction of specific foods	1–2 servings (a serving is 1 egg; or 1 oz meat, poultry, fish; or ¼ cup cooked beans)	1–3 servings	1–3 servings
FRUITS & VEGETABLES (FOR VITAMINS)			
See Chapter 9 on introduction of specific foods	½–1 cup. See Chapter 10 for specific foods.	¾–1¼ cups	1–1½ cups
CARBOHYDRATES (FOR ENERGY, MINERALS, AND VITAMINS)			
See Chapter 9 on introduction of specific foods	According to appetite, refined and whole-grain items	According to appetite, refined and whole-grain items	According to appetite, increasing amounts of whole-grain items
FATS, OILS, & SWEETS			
Contained in breast milk and formula	Oils such as canola, corn, olive, peanut, and sunflower in cooking Butter, desserts, and candy limited	Same as 12–21 months	Same as 12–21 months
MULTIVITAMIN/MINERAL SUPPLEMENT			
Recommended for nursing infants; not necessary for bottle-fed babies	Recommended	Recommended	Not necessary with consistently good diet but still a good idea

* 1 oz cheese = 6 oz milk; yogurt (plain or fruit flavor) can exchange 1:1 with milk.

Adults
Servings:
2–3 servings (1 serving = 1 cup low-fat or skim milk or yogurt, or 1 1/2 oz cheese)
2–3 small servings (a serving is 3 oz meat, fish, poultry; or 1/2 cup cooked beans; or 1 egg)
2 1/2 – 4 1/2 cups
6–11 servings according to energy needs, primarily from whole-grain items (a serving is 1 slice bread, 1 oz dry cereal, or 1/2 cup cooked cereal, pasta, etc.)
Eat sparingly
Not necessary with consistently good diet (except pregnant and lactating women)

eggs actually contain about 20 percent less cholesterol than previously suggested). In addition to iron and zinc, a single egg contains more than a third of a two-year-old's daily requirement of vitamins A, B_{12}, and K, riboflavin, pantothenic acid, iodine, phosphorus, and selenium as well as a generous helping of essential fatty acids! Barring a family medical history suggesting otherwise, eggs in recipes are fine, and if you want a few meals a week of eggs or red meat, that is fine, too. Provided that you also generally avoid the sources of saturated fat that have few essential nutrients (such as butter, cream, fatty meats, ice cream, and foods containing coconut and palm oils) your child's overall diet will be nutritious *and* relatively low in saturated fat.

6. *Give your child a multivitamin/mineral supplement.* Many parenting books say that supplements aren't necessary, but nutrition surveys show that most children older than six months are short of several vitamins and minerals unless they take a supplement. Furthermore, most young children don't eat enough food to make getting all the RDAs easy, even if they generally eat healthy foods.

PRACTICAL STEPS FOR EASY MEALS

Here are three ways to minimize kitchen time:

1. *Batch and store.* Provided that you know that the food is popular, cooking several portions at once—and freezing what you don't eat immediately—is your best technique for maintaining a varied family diet

of good food without too much effort. Batching and freezing works well for dinner entrees, some carbohydrates, some breakfasts, and many baby dinners. If you are really organized, you can cook one big entree and a carbohydrate food such as rice or pasta each week, freeze most of it, and enjoy something different four or five nights a week simply by heating up a different batch. Freshly cooked vegetables are better than frozen or reheated, and they usually take only a few minutes to prepare while you are defrosting an entree.

2. *Save leftovers.* It is surprising how tidbits left from tonight's dinner can become a whole meal for a small child. Refrigerate or freeze leftovers promptly in child-sized containers.

3. *Try to keep some basics in your refrigerator, freezer, and cupboards that will make more than one different meal.* We like to keep cooked rice and hardy vegetables such as carrots, broccoli, onions, and celery readily available. With a little steak or chicken from the freezer, you can whip up a quick stir-fry. The same meats can be served at another meal with mashed potatoes and steamed carrots and broccoli, while the vegetables can combine with a little oil or some spaghetti sauce and a sprinkle of cheese to go over pasta. A basic vinaigrette and other dipping sauces are also useful to go with cut-up veggies at dinner—or before, if the kids are ravenous. It's a good way to stave off hunger while dinner is being fixed.

HOW SAFE IS OUR FOOD?

Irene, mother of three-year-old Roger, has been talking with nutrition-conscious parents at preschool who tell her she should shop at the more expensive organic health food store rather than at her local supermarket. Her doctor has reassured her that she doesn't need to, but Irene still wonders if she is doing the right thing.

Organic fruits, vegetables, and meat—raised without pesticides (which primarily control insects, fungi, and plant diseases), herbicides (which control weeds), hormones (which control growth and productivity), and chemicals to boost shelf life—are increasingly available, and are widely viewed as superior choices despite often substantially increased costs. However, the issue is not so simple, and decisions about organic versus conventional need to be made by each family after they have considered the facts.

Organic produce actually often does contain some pesticides and other chemicals. Because organic farmers are allowed to use some "natural" chemicals, and because the definition of what chemicals are natural is regulated at the state level, different parts of the country have different standards. Having said this, organic products certainly contain fewer pesticide, herbicide, and hormone residues than conventionally produced foods. A recent survey found residues in 25 percent of organic produce compared to 77 percent in conventional produce, and the organic produce also had smaller amounts of generally less harmful chemicals.

One of the biggest concerns with conventional produce is that some of the chemicals used in farming today may be more harmful than suspected when existing regulations were developed (often based on studies in rodent species, which may not have the same chemical sensitivity as humans). There is certainly precedence for this concern—DDT (dichlorodiphenyl-tricholorethane), for example, was once thought to be safe, but was subsequently banned after being linked to cancer. Unfortunately, DDT continues to lurk in rivers and streams because it is undegradable, which makes eating several species of fish a possible risk (see page 75).

On the other hand, sometimes chemicals are withdrawn from use needlessly. Alar (daminozide), a pesticide used to improve apple quality, was taken off the market in response to a media frenzy generated by an environmental action group. This happened even though the best evidence showed that adults would have to eat *fifty thousand Alar-treated apples every day* to suffer any measurable adverse consequences! Alar is now gone, but some food safety experts worry that the alternative pesticides that have replaced it may be less safe than Alar.

One of the main factors giving rise to uncertainty over pesticides and herbicides is that there are so many chemicals—*currently six hundred*—that farmers are legally allowed to use on their produce. Because of the complexity of the data needed to assess the risks of each one, it is unlikely that all of these chemicals are optimally regulated. The Environmental Protection Agency is currently re-reviewing its safety limits on agricultural chemicals but, because of the volume of work, is not expected to complete the report until the year 2006.

There is also a positive side to pesticides. Many are used for a good reason—namely, to kill pests! The average American unknowingly eats *1 pound* of insects every year (in commercial products such as jam, peanut butter,

HOW TO MINIMIZE CHEMICAL RESIDUES IN NONORGANIC PRODUCE

1. Wash produce thoroughly with water before use, using a vegetable brush on less delicate items. You reduce pesticide residues in most produce by 25 to 50 percent when you do this, and up to 80 percent in some items such as tomatoes.

2. Know the top five fruits and vegetables with high chemical residues (strawberries, red and green peppers, spinach, cherries, and peaches) and either wash these foods particularly well, avoid eating large amounts, or consider buying organic for just these items.

and tomato paste), not to mention bacteria and fungi. This is not actually harmful (they are cooked and sterilized!) but we will undoubtedly eat even more if organic produce becomes common. The public desire for no pesticides *and* no pests is a difficult—if not impossible—standard to meet. Many (though not all) agricultural chemicals currently in use prevent dangerous bacterial and fungal contaminations that can cause food poisoning as well as longer-term problems (such as liver disease and cancer in the case of aflatoxin mold on corn and peanuts). In the past (and until as recently as 1920), whole villages and towns were occasionally wiped out by food contaminations such as ergot poisoning (a fungus growing on grains and causing gangrene and convulsions). The risks of pesticides and other chemicals used in farming need to be balanced against the benefits they bring.

Cost is another consideration. On average, organic produce costs 57 percent more than conventional produce. If you buy fewer fruits and vegetables because organic ones are more expensive, this is unquestionably a bad bargain for your health. There are major long-term health benefits from eating more fruits and vegetables (organic or otherwise), and anything that would make you eat less should be avoided.

The antibiotics and hormones fed to nonorganically raised animals and poultry to increase yields are another potential area of concern. And because they offer fewer potential safety benefits to counterbalance the negatives, antibiotics and hormones are perhaps the clearest case where organic products have possible advantages without possible disadvantages.

Several studies have raised the concern that antibiotic-resistant strains of bacteria can develop in farm animals and then be transferred to people. In addition, those same antibiotics and hormones have the potential to be unpredictable regulators of human cell metabolism and growth. Like pesticides and herbicides, these chemicals are certainly good for farm productivity. However, some of the ones currently in use reduce the ability of human antibiotics to be a safety net against otherwise-untreatable diseases, and whether they are all completely safe remains to be conclusively established. The FDA recently announced plans to tighten rules on the types of antibiotics that can be used in farm animals, which is a welcome step, but translating those plans into regulations will take time.

WHAT ABOUT IRRADIATED FOODS?

Despite the many frightening stories about food safety, our food supply is now actually safer than at any other time in history. The major food contaminants are now bacteria such as *E. coli* (including the lethal O157:H7 strain occasionally found in hamburger, fresh apple cider, and other produce), *Salmonella, Campylobacter jejuni,* and *Shigella.* Previously there were many more microbes that threatened the immediate safety and long-term health of children and adults alike.

So why do we need irradiation—a form of "cold pasteurization" in which gamma rays (similar to X rays) are passed through food to destroy all the DNA—including that of any live bacteria and fungi?

The main reason is that, although our food supply is much safer than it was, today's microbes continue to cause an estimated eight million cases of sickness nationwide every year, and nine thousand of these cases result in death. The sicknesses, incidentally, are not just intestinal. Food bacteria can cause wide-ranging symptoms including fever, headaches, and nausea as well as diarrhea and abdominal pain. Repeated *Shigella* infections have also been linked to chronic rheumatoid arthritis in childhood. Irradiation considerably reduces the risk of food poisoning and at the same time extends shelf life, improves the quality of fresh foods such as fruits, and can replace previously used chemical preservatives.

On the down side, there remains some uncertainty over whether irradiated foods are as completely healthful as nonirradiated foods if the issue of bacterial contamination is set aside. Although forty years of animal studies have failed to turn up any specific dangerous effects (and, contrary to popular belief, irradiated food *does not* result in radiation exposure to the people who eat it), irradiation does somewhat reduce the vitamin content of

GENERAL GUIDELINES FOR FOOD SAFETY IN THE KITCHEN

1. **Maintain a clean environment.** Wash your hands before you start cooking, and keep all equipment scrupulously clean. Use a dishwasher (with the heated drying cycle) for dishes and utensils if possible. If you don't have a dishwasher, paper towels and freshly laundered dishtowels reduce contamination compared to dishtowels that have been in the kitchen for several days. *For babies under one year,* nipples and nipple rings should be sterilized in boiling water for five minutes. This is important because infants (especially bottle-fed ones) are particularly susceptible to intestinal infections.

2. **Be careful with high-protein foods.** Fish, ground beef, poultry, and similar high-protein foods should be transported home rapidly, refrigerated immediately, and either cooked by their sell-by date or frozen for later use. Keep all raw and cooking meats away from other food, wash up well after handling them, and cook all items for children to the well-done stage (165°F internal temperature for most ground and whole meats, 175°F for poultry, with thermometer inserted into meat after the initial searing of the outside to prevent internal contamination by surface bacteria). If you marinate, keep the mixture in the refrigerator prior to cooking.

3. **Be extra careful with eggs, too.** If you can, buy pasteurized eggs (which are new to the market) because they are much safer and you can use them any way you want. Like poultry, the unpasteurized eggs found in most stores may harbor *Salmonella* and need to be used with care. Buy only refrigerated cartons of uncracked eggs and store in your refrigerator. If you can find only unpasteurized eggs, avoid serving them raw or partly cooked

food (especially the antioxidant vitamins). With their extended shelf life, irradiated foods have even fewer vitamins by the time they are actually put on the table. In addition, because irradiation is so effective in reducing microbial contamination, there is potential for commercial abuse if traditional sanitary practices are scaled back to produce sterile but unclean foods.

For these reasons, the current government policy of limiting irradiation to specific foods at high risk of bacterial contamination (including pork, (including soft-boiled ones). Licking the bowl is, alas, unsafe when raw eggs are in the batter.

4. **Inspect produce carefully before buying and wash well before use.** Wash all fruits and vegetables—organic and conventional alike—with warm water (exception: prewashed ones in sealed bags, which are thought to be safe contrary to a mistaken recent report), scrubbing skins with a brush as appropriate. Using bleach is not recommended because of potential residues. Throw out all fruit with cracked skins, all outside leaves, and all spoiled parts (including green bits on potatoes and any mushy parts of melons). Cartons of raspberries and blackberries that have any moldy ones should be left on the supermarket shelf, or thrown out if you bought them accidentally.

5. **Avoid unpasteurized juice.** *E. coli* O157:H7 makes this a risky treat.

6. **Refrigerate or freeze leftovers immediately after you finish the meal.** Use shallow containers to ensure rapid cooling. In the case of baby foods, make sure that they were not contaminated with a used spoon (in which case the whole portion should be discarded).

7. **Deal firmly with unwanted guests.** If you find any moldy food in your refrigerator or cupboard, throw it out immediately, being careful to avoid letting the bacteria or mold spores leak into the atmosphere while you are doing it. The one exception to this rule is hard cheese: microscopic mold growth is thought to penetrate $1\frac{1}{2}$ inches (but no further) into hard cheese. Cut off a 2-inch strip from each side that shows any mold.

potatoes, and fruits, with possible future approval of ground beef, seafood, and eggs) is appropriate, as is favoring the new oxygen-free, cold-dose irradiation techniques that minimize the loss of vitamins and the formation of free radicals, and labeling irradiated products (though not mixed products containing some irradiated items) with the Radura symbol and the words "treated by irradiation." On your side, don't allow the extended keeping qualities of irradiated items to lull you into shopping less frequently. If you store irradiated items for no longer than you would nonirradiated ones, you will minimize storage-related vitamin losses (which can be substantial—up to 50 percent for some vitamins in some produce during extended storage).

VEGETARIAN AND MACROBIOTIC DIETS

About 14 percent of American households now have at least one vegetarian family member. If you are a vegetarian, can you feed your child the same food that you eat?

If your household is lacto-ovo-vegetarian—eating dairy products and eggs, but not meat, fish, or poultry—the short answer is yes, with care. There are certain nutrients you need to be careful about—vitamin B_{12} and iron in particular. But provided that your child does drink milk, eats eggs, and receives a daily multivitamin/mineral supplement, there is no reason why she cannot eat the same foods as you.

If you avoid eggs and milk products in addition to meat, fish, and poultry, you are eating a vegan, or strict vegetarian, diet. Macrobiotic diets may include fish but are often vegan. To feed your child a vegan diet and keep her in the best of health is very challenging. Even if you breast-feed your child, iron deficiency leading to impaired mental function is a real risk, as are vitamin B_{12} and calcium deficiencies. For these reasons we recommend against strict vegetarian diets until your child is at least six years old. Instead the family diet should be supplemented to include the recommended amounts of milk, milk products such as cheese and yogurt, eggs, and a children's multivitamin with minerals. If, despite the concerns, you definitely want to feed your child a vegan diet, enlist your pediatrician's help to minimize risks to development.

FOODS TO AVOID OR STRICTLY LIMIT

Almost no common food is dangerous enough—barring allergic reactions and excluding alcohol—that your child can't have a small amount occasionally. In fact, being extremely restrictive can actually backfire when he starts mingling in the outside world and sees other children eating such foods. This said, avoid the following foods as a general rule because of health risks now or in the future, and to prevent your child from developing strong preferences for them. There are also specific foods you need to exclude for immediate safety reasons during the first year of life, as described in Chapter 9.

- **Alcohol.** Children are very susceptible to the toxic effects of alcohol, and regular amounts that would be small for a grown-up can lead to permanent brain and liver damage.

- **Caffeine in soda, coffee, and tea.** Caffeine is an addictive stimulant (probably a major reason why soda manufacturers put this tasteless chemical in their products) and directly affects the nervous system, kidneys, and other body tissues. In addition, caffeine reduces calcium availability for bone and tooth formation. The tannins present in caffeine-containing teas also increase the risk of iron deficiency by reducing iron absorption (see Chapter 9).

- **High-nitrite foods such as hot dogs, ham, bologna, and bacon.** As described in Chapter 1, some recent research suggests that high-nitrite foods may increase the risk of childhood cancers (as little as one regular hot dog a week is linked to double the risk). Nitrites themselves are harmless, but they can be converted into nitrosamines and nitrosamides in the body, which are powerful carcinogens (about five million times more powerful than saccharin, for example). Further research is needed on the nitrite issue, and may possibly show that nitrites are not as harmful as currently suspected. In the meantime, we consider regular portions of high-nitrite foods an unnecessary risk because there are so many good and healthy no-nitrite alternatives. Hot dogs and processed meats have also recently been linked to the disease listeriosis, which can cause flu-like and mononucleosis-like symptoms and even meningitis in babies and young children. The bacteria *Listeria monocytogenes* is responsible for listeriosis, and grows undetected in foods contaminated by traditional sources such as animal feces. This says a lot about the quality of meat used in some meat processing plants.

- **Potentially contaminated foods such as game fish, lake fish, and organ meats from nonorganically raised animals.** As described in Chapter 5, these foods are potentially concentrated sources of dangerous neurotoxic pesticides and heavy metals and so shouldn't be consumed too regularly. Check with your state fishing advisory board for recommended limits on fish in your area.

- **High-salt foods.** About 6 percent of individuals (and 60 percent of individuals diagnosed with hypertension) are "salt-sensitive," meaning that high-salt diets increase blood pressure and so promote premature heart disease. There is no easy way to tell if your children are salt-sensitive or not, but since our perception of saltiness depends on how much we eat, you can give your family a low-salt diet and it will taste just as "salty" as a high-salt diet after you have all adapted (this takes about eight weeks). Reducing salt intake is as simple as using fewer commercially prepared foods (80 percent of salt intake comes from items such as chips, soup, sauces, and fast food), reducing salt in recipes to a quarter or half of the amount listed, and keeping the salt shaker off the table.

- **High-calorie sodas and fruit drinks.** From the perspective of their metabolic effects, all sugars (including regular white sugar, brown sugar, and honey) are similar to white bread or potatoes. And contrary to previous speculation, sugar actually doesn't seem to cause behavior problems (see Chapter 17). However, America now produces enough sugar to provide every man, woman, and child with *3 pounds of sugar a week,* a 20 percent increase over ten years ago. Sodas and fruit drinks (which usually contain *very* little juice and few nutrients) are the single largest source of this sugar, which promotes overeating and displaces the healthy foods your child needs for growth and development. Twenty years ago American children drank twice as much milk as soda; today they drink twice as much soda as milk (an average of a gallon a week!) and are suffering nutritionally in consequence. It is a trend that desperately needs to be reversed, and can be—one family at a time.

  Water is the healthiest replacement for sodas and fruit drinks (after milk up to the amount recommended for your child's age), and children love it if they are used to it. Juice is also fine in small amounts (the more micronutrient-dense types such as orange are best, up to 4 ounces daily) but is a problem in large quantities because it replaces a healthier balance of different foods. Apple juice, in particular, is very weak in micronutrients and could almost be classed as soda from the perspective of vitamins and minerals.

- **Candy.** Like soda, it contains almost nothing but calories, replaces healthful foods, and causes overeating.

WHAT ABOUT DESSERTS, COOKIES, AND CAKES?

Desserts, cookies, and cakes are among the most calorically dense foods we eat. Sugar technically contains only the same number of calories as starch (4 calories per gram). However, because sugar contains no moisture it is actually about four times as calorically dense as water-containing starches such as cooked potatoes, pasta, and rice. Baked goods and desserts are even worse, because of the extra calories from fat (to say nothing of saturated fat and trans fatty acids). And caloric density is important. As explained in Chapter 15, research studies have shown that calorically dense foods are easier to overeat than other foods, making them an important cause of excess weight gain in adults and children alike.

Another problem with desserts is that they tend to displace healthier items from your child's diet. If your child regularly eats a dessert with dinner, for example, she will be less likely to eat healthy amounts of vegetables, fruits, and meat at the same meal, and will also be more likely to carry the dessert habit into adulthood.

So what is a parent to do? We like the widespread European custom of having fresh fruit rather than sweets for dessert. It's a much healthier way to eat, and much easier to live with because you won't have to deal with the issue of what gets eaten during the meal's main course. If, like us, you grew up with regular rich desserts, it will take a while to get used to, but when you do it comes to feel like a good way to end a meal. Meanwhile, if you have a sweet tooth, consider a compromise. You and your child can enjoy a dessertlike snack such as frozen yogurt or a muffin with milk for a morning or afternoon snack, and a moderate-sized portion will not interfere with meat and vegetables eaten at meals.

WHAT ABOUT FAST FOOD AND CONVENIENCE FOOD?

We are not great fans of fast-food restaurants, for the reason that homemade food tastes better and is usually healthier, too. Fortunately, you can prevent fast food from becoming one of your child's favorites.

If you visit fast-food restaurants only very occasionally and don't make it a big deal when you do go, fast food will probably never feel like proper food to your child, and when he gets older he will seldom think of asking for it. Going out for fast food once in a while is fine; your child will experience this normal part of American life with you there and will not look on it as something special when his friends talk about it.

Convenience food is a rather different issue. If you can keep home-prepared meals in your freezer, you will never need commercial convenience meals because you will always have something equally convenient—and healthier and better-tasting, too. But when you are busy, a frozen store-bought backup can seem like a lifesaver. Make sure you read the labels and avoid those high in additives or fat, and you will be on the right track.

WHAT ABOUT FAT-FREE FOODS, LITE FOODS, AND FAT SUBSTITUTES?

As we have pointed out, diets very low in fat are not safe for infants and young children because they can impair development. But individual low-fat, lite, and even fat-free products can be fine if your child's overall diet is kept at the right level of fat for her developmental age, and many contain less saturated fat than the regular product.

Be aware, however, that many low-fat foods are *not* low in calories. A recent supermarket survey showed that some low-fat soups, prepared meats, crackers, french fries, and peanut butters have just as many calories as the manufacturers' regular brand.

When it comes to the safety of fat substitutes, it really depends on what the substitute is. Often water is used to make a food fat-free (for example, in salad dressings). Then the only question—as long as your child is getting enough fat overall—is whether the food in question tastes good enough for her to want to eat it.

But fat substitutes such as olestra (brand name Olean), a nonabsorbable fat substitute, are a completely different matter. Our personal recommendation is to avoid giving foods containing olestra to children under six years, because of some consumer complaints that large amounts cause digestive upsets and, more important, the fact that it interferes with the absorption of vital fat-soluble nutrients usually absorbed by the body along with fat. While extra amounts of fat-soluble nutrients such as vitamins A, D, and E are added to foods containing olestra to counterbalance the absorption problem, that's not the case for fat-soluble phytochemicals not yet considered to be nutrients. Research is increasingly showing that many foods are more than the sum of their individual known nutrients.

WHAT ABOUT ARTIFICIAL SWEETENERS?

From the perspective of health, aspartame (NutraSweet) is generally considered safer than saccharin (exception: the rare individuals with hereditary phenylketonuria, who shouldn't take aspartame at all). It has been extensively tested and doesn't measurably increase the risk of either cancer in the long term or behavior problems in the short term. Saccharin, on the other hand, has been shown to cause cancer in animals when consumed at much higher levels than ever found in a human diet. It is generally considered risk-free when consumed in the small amounts typical for children and adults, but whether this means it is completely risk-free or mostly risk-free is not entirely certain.

For this reason it is best to avoid giving your child regular portions of foods and drinks containing saccharin. Sweet'n Low contains saccharin, as do some sodas, jams, canned fruit, candy, dessert toppings, and salad dressings.

But what about aspartame? Even if aspartame appears to be risk-free, this doesn't mean that you should necessarily encourage your child to eat it. You don't need to particularly avoid it, but regular consumption of sweet foods encourages a sweet tooth whatever the origin of the sweet flavor, and so builds a liking for the sugar and excess calories that you want your child to avoid.

HELPING BABY-SITTERS
TO FEED YOUR CHILD RIGHT

Many parents, including ourselves, rely on people outside the immediate family for help with child care, and part of that care, of course, is feeding. Just as you expect the person or people who look after your child to discipline him in a way you find acceptable, it is also reasonable to expect them to feed the right foods in the right way. And in the same way that you might spell out your discipline policy to a new helper or inquire after the discipline policy of a day-care center you are thinking of using, the best way to ensure good results when it comes to food is to be proactive.

BABY-SITTERS, NANNIES, AND HOUSEKEEPERS

These caretakers will benefit from being left some prepared (by you) foods and/or a simple list of instructions. It is surprising how poorly many peo-

ple feed small children, and you can head off problems by stating your expectations clearly. Experienced baby-sitters are used to dealing with family differences and shouldn't be fazed by a list of instructions. Young
baby-sitters will usually be grateful for the help.

As you prepare the meal or snack, or a general suggestion list, make sure
to include tried and tested items you know your child enjoys, saving less
popular items or new foods for meals when you are home. As a general
rule, try to provide a quarter more total food than you expect your child
will eat (plus some for the baby-sitter) and tell your baby-sitter that your
child is unlikely to want it all—and that that's fine.

Sometimes an otherwise wonderful baby-sitter will do some things that
make you cringe. Maybe she persistently tries to overfeed your nine-
month-old baby when he is clearly full, because she firmly believes she
knows best about how much babies need to eat—or keeps putting your
four-year-old off different vegetables by educating him about how healthy
they are. Good child care is hard to find, and you probably won't want to
replace your sitter just because she or he is in a different place from you
when it comes to eating.

If clear instructions don't help, reduce the amount of food you leave (to
prevent overfeeding) and shift the makeup of individual meals so that the
most important foods get eaten only when you are there. In particular,
fruits and vegetables are foods you want your child to like, because it is
hard to make a healthy diet without them.

Let's say your baby-sitter gives your child lunch and snacks. Make
breakfast and dinner the two meals that count most. Fresh fruit with
breakfast every day, fruit and vegetables with dinner at night, and all
these items on weekends, too, will go a long way toward preventing
your baby-sitter from creating unnecessary aversions. Lunch and snacks
can be familiar items—either without fruit or vegetables, or perhaps let
your baby-sitter offer just one or two favorite fruits. Alternatives such as
soup, sandwiches, and cookies can always be replaced with other foods if
dislikes begin to set in.

FRIENDS AND RELATIVES

Some neighbors and members of your extended family are wonderful
about food. But others, however much you love them, can drive you crazy.
And it can be hard to confront the problem, since after all they are family

and friends. The elderly neighbor who gives your child brownies just before dinner and the relatives who come for a weekly meal with a large chocolate cake and a two-pound box of chocolates are equally frustrating. It is not that they are trying to wreck the nutrition plans you've carefully laid for your child. Rather, they may come from a background where showing love with rich sweets was accepted and normal.

If it happens only occasionally, your best defense is simply to ignore it. You don't need perfect nutrition every day for your child to have an overall good diet. Your child doesn't want dinner because of the M&M's he just ate next door? Simply require him to sit at the table with the rest of the family, as normal, and tell him he doesn't have to eat anything if he is not hungry. This way he never gets to learn that eating M&M's is something special that you don't want him to do. As for the weekly chocolate cakes, if you can't bring yourself to stop them from being brought, throw out the remainder when the guests are gone.

If visiting your neighbor to get cookies at 5 P.M. becomes a regular habit, with your child as a willing accomplice, simply tell them both that you want it to stop because it spoils his appetite for dinner. If you don't want to take away the pleasure of the visit, you can perhaps suggest it as an earlier snack-time routine instead, and set firm limits on how many cookies or whatever can be offered.

DAY-CARE CENTERS AND FAMILY DAY CARE

These valuable resources vary quite a lot about food. Larger day-care centers often ask parents to send their young children in with all milk and food. In this case, you can use our suggestions for preschool lunches (page 222), tailored to your child's age, to help you pack appropriate items.

For older children, both large day-care centers and family day care often provide snacks and lunch. If snack foods are provided, they are usually juice with plain cookies or crackers. Since apple juice is low in nutrients, you may wish to consider requesting that more nutritious drinks be served, such as milk or orange juice. Plain cookies are not actually bad food when eaten in moderation, but if your center serves nothing else they may be receptive to suggested alternatives such as crackers (especially the lower-fat brands containing some fiber), served plain or with a spread such as cream cheese or peanut butter, and fresh fruit.

The quality of lunches cooked by a center can vary a lot. However, most centers that supply lunch also provide the parents with their weekly menu, so you can see what your child is getting. If your center cooks hot dogs, for example—which you don't want your child to eat because of the nitrites— you will need to explain. Most day-care centers are enthusiastic about serving healthy food, and the director may be glad to share our list of foods to avoid (pages 124–126).

CHAPTER 9

❖

Four to Twelve Months

The Big Transition to Solid Food

Anna has been showing signs of being ready to try solid foods, and today's the big day. The first offering will be infant cereal, and Anna's mom is trying to go slow and talking about the food as she guides the spoon to Anna's lips. Anna tastes . . . blinks . . . and tries to swallow—not very successfully. Her mom can't help it—she laughs, and so does Anna. The big transition has begun!

Your baby is now between four and six months old and has changed dramatically since birth, nearly doubling her birth weight and making great developmental strides. But many more dramatic things will happen soon. At four months she is fundamentally still a helpless infant. By her first birthday, however, your baby will be transformed. Sitting, crawling, using fingers and thumbs for delicate tasks, understanding many things you say, and perhaps saying a few words herself are all developmental landmarks she will have achieved. She will also be walking, or well on the way to it, and will have figured out the best ways of influencing you, her beloved parent and provider.

You will soon begin to notice changes in some of your baby's instinctive behaviors that start to prepare her for the transition to solid food. At around four months she loses the "extrusion reflex" that pushed everything out of her mouth except for a nipple and maybe your finger. She will also start to show an intense desire to chew, especially when teething begins. She can show if she is hungry, too—by looking eager, opening her mouth, and leaning forward to be fed.

Another important change is your baby's increasingly powerful drive to put everything—not just food—into her mouth. This natural behavior may drive you crazy because of the new level of watchfulness it requires. But it is precisely these mouthing and chewing instincts that can help you in the transition to solid food. Your child wants to put something in her mouth. You offer her food—and she is on the road to weaning! Of course, there are important things you need to know about the right ways to offer her food, but working with your baby's instincts can make the process easy and natural.

Feeding skills advance rapidly during these transitional months. At four months your baby can merely—sometimes barely—swallow spoonfuls you offer. By six to seven months she can sit in a high chair and get food into her own mouth by dipping her fingers and fists into it. She can't really use a spoon or a cup, but enjoys playing with them. By seven to eight months she will probably be able to pick up and eat the "finger foods" her emerging teeth are nearly ready for, and nine to eleven months sees the first unaided use of a cup and spoon.

Your infant is also undergoing dramatic metabolic developments. Around four months her immune function, digestive system, and kidneys will have matured to the critical point where some solid foods can be eaten with relative safety; by twelve months her metabolism will be essentially that of an adult and she will be ready to eat almost anything you put on the table. And it is important that she does. From six months on, breast milk or formula can no longer supply enough calories or the balance of nutrients most infants need. At the same time, the physical act of eating solid foods prepares her facial muscles for talking and lets her practice her fine motor skills. In fact, your child begins to *need* solid foods at just the time she becomes physically and metabolically ready to eat them.

OPPORTUNITIES AND GOALS FOR FEEDING FROM FOUR TO TWELVE MONTHS

Keep these basics in mind as your baby makes the big transition:

- *Continue to give your baby breast milk or formula.* Make breast milk or formula the only milks your baby gets before twelve months, to promote healthy growth and help her avoid the allergies and gastrointestinal damage that are still a risk with cow's milk at this time. Although milk is not adequate as a sole diet after six months, it provides nutrients that complement those in solid foods, especially milk fat for essential brain development and calcium to build strong teeth and bones. The strength of your baby's first set of teeth is largely determined by eleven months, and dental hypoplasia (poorly formed enamel due to inadequate calcium) will encourage rapid tooth decay.

- *Ensure adequate iron intake.* Before one year, solid foods—even if they are iron-fortified—simply don't provide enough iron to reliably prevent developmental impairments and anemia. Give your child a multivitamin with iron if you are nursing, or use a "with-iron" formula if you are bottle-feeding.

- *Introduce solid foods between four and six months.* Later in this chapter you'll find a list of safe solid foods and the ages at which you can introduce them. By twelve months your baby can have learned to enjoy forty to sixty different items. Major illnesses during the first months, developmental problems, or a strong family history of food allergies are the only major reasons to delay solids (see Chapter 16 for more information on allergies).

- *Allow your baby to become an independent feeder at her own pace, and encourage self-regulation of how much gets eaten.* By letting her have some control over how much and when she eats, even at this early age, you help prevent picky eating and future weight problems.

WHEN SHOULD YOU START?

I remember buying my daughter's first box of infant cereal. I couldn't wait to get home and give it a try. Like me, you may be excited and eager to get started, but how do you know if your baby is ready? Between four and six months he will probably show you one or more of these signs:

- Whether your baby is breast-fed or bottle-fed, are there some meals when he is not satisfied at the end of the feeding? Does he cry or continue to suck hard?
- Have you had to increase the frequency with which you feed him to two hours or less between many feedings?
- If bottle-fed, does he take more than 40 ounces of formula a day?

- Is he showing an interest in your food at the table—crying for some, opening his mouth, or trying to reach for it? Even if he is still satisfied by milk, this is a sign that he is developmentally ready, provided that he also has good head control and can sit up with support.

You don't, by the way, have to wait until your baby gets his first teeth. The time at which babies cut their first teeth is very variable—as late as eighteen months in some cases. Long before that time, their hard gums are ready to deal with solid foods.

FIRST SPOONFULS: WHAT, AND HOW MUCH?

The fortified infant rice cereal you'll find at the supermarket is a good place to start. Although the occasional baby is sensitive to it, rice cereal has the lowest risk of causing a reaction. Mix it with breast milk or formula to a fairly liquid consistency for the first feedings. The amount can be determined by his interest, ranging from less than a teaspoon per meal to two tablespoons.

FIRST SPOONFULS, STEP BY STEP

You are now ready! Remember that your main goal is to let your child enjoy solid foods, rather than trying to get a particular amount in.

1. Pick one meal a day when your baby is hungry but not ravenous and irritable. If he is still waking at night, try dinner first. Research has not borne out the widespread belief that solids at dinnertime help babies sleep through the night, but our experience as parents is that they sometimes work.

2. If you are nursing, give your baby a breast-feeding first to prevent breast milk production decreasing. If you are feeding formula, start with solids, because solids are sometimes harder to introduce to formula-fed babies and this can encourage popularity. A six-month-old may be ready to sit up in a high chair, but if your child is younger or is not happy in a high chair, cuddle him on your lap with his body turned toward you.

3. Use a small, soft (plastic-coated) spoon, and put a very small amount on the end. At first your baby will probably not realize that he has to

open his mouth for food, so you have to wait for an opening, or put a little on his lip. He also will not know, initially, how to swallow this new food. Most babies learn within a few days, but in the meantime most of what goes in will dribble out. Just use a bib (unfolded cotton diapers work well in this capacity) and scoop up the excess so that he's comfortable.

4. Don't rush. Wait until he has dealt with one spoonful before offering another. Let him tell you how long to make these first feedings.

5. When your baby looks as if he has had enough, or is getting frustrated, stop feeding and offer another breast-feeding or formula to finish off the meal. This is important. If he comes away with a sense of comfort and satisfaction, he will want to repeat the experience.

Try cereal at about the same time every day for a week. If he hasn't got the hang of swallowing it, or seems uninterested, stop for two or three weeks, then try again. Formula-fed babies often get off to a slower start with solids than breast-fed babies. Formula—unlike breast milk—tastes the same every day and so doesn't prepare babies for the very different taste of solid food.

If he seems to want more, you can increase portions to 2 tablespoons of dry cereal mixed with formula or breast milk, and move on after a week or two to a second daily meal. You can also try baby barley cereal and baby oatmeal, leaving three to five days between each new introduction so that any problems can be easily traced (because of the risk of allergies, avoid any cereal containing wheat until eight months).

After one month of solids, or five months of age (whichever comes sooner), cooked apple and pear purees are safe fruit choices your baby will probably enjoy. If your baby is on formula, you may also want to try a daily tablespoon of prune puree, which can solve a constipation problem in short order. Unless you have a particular urge to try your baby on vegetables (in which case the commercial jars of squash and carrots are safe options), we recommend saving other solids for after six months, when your baby's immune system, gastrointestinal tract, and metabolism will be ready for greater diversity.

BREAST MILK OR FORMULA
CONTINUES TO BE IMPORTANT

At twelve months your baby still needs at least half her calories from breast milk or formula.

BREAST MILK

If you have been breast-feeding, you can continue for as long as you and your baby want. Many babies wean themselves between nine and twelve months, as they become more independent in their feeding. However, research worldwide has shown that mothers can supplement their children's diet with breast milk almost indefinitely.

If you are working full time, you can express milk at work and bring it home for feeds when you are away (see Chapter 5). If you find your milk supply dwindling, you can move to a regimen of both breast-feeding and formula. Provided you continue to nurse at least four times a day for fifteen or more minutes a feeding, and use formula only one or two times a day, you will probably be able to nurse up to eight or nine months, and perhaps longer. When she gets ready, your baby will wean herself naturally and easily.

FORMULA

As formula-fed babies make the transition to solid foods, the amount of formula they drink can be decreased gradually from 28 to 38 ounces per day at four to six months to 20 to 30 ounces at twelve months. During that time, you might move from five 6-ounce bottles daily to three 8-ounce bottles. Make sure to offer your baby 2 to 4 ounces of water (or more according to thirst) every day to make up for the liquid lost as formula is reduced.

If a particular formula has been working well up to now, you can continue it until your baby is one year old, when you can safely make the transition to whole cow's milk. There's one exception: If, for any reason, you have been using a low-iron formula, you need to switch to a with-iron variety immediately. By four to six months your baby's inborn iron stores have been depleted, and a good supply of this mineral is essential for brain development and other functions.

And when do you move to a cup instead of a bottle? Not too soon—and slowly when you do. Many infants are physically able to hold and use a cup by nine months or even earlier, but many still have an emotional need for sucking. If your baby seems interested, offer a cup for a single feeding every day starting at around nine months. Most babies are developmentally less in need of sucking by fourteen to seventeen months, and a gradual switch to a cup comes more naturally.

Lunchtime, when everyone is awake and feeling a bit independent, is a good meal at which to start cup feeding. A "sippy cup," with a shallow mouthpiece, two handles, and (if you can find one) a weighted bottom, will be easiest for your baby to use. If you normally give her formula with lunch, simply put a little formula in the cup (refilling as necessary) and put it on the tray where she can reach it. Hold the cup for her when she wants to drink during the meal, and sit her on your lap to finish it when she is done with solid food. Over a period of a few weeks she will want to take over from you, especially if you show her how to hold it and move it to her mouth. If you are nursing and want to use a cup for water, expressed milk, or juice, again put the cup on her tray within easy reach, and help her for as long as she seems to want help.

To make the complete transition to a cup easier, don't encourage your baby to hold her own bottle. She will be more willing to give up the bottle when she becomes mobile if she associates it with cuddling in your lap. Allowing a baby to hold her own bottle for extended periods also increases the risk of cavities, because milk fed this way tends to pool against emerging teeth.

SHOULD MILK COME FIRST OR SECOND IN A MEAL?

As noted above, if your baby drinks formula, he should start most meals with solid foods and finish off with formula. This teaches him to like solids because he associates them with relief from hunger. However, if you want to continue nursing, start your baby's meals with a breast-feeding so that your milk supply doesn't decline from reduced demand.

Milk should be given with all meals up to about nine months; otherwise it is hard for your baby to eat enough calories. After nine months, provided that the total daily milk volume is right for his age, you can drop milk from dinner or perhaps one snack, and offer water instead, so that there are times during the day when he eats food with milk and times when he does not. This will pave the way, after twelve months, for moving onto a schedule in which he has milk only two or three times a day.

GOOD SOLID FOODS TO TRY

4–6 months	6–7 months	8 months	9–12 months
	add now:	*add now:*	*add now:*
CARBOHYDRATES			
Fortified baby rice, barley, and oatmeal cereals		Plain unsweetened breakfast cereals such as oatmeal, Cream of Wheat, Cheerios, Rice Krispies, and multigrain flakes Crackers, rice and pasta, bread and bagels	
FRUITS			
Apple, pear, and prune purees	Cooked puree, strained, or small cooked pieces of fruits such as apple, pear, blueberry, prune, plum, peach, and kiwi; raw mashed banana (very ripe)	Thin strips of all kinds of cooked fruits, and soft raw fruits such as pineapple, mango, and papaya	Thin strips of harder raw fruits such as apple
VEGETABLES			
	Home-cooked purees of low-nitrate vegetables such as peas, potatoes, broccoli, and yams, and commercial baby food purees of other vegetables such as carrots (which are screened for nitrate levels)	Pieces of well-cooked vegetables such as string beans, snow peas, winter squash, zucchini, asparagus, broccoli, cauliflower, potatoes; ripe avocadoes	Tiny strips of the softer raw vegetables such as green and red peppers, cucumbers (a vegetable peeler makes nice thin slices), and lettuce

4–6 months	6–7 months	8 months	9–12 months
	add now:	*add now:*	*add now:*
MEATS AND OTHER PROTEINS			
		Pureed mixed entrees with lean beef or chicken, and hard-boiled egg yolks	Small pieces of well-cooked meat, and entrees cut up into small pieces or pureed. Beans (without skins) and soy products, yogurt, and cheese are fine to try now, (but avoid cow's milk itself until 12 months)
JUICES			
		Fruit juices such as apple, pear, grape, and cherry (maximum 3–4 oz per day)	

MOVING ON TO A MIXED DIET

INTRODUCING NEW FOODS

Up to six months it is good to be conservative about what you feed your baby, but *between six and eight months* you will probably both be ready to move on to more exciting foods. Purees and small pieces of all kinds of soft cooked fruits are good from six months, and ripe mashed banana and avocado are usually popular. Avoid very acidic fruits such as oranges, grapefruits, strawberries, and tomatoes, which can upset delicate stomachs and promote diaper rash. Low-nitrate vegetables such as potatoes, peas, broccoli, and yams are also safe to home-prepare starting at six months (though broccoli may be gas-producing in some babies). For vegetables containing more nitrates, such as spinach, squash, string beans, and beets, use only commercial baby food before eight months. (See Caution! on page 144.)

Parents are sometimes advised to introduce yellow and orange vegetables before green, but there is no important health reason to do so. Be aware that more than 2 to 3 ounces per day of orange and yellow vegetables such as carrots or winter squash (or two large jars of commercial vegetable purees, which usually contain a lot of orange vegetables) consumed regularly before one year may give your baby's skin an orange tinge. This unsightly but harmless condition, known as hypercarotenemia, is caused by orange-pigmented carotenes.

From eight months, your baby can safely try adult cereals (including those containing wheat) softened with formula or breast milk, small pieces of well-cooked fruit and vegetable, plain unsweetened cereals such as Cheerios that can be given without a choking risk, hard boiled egg yolks, and pureed mixed meals of vegetables and lean meat. Approximately equal quantities of cereal (mixed with formula or breast milk), fruit, and vegetables are a good balance. Do continue to avoid adding salt and sugar to mixed dishes; your baby doesn't need them, and research has shown she will be less likely to love them in the future if she doesn't get used to them now.

A few foods should still be avoided until nine months. These are soy products such as tofu, pieces of meat (still difficult to chew), and the harder raw fruits (a choking hazard).

At nine months, the only major foods still excluded are cow's milk, egg whites, fish, shellfish, nuts, chocolate, a few fruits (citrus, strawberries, and tomatoes), and most raw vegetables (again, to prevent choking). Most of these will be added after about twelve months.

HOW QUICKLY CAN YOU DIVERSIFY YOUR BABY'S DIET?

Traditionally parents were told to introduce just one new food per week until one year. However, unless you have a family history of allergies, you can safely introduce a new food every three to four days. If your baby shows signs of intolerance or allergy, including vomiting, diarrhea, or a diaper or general skin rash, take any foods introduced within the five previous days out of his diet. Introduce them again one at a time with at least five days between each one. In this way, you will be able to pinpoint whether there's a problem with a specific food.

Don't, by the way, assume that every stomach upset, vomiting attack, or diaper rash is caused by a food allergy. It's more likely to be an infection of some kind. Repeating the food exposure after your baby has recovered is an important step that will show you whether there is really a problem.

Some skin and bottom changes are a normal consequence of introducing solid food. A mild rash on your baby's face with no other symptoms, for example, may mean nothing more than a local irritation on delicate skin. Try to keep food smears to a minimum for a day or two and rinse his face well after each meal. Some stool changes are usual, too, such as the increasingly adult odor. You may also see what appear to be undigested lumps of vegetables and variations in color that reflect what was eaten yesterday. This is all perfectly normal for the next several months, until his immature digestive system learns to cope with adult foods.

SOLID FOODS AND MILK: WHAT'S A HEALTHY BALANCE?

Many parents worry that their six- to twelve-month-old is eating too little solid food compared with what they've read or been told a baby that age should eat. This can lead to overencouraging babies to eat more than they want. A few parents worry that solid foods are starting to eclipse milk, and they try to hold back. Both these scenarios can set the scene for unnecessary future food battles.

The following recommendations for milk and solid foods are based on measurements of what healthy infants *actually eat.* They are lower in calories than past recommendations, because recent research has shown that most babies and children simply don't need as many calories as was suggested for decades.

Solid Foods and Breast Milk or Formula: What's Usual?

AGE	TYPICAL NURSING TIMES (ON DEMAND TO 1 YEAR)	FORMULA	SOLID FOODS
6 months	50 min.–2$^{1}/_{2}$ hrs. per day	28–38 oz	0–100 calories
9 months	40 min.–2 hrs. per day	24–34 oz	200–300 calories
12 months	10 min.–1$^{1}/_{2}$ hrs. per day	20–30 oz	300–500 calories

---

Fortified cereal has 15 calories per dry tablespoon

Pureed and strained fruits typically offer 50–70 calories per 2$^{2}/_{3}$ oz jar

Pureed and strained vegetables offer 20–50 calories per 2$^{2}/_{3}$ oz jar

The number of different solid foods you offer your baby at any one meal (in addition to milk) can vary depending on what you are cooking, but a single food at breakfast, two with lunch, and two with dinner is a good goal for babies up to nine months. After that time, as your baby progresses to eating more table foods, one or two foods with breakfast and two or three with lunch and dinner will provide the variety and balance that are needed.

Total amounts of solids and milk can vary widely from day to day and meal to meal—that's absolutely normal. And although smaller babies will tend to consume less than heavier ones, no baby is typical. Yours may need more or less than the average to grow normally. And it is fine for your baby to eat less solids than indicated as long as he is showing normal growth and progressing toward a balance of milk and solid food.

CAUTION! FOODS TO AVOID

- *Choking hazards:* Pieces of hot dogs, whole grapes, nuts, lumps of peanut butter and similarly viscous spreads, popcorn, and anything large or round can get stuck in a small airway. Pieces of hard raw vegetables are also a potential hazard, so introduce these only as thin strips and after your baby has molars and is using them to chew his food. *Watch your baby at all times when he is eating, because even "safe" foods can cause choking in an unattended child.*

- *Common allergens:* Avoid meat and egg yolks before eight months, soy products, beans, yogurt, and cheese before nine months, and cow's milk, egg whites, fish, nuts, chocolate, citrus fruits, tomatoes, and strawberries before twelve months.

- *High-nitrite meats:* Most hot dogs, hams, sausages, bologna, and bacon contain nitrites. This is a problem not only because of the possible long-term cancer risk linked to nitrites, but also because nitrites can cause a life-threatening form of anemia called *methemoglobinemia* before six months of age. The nitrites transform your baby's immature hemoglobin into methemoglobin, which is unable to transport life-sustaining oxygen around the body. One of the early signs of methemoglobinemia is an intermittent bluish tinge around the lips, nose, and ears, revealing the lack of bright red oxygenated blood under the skin.

- *High-nitrate vegetables:* Beets, carrots, green beans, squash, turnips, spinach, and collard greens should not be home-prepared before eight months. High-nitrate vegetables are as much of a concern as high-nitrite hot dogs when it comes to methemoglobinemia, because young babies' stomachs convert nitrates to nitrites. Commercial baby foods made with vegetables are less of a concern than home-prepared items because the manufacturers buy their produce from areas where nitrate levels are low, and check the produce before use.

- *High-nitrate water:* The government has mandated a safe limit of 45 milligrams of nitrate per liter, but an increasing number of water supplies—especially in rural areas—fail to meet this standard because of the widespread use of high-nitrogen fertilizers. If you live in a high-risk area, use bottled water for the first eight months, or check with your local water authority about getting your water tested.

- *Honey:* One of the most frequent causes of infant botulism is honey, responsible for about a third of all cases in children under six months. Before twelve months your baby's intestinal tract doesn't have the adult secretions and complex "good" bacterial flora that can minimize the growth of *Clostridium botulinum,* which is commonly found in honey, even in heat-treated commercial brands. Just a tiny amount of honey—used to sweeten a pacifier, for instance—can contain enough spores to cause a problem. Corn syrup, once suspected of carrying the spores, is now believed to be fine.

- *Tea:* Tannins contained in green and black tea inhibit iron absorption and so increase the risk of iron deficiency. The caffeine in tea may also cause calcium to be lost, making it harder to build tooth and bone strength. Herb teas should also be avoided, because many contain pharmacologically active plant extracts whose effects have not been documented in young babies.

- *Frequent servings of products containing trans fatty acids:* Margarine, commercial baked goods containing margarine, such as cakes, cookies, and pastries, and any food listing partially hydrogenated vegetable oil. As explained in Chapter 3, trans fatty acids have the potential to inhibit the synthesis of essential fatty acids needed for brain development.

SAMPLE MENU FOR A BREAST- AND FORMULA-FED BABY AT SIX MONTHS (MOTHER WORKING)

6:00 A.M.	Breast-feeding
8:30 A.M.	Breast-feeding before work
11:00 A.M.—lunch	6 oz expressed breast milk or formula 2 tbsp dry baby oatmeal mixed with 1 oz formula
1:00 P.M.—drink	2 oz water
3:00 P.M.—snack	6 oz expressed breast milk or formula
5:30 P.M.—dinner	Breast-feeding when Mom returns from work 1½ oz apple puree mixed with 1 tbsp dry oatmeal cereal 1 oz water
6:00 to 9:30 P.M.— snack	1 or 2 breast-feedings before bedtime

MENUS AND SCHEDULES

It's very important to continue to feed your baby mostly on demand before twelve months. If he is forced to eat when he's full and prevented from eating when he's hungry, it makes life harder for everybody. At the same time it sends the message that eating is not related to hunger. It's a mistake to interfere with this basic biological need, of course—when we think about it this way, it seems so obvious. Yet several generations of Americans were raised on the "scheduled feeding" system, and one result of that has been a nation metabolically misprogrammed to eat at any time and to ignore bodily signs of hunger and fullness. It is not surprising, really, that we are plagued by obesity and eating disorders.

Even with feeding on demand, from about six months on you can gradually adjust your baby's feeding schedule to resemble the rest of the family's. Simply provide solid foods at your normal meal and snack times, and generally only milk and water and occasionally juice at other times. Breakfast is an easy meal to start with. Feed your baby breast milk or formula with cereal, and perhaps some fruit puree, to make a good start to the day. Where you go from there will depend very much on him. Some still want four or even five evenly spaced formula meals, or six to eight breast-

SAMPLE MENU FOR A FORMULA-FED BABY AT ELEVEN MONTHS

8:00 A.M.—breakfast	6 oz formula
	3 tbsp fortified cereal
	3.5 oz apple puree
11:00 A.M.—lunch	1 slice oatmeal bread with melted mozzarella
	Small strips of cooked carrot
	$^1/_4$ banana, mashed or cut into slices
	5 oz formula
	Water
2:00 P.M.—snack	6 oz formula
	1 saltine cracker
5:00 P.M.—dinner	$^1/_2$ oz roast chicken pieces
	$^1/_4$ cup mashed potato (made with water and butter, not milk)
	1 tbsp cooked broccoli
	4 oz formula
	1 oz cantaloupe slices
	Water
8:00 P.M.—snack	4 oz formula

milk meals—similar to the milk-only pattern of the first few months, but with a little solid food added at "lunch" and "dinner." This is absolutely fine. As you find your baby taking an increased interest in solid food, he will move naturally toward a regimen of larger meals and smaller snacks. By the time he is nine to twelve months old, chances are he will have shifted to a pattern of three meals plus two or three snacks per day; this routine will last him right up to kindergarten.

Even the most flexible baby will sometimes be ready for dinner before it is cooked, especially when he is having a growth spurt. At these times, simply give him a cracker or two, a little cooked fruit or vegetable if it is ready, or a small portion of cereal. Then seat him at the table when dinner is ready. He may eat less than normal, but he'll enjoy the company and his appetite will tell him how much he needs.

SAMPLE MENU FOR A BREAST-FED BABY WITH FORMULA SUPPLEMENT AT ELEVEN MONTHS

7:00 A.M.—breakfast	15-minute breast-feeding 2 tbsp baby rice cereal mixed with water and 3.5 oz pear puree
9:30 A.M.—snack	6 oz formula
Noon—lunch	15-minute breast-feeding 1 slice bread, spread with a little butter 1 hard-boiled egg yolk, in pieces Thin strips of cucumber Water
3:00 P.M.—snack	15-minute breast-feeding ½ kiwi in slices
5:30 P.M.—dinner	15-minute breast-feeding ¼ cup pasta shells with a drizzle of olive oil 1 tbsp squash 1 tbsp cooked, mashed beans Water
8:00 P.M.—snack	15-minute breast-feeding

WHAT ABOUT COMMERCIAL BABY FOOD?

Commercial ready-to-feed baby foods can seem wonderful when your baby is hungry for dinner and you have only just come home from work, or when the adults crave spicy chili con carne with corn bread and salad. Commercial baby foods also come with guaranteed sterility, controlled levels of nitrates, lower salt and sugar content than adult foods, and no additives.

The big drawback is that many of them bear little relation to the real thing. Although many of the fruit purees taste fine, the vegetables and mixed entrees often leave a lot to be desired, and your baby may reject them out of hand. Even if she eats them now, you may miss your opportunity to introduce her to foods you want her to enjoy later, when she will naturally become more resistant.

We recommend reserving commercial baby food for first introductions before six months, for high-nitrate vegetables between six and eight months, and when you need the convenience later. For regular meals, puree her fruit, the veggie du jour, or any entree from the family menu that has safe ingredients, taking her age into account. If you freeze leftover puree in ice-cube trays, you will always have a home-cooked "instant" meal when you need it.

Caution: Don't feed directly from the baby food jar unless you are prepared to throw leftovers away. Saliva contaminates the jar and encourages bacterial growth. If you use a clean spoon to put a portion into your child's bowl, you can refrigerate the remainder for a day or two. Also, be sure that unopened jars are safe by checking the sell-by date and making sure the pressure button in the cap is down before you open it.

EATING OUT

If you enjoy eating out, pick a casual restaurant and take your baby! Many parents find that a baby under seven months is easier to take than any other age (many will nod off if you take them in something they can sleep in). Commercial baby food really comes into its own when you are at a restaurant. Rather than worrying about what every dish contains, simply take a jar or two of usually popular items and a bottle of milk or water. It's a great way to relax and feel as though life is returning to normal.

SUPPLEMENTS: DOES YOUR BABY NEED THEM?

If your baby is drinking formula with iron, a multivitamin/mineral supplement is not necessary. Formula is fortified and will supply most of what is needed, whether or not he is eating many solids.

For breast-fed babies who receive no additional formula, an infant multivitamin/mineral supplement can be prescribed by your pediatrician. This supplement is needed because of the decreasing levels of micronutrients in breast milk after four months. Although solid foods can potentially fill the gap, most babies don't eat enough to ensure this.

Fluoride (a total of 0.5 milligrams per day) is recommended for babies six months and older because it dramatically strengthens emerging teeth and has no harmful side effects when taken in recommended amounts. Some fluoride is present in food, so a small supplement (0.25 milligrams per day) is recommended only for babies who don't drink any fluoridated water daily (either in formula or by itself for thirst). Breast milk contains

COMMERCIAL BABY FOOD: A CRITICAL LOOK AT WHAT'S ON THE MARKET

- **Dry baby cereals.** Rice, oatmeal, barley, and mixed cereals are well worth keeping in your cupboard. They are fortified with iron, and their powdery form makes a smooth paste when mixed with breast milk, formula, water, or fruit puree, no cooking needed. Use until eight to nine months, or when your baby makes the transition to fortified adult cereals. The jars of premixed cereal offer no advantages over dry cereal except when you are away from home and need an instant meal-in-a-bottle.

- **First- and second-stage baby food.** Smooth purees of individual fruits and vegetables and some mixed dishes come in small and larger sizes for young babies with different appetites. Some of the fruit purees, and the vegetable mixtures marketed by the organic companies, can taste quite good, others much less so. These are useful in the early months, when you want to supplement or replace a family dinner, if you take a trip, or when you get caught short without anything suitable in the refrigerator or freezer.

- **Follow-up (or third-stage) baby foods.** Marketed for babies who are old enough to eat almost anything, these usually mixed dishes typically have a mashed texture and a taste that is remarkably uniform, whether the label says "chicken noodle casserole" or "ham and tomato delight." Your own mashed dinners will make the transition to adult foods easier, and will taste better, too.

very little fluoride (irrespective of whether your water supply is fluoridated), so babies still receiving the majority of their fluid from nursing should have a supplement also.

SMART STRATEGIES FOR FEEDING BABIES FOUR TO TWELVE MONTHS OLD

1. ALLOW YOUR BABY TO ENJOY SOLIDS

Letting your child enjoy solid foods is much more important at this age than monitoring how much gets eaten at any given meal. It really doesn't

- **Baby crackers.** Zwieback toasts and similar items provide good chewing practice from about eight months on, provided you supervise carefully to prevent choking. Pieces of lightly toasted chewy bread crust and bagels work well, too, and are often enjoyed at least as much. Frozen bagels are also worth a try to relieve the teething pain common at this age.

- **Baby cookies.** They have less salt, sugar, and additives than the adult kind, but your baby needs no extra encouragement!

- **Baby chicken/meat sticks.** Looking and tasting rather like anemic hot dogs, these high-protein finger foods are best left on the supermarket shelf. Your baby is getting plenty of protein from milk right now, and doesn't need any encouragement to form an attachment to their nitrite-laden cousins.

- **Meals in a bottle.** Tasteless chicken pieces and squares of carrot floating in a watery fluid typify these gastronomic nightmares. Any baby old enough for these will prefer real food.

- **Baby juice.** Packaged in convenient 4-ounce bottles, baby juice comes in several flavors that your baby will enjoy. *But* they are expensive, introduce a liking for something you will want to control in the future, and contain almost nothing but calories. Use them sparingly if at all.

matter if your baby doesn't want to try squash today—so avoid all coercion and encouragements such as "Just one more for Mama!" Let him have a breast-feeding or bottle instead, or another solid food if he seems eager, and try again another day. When you take this approach, you start teaching him that healthy food is something to be enjoyed.

2. LEARN TO RECOGNIZE HUNGRY VERSUS FULL

At four months, looking distressed and crying are still your infant's best ways of letting you know something's wrong: He's hungry, thirsty, tired, wet, or bored. By now, you may even be able to figure out from the cry what the problem is, especially if the crying is coupled with fist chewing or

A NOTE OF CAUTION ABOUT FRUIT AND VEGETABLE JUICES

Some research studies have shown that large amounts of fruit juice stop infants from gaining weight and height normally. Fruit juice fills the calorie gap and replaces foods that would offer the balance of nutrients needed for healthy growth. It also contains lots of the fruit sugars fructose and sorbitol, which can cause abdominal cramps, bloating, and diarrhea, and also encourage cavities in emerging teeth if fed by bottle.

So make a conscious decision about whether to start your baby on fruit juice. It isn't necessary for vitamins if your baby is eating fruit regularly. If you do offer juice, set a limit of 3 to 4 ounces daily and choose juices with some nutritional value, such as red grape or pineapple (apple juice, in particular, contains little but carbohydrates, and citrus juices shouldn't be given until twelve months). You can give juice undiluted, or add water if you prefer. Just tight line make sure that your baby also gets used to having plain water daily, so that he doesn't come to rely on drinks with unnecessary calories to quench his thirst.

Vegetable juices such as carrot can be served from the same age as vegetables themselves, but again are best used sparingly. They don't give your baby practice with eating solid food and, because they replace vegetables, make it less likely your baby will learn to like the real thing. As a general rule, restrict vegetable juices to at most 1 ounce per day before eight months, and 2 ounces per day afterward. If you do give your child vegetable juice, reduce the amount of fruit juice you give so that the total does not exceed 3 to 4 ounces daily.

ravenous looks. Soon he will likely also develop the habit—which will both amuse and sometimes frustrate you—of turning his head decisively away from the nipple after a good feed. "Enough," he seems to say, "I'm full." By six months he may sometimes show that mouth-shut, head-turned demeanor toward the end of a meal of cereal, but you will see his lack of interest even earlier, when he opens his mouth just wide enough for the spoon, takes only a little, and swallows slowly. By eight or nine months he will learn how to actually push the food away!

Reading your baby's food signals will help you to organize his feedings so that he eats when he is hungry, stops when he is full, and doesn't constantly demand snacks. If your six-month-old is acting hungry and it is not yet dinnertime, stop and think whether he ate within the last two or three hours. If he did, offer play or some other nonfood option before trying food. If it's been two to three hours, offer milk or food. Maybe he is hungry, either because his last meal was small or because he is having a growth spurt. If he sucks only briefly or just plays with his food, he's not really hungry. The absence of a usually healthy appetite most often means that something has changed—maybe he is cutting a tooth, or perhaps he's coming down with something and you'll see a fever or symptoms of a cold later in the day.

3. LET YOUR BABY LEAD THE WAY

Offer small portions (you can always give more), use a soft baby spoon, and wait while your baby finishes each mouthful completely before offering more. Because your baby will prefer being fed this gentle way, the whole process will be easier, quicker, and more enjoyable. Try to resist the urge to overfill his spoon in an attempt to speed things up—the resulting ooze that comes back out, and the twisting and mouth contortions he goes through, will actually slow things down.

Letting him lead the way also means letting him take over the job of feeding as his skills develop. At first this may mostly take the form of smearing food gleefully around his mouth. He'll soon move on to finger feeding, and will eventually want to take that spoon away from you. It's part of the miracle of development that, as parents, we are privileged to watch and participate in.

4. TRY TO MAKE MEALTIMES RELAXED AND ENJOYABLE

Especially at this age, extended meals need to be a way of life, so try to see them as an enricher of family life and a time when your child can practice his new physical prowess at the table. It will take your child about four years to become a competent consumer of adult foods. Meanwhile, mealtimes of forty-five minutes or more are not unusual, and foods will get eaten more readily if the atmosphere is relaxed and cheerful. Some patience is helpful! When you have finished your own meal and are ready to clear up, your baby may still be busy with his food. By all means see if he is receptive to your offering him a spoonful between his own attempts. If he is frustrated and hungry, he will be glad for your help.

5. PRACTICE VARIETY—AND REPETITION

Variety and repetition will both become important by about seven months. Does this sound like a contradiction? It's really not. Repetition is what gets your baby used to the foods you want her to accept. Variety, though somewhat limited at this age, is what keeps food interesting and will be crucial for preventing eating problems in the coming years. And although your real window of opportunity for introducing your child to all the adult foods you want her to like begins at twelve months, you can nevertheless get a jump start on those introductions now.

Before seven months it's too early to think about variety because your baby lacks the ability to compare past events and present ones—an essential developmental step for appreciating the difference between yesterday's meals and today's. After seven months, however, keep trying out new foods every three to four days, while continuing to offer old favorites every three to fourteen days, and cereal and milk as daily staples. If you keep this up, by the time your baby is ten months old she'll have tried thirty to forty different items! Some of these will be instantly popular, while others will either take more familiarity before they are accepted or will join a short list of things that simply don't make the cut.

6. AVOID GIVING YOUR INFANT FOODS YOU DON'T WANT HIM TO LOVE WHEN HE'S OLDER

One baby we know ate fast food from the age of six months because his busy parents wanted easy meals, planning to clean up their act later. By nine months french fries were this baby's favorite food! Occasional experiences are fine, but regular repetition of foods your child likes makes them strong favorites that are hard to eliminate later.

7. BALANCE FOODS AND LIFE

Try to give your baby as much good-quality attention at nonmeal times as when you feed her. Being talked to, cuddled, played with, and taken on walks are all ways she will love spending time with you now. When you give her attention in these ways as well as when you feed her, you send the signal that your love is unrelated to what she eats. This helps her maintain the self-confidence and instinctive self-regulating abilities that will stand her in good stead in the future.

8. BE A FOOD ROLE MODEL

If you eat Grasshopper cookies (my personal favorite, alas) after dinner, by the time your child gets to about nine months, she will want to as well.

COMMON PROBLEMS AND FREQUENTLY ASKED QUESTIONS

At nine months Davey is still living primarily on formula. He eats like a bird when it comes to solid food, and has barely gained weight since he was six months old. His parents are worried that something is wrong.

It's normal for parents of six- to twelve-month-olds to feel their babies aren't eating and aren't growing. The enormous growth spurts of the first months of life make for huge appetites, and the much slower growth later in the first year makes food requirements proportionately smaller. Also, breast-fed babies often grow particularly fast early on, with a compensatory slowdown later. Formula-fed babies seem to "lag behind" at first, and then catch up. It all evens out between one and two years. If Davey is gaining height normally and gaining a little weight (even if not much), his parents should focus on letting their son control how much he eats, and stop worrying. In fact, if they overencourage now, they may be letting themselves in for picky eating and food battles later on. To prompt Davey to eat more solid foods, they can limit his formula consumption to 24 ounces per day and offer a plentiful variety of solid foods. A pediatrician's assessment is essential, however, for babies who stop gaining any weight at all.

Ten-month-old Jamie makes a huge mess whenever she eats. Lunch gets smeared in her hair and dropped on the floor, and she needs a bath after every meal.

If your child is like Jamie and you don't mind mess—and have a place where it can be cleaned up easily—by all means let her make a mess and give her a bath afterward. She will learn to eat by herself more quickly this way and have lots of fun in the process. But if you need to, you can take more control and things will still work out fine. Give her a spoon and let her try to feed herself from a bowl and with a few pieces on the tray. Take them away when she starts to make a mess deliberately. Give them back nicely in a few seconds, and tell her she can have them if she tries not to make a mess. She won't understand at first, of course, but with repetition and good humor she'll get the idea quickly, and you'll both end up happier.

Sarah's mom feels ready to give up nursing but Sarah—at eight months— refuses formula. She'll drink water from a cup or a bottle but won't touch formula no matter how it is offered.

If her mom wants to give up nursing, getting Sarah to like formula is important. There are several ways to go about it. Starting with a feed when Sarah is lively, her mom can nurse for half as long as usual and then offer Sarah a bottle of body-temperature breast milk that has been expressed. This helps Sarah get used to milk in a bottle. After a few days, when she is comfortable with that idea, the expressed milk can be mixed with formula half and half, moving to 100 percent formula gradually. Over a few weeks, nursing can be replaced with formula one feeding at a time, leaving the early-morning and late-night feedings as the last to change.

Another approach is to have Sarah's dad feed Sarah formula when her mom is out of the house. This helps by introducing the formula when the familiar association of Mom and nursing are out of the picture for the moment. Of course, any of these strategies can be combined.

Ashley, six months, is just starting to cut her first tooth. Her mother is wondering if this is the time to stop nursing, so she doesn't get bitten during feedings.

Very few babies think of biting when they nurse, so chances are Ashley's mom has nothing to worry about. If Ashley is one of the few that does try, her mom can stop the feed immediately and say no nicely but very seriously before resuming. Once or twice will probably be all it takes for Ashley to keep her teeth well hidden.

At seven months Robert is a confirmed grazer. He picks at his breakfast, only to need milk one hour later, and then another snack or even two before lunch. The rest of the day is just as bad. His parents want to fix the problem but are reluctant to starve him into submission.

Some babies don't seem to make an automatic transition to three meals and two snacks and instead want to "graze," with perhaps as many as ten meals a day. This can be very hard on their parents, especially if the mom is still nursing.

Usually this happens when the family gets into a vicious cycle where the baby eats when he is not yet hungry, then doesn't eat enough, and then very soon feels hungry again. It doesn't matter a great deal to the baby, for whom eating and sleeping are primary activities anyway. But for the household, and for the child's eating habits in the long run, it's better to gently nudge him toward longer times between feeds.

Robert's parents can start by simply taking their time. When he wakes in the morning, they shouldn't rush to feed him, but wait until he cries for milk. If he gets bored after a few minutes, they may stroke and encourage him to take some more—without forcing the meal—and then move on to cereal and fruit as well. If he shows signs of hunger before three hours have passed, they can offer a little drink of water, a game, a walk, or a bath. With some persistence over a few days, his stomach will adapt to going longer between meals and snacks.

They can also start to employ the variety principle. Instead of milk and one other food for breakfast, Robert's parents can offer milk plus *three* foods (for example, cereal and apple puree and banana slices, followed by milk). Rather than mixing it all up, they should wait for him to stop eating one and then offer the next. The extra interest will probably encourage him to eat more, and it will take him longer to get hungry again.

Ten-month-old Monica has four fine new teeth. Her parents would like to know when to start brushing them.

Different dentists have different opinions on this issue. Some will tell you to start brushing even before the first tooth appears; others will say it is okay to wait to start brushing until two years, and that until this age wiping your baby's teeth with a soft cloth works fine. If Monica is happy to have her teeth brushed with a soft baby brush, then now is a good time to start. If it seems to frighten her, wiping with a soft cloth now and graduating to a brush around one year will be fine, too. Whatever decision is made about brushing, most dentists recommend using a very tiny amount of toothpaste or even holding off until two years (because large amounts need to be spat out, not swallowed, to avoid excess fluoride).

CHAPTER 10

❖

Twelve to Twenty-one Months

A Nine-month Window of Opportunity

Diane is so proud of her one-year-old son, Timmy, because he eats anything she puts on the table. "The weekend of Timmy's birthday," she says, "we had lunch at a Chinese restaurant and there were snails on the buffet—he even tried those!" Her friend Paula comments, "Enjoy it while you can! Russell was just the same—until he was about two. Now he won't even eat pizza if it doesn't come from our usual pizzeria!"

First birthdays are a defining moment in the lives of mothers and fathers. You look back and remember with amazement how only a year and a day ago you were without this wonderful child who has so changed your life. You think, too, how much he has grown from an infant into a real person with a real personality. It hasn't always been easy, certainly, but your life has been enriched and expanded in ways that you never imagined.

First birthdays are a defining moment for your child, too. He is now ready to conquer the world! Walking, running, and talking are all developmental milestones that he will master before his second birthday. From being a baby you still have to help at meals, he'll soon arrive at some real independence, competently feeding himself with a spoon and cup. He will also make the transition from a diet containing many "baby" foods to an almost exclusively adult menu.

Sometime between fifteen and twenty-one months most children become conscious that they have some very different goals in life from their parents. They learn to say no. Even before your child purposefully uses the word to defy you, he may start "saying" it with fine-tuned negative behavior.

But with an angelic one-year-old sitting on your lap, that big transition to the "terrible twos" is off on the horizon. What you have ahead of you at this moment is an important opportunity, which usually lasts from one year until twenty-one months or a little longer.

It's a time when physical development, metabolic maturity, and natural instincts converge to encourage adventurous eating. Your child wants to eat like you, is metabolically and physically able to do so, and has not yet become cautious about trying new foods. Provided you are low-key and don't actively push the foods you want your child to like, this window of opportunity allows you to get your toddler settled into a diverse diet of adult foods in a natural progression.

Three toddler instincts are especially helpful in this transition. First, as you've no doubt noticed, your child is still compelled to put things in his mouth. He'll continue to display this instinct until feeding has become a completely easy process.

Second, your child has an increasing urge to "do it himself." Being able to control what goes in his mouth is one of the first steps in this budding independence. Of course, simply maneuvering a spoon is a challenging job for a toddler, and feeding will be a communal project for some months yet. But you will save yourself some future battles by letting him take the lead.

Third, your child has a deep instinct to copy you. Imitation is how children learn—long before they realize they are learning. Especially toward the end of these nine months, they are programmed to copy everything we do and everything we eat. Setting a good example yourself is one of the important keys to raising a healthy eater.

OPPORTUNITIES AND GOALS FOR FEEDING FROM TWELVE TO TWENTY-ONE MONTHS

Foods your child eats at this time—and how she eats them—continue to program her for strong bones and teeth, a healthy metabolism, and optimum development. At the same time, your child is still busy forming the subconscious feelings that will last a lifetime. When she enjoys eating fruits, vegetables, legumes, and dairy products, she creates an internal blueprint for the foods she will feel good about eating in years to come. Keep the following points in mind:

- *Maintain your toddler's milk consumption at 16 to 24 ounces per day, or ensure an adequate calcium intake from other dairy foods.* Whole cow's milk is now a safe alternative to formula or breast milk. If for some reason your child cannot or will not drink milk, turn to page 202 for information on other rich sources.

- *Introduce your toddler to the full range of healthy adult foods you want her to enjoy in the future.* By twenty-one months she can be familiar with as many as two hundred foods and will consume between 40 and 60 percent of her daily calories from foods other than milk. Even though your child can now eat adult foods, she still needs a diet with relatively more fat, less fiber, and more essential nutrients than a grown-up.

- *Move gradually toward a schedule of three meals and two snacks per day, while encouraging self-feeding and self-regulation of amounts eaten.* When you allow your toddler to eat the amount she wants at her own pace, you head off bad habits such as fussiness, grazing, and food refusals before they have a chance to set in.

Now is also the time to take a first look at your family medical history to see if your child's diet needs extra consideration. If there is a family history of premature heart disease, long-term prevention starts with some dietary modifications now (see "Exceptions to the Whole-Milk Rule," page 165). Likewise, if your child is overweight, some changes now can nip a serious problem in the bud (see Chapter 15).

WHAT YOUR CHILD EATS

Now that your child is one year old, he can eat almost anything you do if it is cut up into small pieces that are safe for him (see page 169 for information on toddler food safety). Although his mineral, vitamin, and fat needs continue to be high in relation to his overall food intake, most of his nutritional needs will be met if his total daily intake includes, on average:

- 16 to 24 ounces milk
- $^1\!/_2$ to 1 cup fresh fruit and vegetables
- 1–2 1-ounce servings of lean meat, poultry, egg, or fish, and/or $^1\!/_2$ cup fortified cereal
- About 200 to 500 calories' worth of other good foods such as cereals, breads, and legumes (beans, peas, peanut butter), as appetite demands (see below)
- Water as desired for thirst

These food amounts may seem rather small. As we mentioned in Chapter 3, recent research has shown that the typical calorie needs of infants and young children are much lower than previously believed. However, it is not necessary for you to count calories for your child: His appetite can be your guide as long as he continues to grow normally.

Your toddler's daily intakes may be increasingly variable as he gets accustomed to the different foods you are offering. Other events also come into play. Teething can decrease appetite for days at a time, though hard cold foods such as frozen bagels, frozen sliced strawberries, and ice pops made with 100 percent juice, consumed under direct supervision, can ease the discomfort of eating. Minor sicknesses may also be frequent, as your toddler has more contact with the outside world. These can decrease his appetite to half or a quarter of normal for a day or two. After your child has cut his tooth or recovered from his cold, he will probably be ravenous for a few days and get right back on his normal growth curve.

Calories in Some Toddler-Sized Portions

FOOD TYPE	AMOUNT	CALORIES
Cold breakfast cereals	$^1\!/_4$ cup	22–37
Hot breakfast cereals	$^1\!/_4$ cup	36
Breads (white, wheat, rye)	$^1\!/_2$ slice	30–45
Bagel	$^1\!/_4$ whole	50
English muffin	$^1\!/_4$ whole	35
Starches (pasta, noodles, rice, mashed potato)	$^1\!/_4$ cup cooked	50
Beans	$^1\!/_4$ cup cooked	55
Peanut butter	1 tablespoon	90

GROWTH PATTERNS BETWEEN ONE AND TWO YEARS

Growth slows down a lot after your child's first birthday—which is one reason why appetite seems to decline so much. In the early months your baby was gaining nearly 2 pounds and over 1 inch in length every month—a pace that, if continued, would bring her to 400 pounds and 21 feet by eighteen years! More moderate growth rates are typical now—a little under half a pound and less than half an inch per month—and will continue into the preschool years.

Nonetheless, your child's occasional growth spurts may continue to amaze you. Maybe he needs new clothes *again,* or your wall chart shows he has added 2 inches between one month and the next.

These growth spurts start in the bones—which is why you may notice your child thinning out during a growth spurt. His bones are lengthening in response to timed growth signals originating in DNA, and his muscles and other tissues follow on as they get tugged into position by the longer bones. With every growth spurt he becomes a little more muscular and a little leaner—the start of the body composition changes that turn most roly-poly one-year-olds into long-limbed four-year-olds.

One predictable time for growth spurts is spring—which makes it a good idea to wait until the last minute to buy summer clothes and shoes. Research studies have documented that children grow more rapidly in spring than at any other time of the year, and growth spurts during this season can add as much as an inch in just a few days. Like the plants that know when it is time to flower, our children's bodies are powerfully connected to nature in ways that even our modern lifestyle can't touch.

MAKING THE TRANSITION TO COW'S MILK

Milk is one of the big transitions for one- to two-year-olds. At this age most children can drink whole cow's milk with minimal risk of allergies, and 16 to 24 ounces daily is an amount that will remain healthy from now until adulthood.

If you are still nursing, you can continue for as long as you want, but be aware that most mothers produce only small amounts of breast milk after one year. If you are nursing for less than forty-five minutes a day, your child needs 8 to 12 ounces of cow's milk as well to ensure enough calcium. You can substitute other milk-based products, such as yogurt and cheese, for some or all of the milk (6 ounces of yogurt or 1 ounce of cheese is the equivalent of 6 ounces of milk).

Whole cow's milk, rather than low-fat milk, is appropriate until age two for most children. The high fat content of whole milk meets continuing high fat needs for myelination of delicate nerves within the brain and throughout the body.

Many children have a problem with the transition from breast-feeding or bottle-feeding to cow's milk in a cup, with the result that they never learn to eat the one food that ensures calcium intake with ease. To make certain the switch is a smooth one, think of it as a two-step process that starts between twelve and thirteen months and lasts between one and five months, with small incremental steps every week or two. It is important to take the process slowly so that your baby doesn't become resistant—but don't start too late. If you wait until fifteen months or later, you may find that your baby has become so attached to her bottle that she won't easily take to drinking milk another way.

For nursing mothers who haven't already started using a cup, simply put it on the high chair at mealtimes and show your baby what to do. You can try both cold and warmed cow's milk—most babies prefer it one way or the other. Provided you don't also put a bottle on the tray, your child will soon learn to enjoy what is in the cup for the refreshment it brings.

For formula-fed babies, start by replacing formula with a mixture of four-fifths formula and one-fifth cow's milk. Use a bottle or cup—whichever the child is accustomed to—and keep the milk the usual temperature. If she resists the change, back off for a week and then try again. After five to seven days you can increase the proportion of cow's milk to a quarter and then to a third the following week. Within two months your baby makes the complete transition.

By the time your baby is fourteen months old she will be ready to move to a cup if she hasn't already—this is actually more difficult than changing milks! Some infants are willing to switch straight over (one meal at a time) if you simply substitute milk in a sippy cup for milk in a bottle. Initially your child will probably be pretty surprised by the change, but if you keep the milk the usual temperature and cuddle her as you usually do when she is

EXCEPTIONS TO THE WHOLE-MILK RULE

The two exceptions are for toddlers who are already overweight (see Chapter 15) and those who have a family history of very early heart disease (before age forty). Both these groups can benefit from moving straight to 2 percent rather than whole milk. In the case of families with heart disease, it is important to make up the loss of fat in milk by offering other foods with healthier fats, such as canola, corn, and olive oils, hummus, peanut butter, and tofu spreads that don't contain partially hydrogenated oils. This way your child will avoid saturated fats and trans fatty acids without going short on total calories.

being given a bottle, very likely she will drink most if not all of her usual amount.

If your child seems resistant, you can start by putting a little water in her sippy cup and leaving it on her tray at one or more mealtimes daily. This way she will get to the cup without the threat of losing her bottle. Then simply substitute a cup of milk for one bottle of milk. Be comforting if she is disturbed, but don't offer a bottle at this feed. She will get used to the change within a few days.

Over the next one or two months you can gradually substitute more cups for bottles. Keep the nighttime feeding and the first morning feeding for a while—they are the ones that your toddler will find hardest to give up. By fifteen to seventeen months she will be much more interested in moving around, and a cozy bottle will have less appeal.

Don't, incidentally, make bottles too attractive in the weeks leading up to the transition. Using them when you don't need to (for example, instead of a cup for water and juice) or offering ones with your child's favorite cartoon character are all ways to inadvertently turn the bottle into a comfort object that will be hard to discard later.

GOOD FOODS TO TRY

This is the year for food adventures! Let your child try everything you can think of, as long as it is not on our "Foods to Avoid" list (Chapter 9) and it is cut up carefully to prevent choking. You'll thank yourself when your child is two to three years old.

TEETH AND YOUR BABY'S DIET

Metabolically programming strong permanent teeth, which are now just beginning to grow and harden within your baby's jaw, is one of the important goals for this year. There are also some simple things you can do to keep those beautiful pearly baby milk teeth (which are only just appearing, but have *already* been programmed for strength) in their current pristine condition.

CAVITY PREVENTION FOR FIRST TEETH

1. Make sure your baby gets enough fluoride—but not too much. Read "Fluoride Facts" (page 181) to determine whether your baby needs a fluoride supplement.

2. Prevent "baby-bottle cavities" by *never* putting your child to sleep with her bottle—filled with either juice or milk. During extended sleepy feeds your baby's mouth bacteria will ferment both fruit sugar (fructose) and milk sugar (lactose) to an acid that literally dissolves tooth enamel. Citrus juices are particularly harmful to teeth and in fact shouldn't even be given by cup more than once per day. One recent study documented a *thirty-seven-fold increase* in the risk of enamel erosion when citrus juice or fruits are consumed three times or more daily.

3. Prevent the breast-feeding version of baby-bottle cavities by not sleeping with your baby after twelve months in order to give lengthy feeds.

4. Prevent regular frequent snacking. Three meals and two or three snacks per day are usually all your child needs now, and more frequent eating leads to excess bacterial acid production.

5. Know the top five cavity-producing food groups: candy, dried fruits, cookies, crackers, and potato chips. Either avoid them completely, serve them early in

Good foods to try include:

- All fresh fruits and vegetables—raw and cooked, plain and dressed. (Note: Save hard raw vegetables such as carrots and celery until your baby is chewing his food, to prevent choking, and start with thin strips cut with a vegetable peeler.)

meals rather than at the end, or brush your child's teeth immediately after the meal. Note that not all these foods contain sucrose (table sugar). All carbohydrates get partly degraded into sugars in the mouth, and the most important determinant of a food's cavity potential is how much it sticks around the teeth.

6. Harness the cavity-preventing benefits of aged cheeses such as cheddar and Swiss. Because their texture encourages saliva flow (which washes away harmful bacteria) and because they contain acid-neutralizing proteins, small amounts of these cheeses eaten at the end of a meal actually stop the harmful effects of very acid-promoting foods eaten just before.

7. Start regular visits with your child's dentist for advice on when to start brushing (most dentists recommend around one year) and other oral hygiene measures.

GROWING STRONG PERMANENT TEETH

Permanent teeth are mineralized between now and eight years. Later, some calcium and fluoride can be absorbed directly onto the topmost layer of the tooth's surface, but the opportunity for packing strengthening minerals into the thick underlying enamel has passed. And because some teeth are mineralized early (between one and two and a half years) and others later (between two and a half and eight years), a regular supply of critical nutrients is what makes every tooth strong enough to last a lifetime.

Along with fluoride, calcium is the major nutrient needed for strong teeth. If your child enjoys cow's milk, it is pretty easy to make sure she gets enough.

- Breads, low-fat crackers, low-sugar cereals, pasta, potatoes, rice, tortillas, and cooked grains. Include regular modest amounts of high-fiber types so your child learns to like them. Just don't expect him to eat large portions, because of his low requirement for fiber at this age.
- All kinds of meats, poultry, fish, and shellfish, except those containing nitrites.

A WINDOW OF OPPORTUNITY FOR VEGETABLES

Older children often reject vegetables because they weren't introduced during this window of opportunity. Focus on variety and freshness to encourage a liking for this important food group in the future.

THINK CRISP: Thin slices of celery or carrot, strips of colorful sweet peppers, snow peas, green beans, and broccoli and cauliflower "trees" can all be served raw, with or without a little dip, from as soon as your toddler is chewing his food nicely. He will enjoy the action of dipping once he gets the hang of it, and you can exploit the variety principle to advantage by varying both the dips and the veggie combinations. Cucumbers, cherry tomatoes, and even bits of crispy lettuce and cabbage (green and red) are good for dipping, too. Crisp cooked vegetables include asparagus tops (trim off tough stems) very lightly steamed and served with a little lemon juice and butter. Broccoli works well with the same approach, and is even better mixed with a crushed clove of garlic and a teaspoon or two of olive oil.

THINK SWEET: Try this recipe for enhancing carrots' appealing sweetness: Peel and slice 1 pound of carrots in 1-inch lengths. Simmer with 1¼ cup water and 2 teaspoons olive oil until tender, about 15 minutes, adding water if needed. At the end of cooking, stir over medium heat to boil off any remaining liquid. The carrots' natural sugars come to the fore in this method.

Also sweet if treated right are fresh beets. Wash and peel 4 to 6 fresh

- All dairy products including milk, eggs, yogurt, and cheese (butter and cream in moderation).
- Beans and peas, and bean products such as tofu. Be aware that bean skins are hard for one-year-olds to digest. This makes many bean recipes better to introduce after fifteen months.
- Foods with small amounts of spices and herbs—even tiny pieces of the herbs themselves to learn their taste.

Aim to progress to adult eating patterns at each meal. For example, breakfast might contain one or two items in addition to milk to drink (for example, cereal with milk and fruit) and lunch and dinner three or four items (a protein food; a starch; a vegetable; and a fruit). As described in Chapter 2, much more variety than this encourages overeating, if the variety comes from high-calorie items, while a very limited variety may result in undereating.

beets, slice very thin, and steam for 10 minutes, with a little chopped onion if desired. Toss with 1 tablespoon rice vinegar or balsamic vinegar and 1 teaspoon butter. Serve warm. Substitute 2 tablespoons yogurt for the vinegar and butter if desired.

THINK COLORFUL: Those bright hues in fresh vegetables actually reveal the presence of healthful phytochemicals. Strips of red, yellow, and green pepper make a delicious salad mixed with a little chopped onion and vinaigrette dressing. Orange-carrot salad, with grated carrots moistened with equal parts orange juice and oil and sprinkled with chopped parsley, is as good to look at as to eat.

EASY SELL: Mixed Chinese vegetables in a stir-fry are crisp and delicious. Slice a small carrot, half a red or green pepper, a small onion, and $1/2$ cup white cabbage, and add similar amounts of snow peas, bean sprouts, or any other vegetables you enjoy. Saute the onion with 1 tablespoon finely chopped fresh ginger and 1 crushed garlic clove for 2 minutes on high heat in 1 tablespoon oil, and then add remaining vegetables and saute briskly. Add 2 teaspoons reduced-sodium soy sauce and $1/2$ cup water mixed with $1/2$ tablespoon cornstarch. Reduce heat, cover, and simmer for 3 minutes.

UNDERAPPRECIATED: Yams (sweet potatoes), baked or boiled and mashed with a little orange juice or butter, are tasty and packed with vitamins and minerals.

CAUTION! SAFETY IS A BIG ISSUE

Now that your child is capable of self-feeding and is also becoming mobile, you need to take vigorous safety measures. If you haven't already done so, childproof everything you can think of, and then look around at child level to see what you forgot.

- **Poisoning.** Most of the items normally kept under the kitchen sink or in the bathroom can be lethal to a one-year-old if they are drunk or eaten, and need to be kept out of reach. Because parents usually focus on obvious dangers such as medicines and cleaning products, seemingly innocent items often cause the accidents. Ingestion of maternal iron supplements is a leading cause of accidental death in infants. Mouthwash is another common hazard.

Even $1/2$ ounce of one of the brands containing alcohol can lead to toxic reactions in a toddler, and about three thousand poisoning cases occur annually in the United States in children under six years.

- **Choking.** Allow food to be eaten only while sitting down under adult supervision. Avoid giving your child spoonfuls of very thick spreads, such as peanut butter, that can get stuck in her throat. Whole grapes and other round objects need to be cut into halves or quarters lengthwise. Hard vegetables and large pieces of food should be cut into thin inch-long strips (not rounds), and all pieces of fish should be minutely inspected for bones. Make sure, too, that all toys are large enough so that they can't be swallowed.

- **Burns.** Toddlers have delicate mouths, so avoid giving any food that is too hot. A rule of thumb: Anything that feels more than moderately warm to you is too hot for your child.

- **Kitchen accidents.** Toddlers are inexhaustibly curious about everything in their kingdom, so get childproof locks for all the cupboards and keep hot pots at the back of the stove (with handles not hanging over the edge where a child might grab them). Never carry pots of hot or boiling food across the kitchen when your toddler is near, put knives in childproof drawers, and move other objects to the back of the counter. Even apparently innocuous items can cause trouble. One boy we know had to have his finger reattached by a plastic surgeon after his twin pulled an opened can of tomatoes off the counter when his mother turned away for a few seconds.

- **Yard and garage hazards.** Nails, drill bits, and safety pins are the kinds of objects that adorn the bulletin boards of the gastroenterologists and throat specialists who are called in to retrieve them. They should be stored well out of reach, along with paints, paint remover, and all garden chemicals. Many plants are also poisonous if consumed. Consider digging up dangerous ones, and teach your child never to eat anything except food you or her other caretakers give her.

*Pretty but Poisonous**

YARD	HOUSE
Azalea	Amaryllis
Boxwood	Chrysanthemum
English ivy	Daffodil
Hydrangea	Hyacinth
Mountain laurel	Iris
Oak (acorns)	Lily-of-the-valley
Rhododendron	Narcissus
Wisteria	Peony

* For more information, including a list of safe plants, visit the Maryland Poison Center Web site (www.pharmacy.ab.umd.edu/webhome/MPC/Plant.html.bak).

FOOD TRAPS TO AVOID

- **Relying on baby food.** We're often asked whether commercial baby food is okay at this age. Our answer is yes, it is okay, but it prevents your exploiting your window of opportunity to introduce new foods. Home-cooked foods can be almost as convenient, can be stocked in the freezer, and are better because they help your child become accustomed to the food that *you* want to eat. They also help to prevent future fussiness—because they taste a little different each time they're prepared.

- **Too much juice.** Limit juice to 4 ounces per day or less. Juice in large amounts can stop children from gaining weight and height normally, because it replaces foods that have a better balance of nutrients. We have also noticed that too much juice seems to stop children liking healthier fresh fruits—perhaps because they are too similar. Water contains no calories or sugar to harm delicate new teeth, and satisfies thirst. If you don't drink water yourself, you might feel guilty giving it to your child instead of flavorful juice. But kids who get used to drinking water often request it before calorie-laden alternatives.

- **Too much sugar.** Contrary to popular wisdom, research studies have shown that children's liking for sweet things is only partly instinctive. You can minimize your child's future sweet tooth by keeping sugar to

A WINDOW OF OPPORTUNITY FOR FISH

Although we don't encourage an overreliance on fried foods, this recipe for crispy cod makes an easy and popular introduction to fish. Serve with ketchup, tartar sauce, or mild rice vinegar, mashed potato, and a favorite vegetable.

Preparation and cooking time: 10–15 minutes

> *Batter:*
> $1/2$ cup flour
> 1 teaspoon baking powder
> $1/4$ teaspoon salt
> $1/2$ cup plus 2 tbsp milk
> 1 teaspoon oil
>
> 1 pound very fresh cod, in $1/2$-inch-thick slices
> Oil for shallow frying

Mix all batter ingredients together with a whisk. Heat oil until a drop of batter fries quickly. Dip cod in batter and put into oil one piece at a time, making sure not to overcrowd pan. Cook on both sides for 3–4 minutes or until golden. Blot well on both sides with several layers of paper towel.

a minimum during this vulnerable year, when his subconscious blueprint about foods is forming. A good rule: Restrict sweet things other than fresh fruit to *once a day or less* on average. Store cookies and other sweets out of your toddler's sight; what he can't see, he probably won't ask for.

MENUS AND SCHEDULES

Page 173 shows four sample menus tailored to a young toddler with typical calorie needs. If yours is a small eater, he may need as little as half the amount of solid food suggested, while very big eaters may need up to twice as much. Expect calorie requirements to increase by about 10 percent between twelve and twenty-one months.

SAMPLE MEALS FOR A TWELVE- TO FOURTEEN-MONTH-OLD TODDLER

Day 1	Day 2	Day 3	Day 4
BREAKFAST			

1 small pancake
1 tbsp maple syrup
1/4 cup straw-
   berries
6 oz whole milk
	1/4 cup oatmeal
	2 tbsp blueberries
	1 tsp sugar
	6 oz whole milk
		1/4 cup fortified
		   cereal
		Piece of melon
		6 oz whole milk
			1/4 cup fortified
			   cereal
			Few sliced grapes
			6 oz whole milk

MORNING SNACK			

4 plain crackers
2 tsp peanut butter
6 oz whole milk
	1 pear
	6 oz whole milk
		1/4 cup plain
		   crackers
		4 oz orange juice
		   diluted with
		   water
			1/2 slice pumper-
			   nickel with
			   cream cheese
			6 oz whole milk

LUNCH			

1/3 cup macaroni
   and cheese
1/2 kiwi
Water
	1/2 cup bean soup
	1/2 slice bread
	1/4 banana
	Water
		Grilled cheese
		   sandwich on 1
		   slice bread
		4 oz yogurt
		Water
			Turkey sandwich
			   on 1 slice bread
			1 carrot, in
			   sticks, with
			   ranch dressing
			Water

AFTERNOON SNACK			
3 dried apricots 4 oz whole milk	1/4 apple 4 oz whole milk	1 plain cookie 4 oz whole milk	1 cheese stick 4 oz whole milk
DINNER			

1 oz chicken
1 tbsp cooked
   spinach
1/4 cup rice
1/4 apple
Water
	1 small slice pizza
	2 slices cucumber
	   with dressing
	1/4 orange
	Water
		1 oz baked fish
		1/4 ear corn
		1/4 cup pasta salad
		1/4 peach
		Water
			1/4 cup meat and
			   vegetable
			   casserole
			1/4 cup mashed
			   potatoes
			1 tbsp peas
			1/4 cup pineapple
			Water

BEDTIME SNACK			
4 oz whole milk	4 oz whole milk	4 oz whole milk	4 oz whole milk

QUICK BREAKFASTS

With the help of your microwave or toaster, many tasty breakfasts can be made in about the time it takes to prepare the grown-ups' coffee or tea.

Fresh fruit

Cold cereal with milk or yogurt

Hot cereal with milk and maple syrup or fruit sauce

Toast, warm rolls, English muffins, or bagels, with cream cheese and other spreads

Pancakes, waffles, or muffins (homemade and stored in your freezer, or check your supermarket freezer section for healthy options)

Omelet, scrambled eggs

Egg and cheese on an English muffin

Now that your child's stomach is bigger, he needs food less frequently and can usually live comfortably with a daily schedule of three meals and two or three snacks that fit with your normal meal routines. Although a bedtime snack of milk is something that many babies like at twelve months, it is no longer necessary. Eliminating it sometime between fourteen and seventeen months as you phase out bottles will prepare the way for dry nights and successful toilet training between the ages of two and three.

Some babies naturally gravitate to this schedule by twelve months, but others need some help. If your baby eats small meals and huge snacks and then is not hungry for his next meal, you need to nudge him in the right direction. Start by making meals more leisurely. Longer mealtimes, perhaps with music to make them more relaxing, mean extra calories. You can add a simple extra food (such as bread and butter) or another course—cottage cheese and crackers, fruit, or yogurt—to encourage consumption with variety. When the next snack time comes around, deliberately reduce the amount by about a quarter. Your child probably won't notice at the time but will be eager for the following meal. Within days you will have established a better schedule without any upheaval or fuss.

WEEKEND SPECIAL: OAT PANCAKES

Oats are among the best whole grains to offer your toddler. Not only are they generally more popular than whole-grain wheat or brown rice, they also lower cholesterol, blood pressure, and unhealthy blood lipid fractions more than equivalent amounts of other grains—good for the whole family! Easy to make and freeze, these pancakes are best with real maple syrup or fruit sauce.

Preparation and cooking time: 15 minutes

   1¼ cups oat flour (see note)
   ¾ teaspoon double-acting baking powder
   ½ teaspoon baking soda
   4 tablespoons buttermilk powder
   1 teaspoon sugar
   ¼ teaspoon salt
   1 egg or 2 egg whites
   1 cup water
   2 teaspoons canola or other oil

Sift all dry ingredients together. With a fork, beat egg and oil until well mixed; stir in water. Mix dry and wet ingredients together with a whisk until just blended. Ladle ¼-cup portions of the batter onto your griddle (which should be a little cooler than for regular pancakes because the oat flour browns quickly) and cook for 1–2 minutes per side until light brown.

Note: Buy oat flour at a health food store or make it yourself by putting rolled oats in a food processor or blender at high speed for 15 to 30 seconds. Buttermilk powder is available in most supermarkets, or you can substitute 1 cup fresh buttermilk and eliminate the water.

Eliminate the late-night bottle before bed by reducing the volume gradually over a few weeks, or by giving the same volume and steadily diluting it every few days until it is all water. You can then reduce the amount of water until it is just a token and is no longer needed. As you do, you may need to add milk at meals to maintain a minimum of 16 ounces per day.

ESTABLISHING A GOOD BREAKFAST HABIT

If you have a big rush in the morning, giving the baby milk or juice is the easy way to get up and out of the house quickly. But by age one your child should have more than milk in the morning. Research studies have shown that breakfast affects school performance, especially in children who are not at the top of their class and who have to concentrate more to do a good job. Kindergarten is a long way off, but establishing the breakfast habit is much easier now than it will be later.

Start on a weekend or vacation when you have more time, and either get your baby up early (with a correspondingly earlier bedtime) or delay breakfast past the normal time, for maybe half an hour. This will ensure that your child is fully awake, hungry, and not rushed—all essential requirements for establishing early morning eating. Then simply provide some foods that your child likes at other times, maybe a favorite cereal, graham crackers, fresh or cooked fruit, or even pancakes or an omelet. At the other end of the day, make sure that you keep snacks and milk after dinner to a minimum so that he is hungry in the morning.

You can try different items over several days to keep your child's interest up. Research has shown that most people, kids included, tend to be more conservative about breakfast than other meals. But do keep an open mind. Fish and tomatoes are popular breakfast items in Israel, and children in China enjoy pickled eggs and pickled vegetables!

SHOULD YOU GIVE YOUR TODDLER A MULTIVITAMIN/MINERAL SUPPLEMENT?

If your baby has not taken a supplement before, now is the time to start. This is important—even if you have heard advice to the contrary. Without daily portions of red meat and eggs (which we don't recommend as a good pattern for the future), it is very hard for toddlers to get enough of essential nutrients such as iron and zinc—even if they are eating what looks like a good diet. Unfortunately, major-brand liquid supplements for children one to two years old do not contain zinc, and the "complete" chewable supplements that do contain zinc are marketed only for kids two years and older. Currently we think the best choice is to use two-thirds of the dose of a two-year-old's complete chewable supplement (that is equal to one-third of a pill for most brands). Read the instructions on the brand you choose very carefully, break off the right amount, crush it, and give it with a little water at dinnertime or before bed. This is not as hard as it might sound, because the pills are somewhat soft and crumbly. By the time your child is twenty-one months old he will probably feel grown-up eating it by itself. For children who don't drink much milk, information on other dietary sources of calcium and calcium supplements is given in Chapter 11 (pages 202–203).

If your water is not fluoridated, or if you use a bottled water that contains less than 0.3 milligrams per liter of fluoride, your pediatrician can prescribe a fluoride supplement from now until your child is six years old.

SMART STRATEGIES FOR FEEDING TODDLERS

Rachel was worried that her fourteen-month-old son, Will, was turning into a picky eater. Although he was growing well and starting to walk, he was not taking to the new foods she was now offering him. Typically he would eat only a spoonful or two of the dishes she prepared, and instead ended most meals with the bowl of cereal and fruit he had been eating since he was seven months old.

We helped Rachel by reminding her of several smart strategies, including the rule of fifteen and the discounting principle described in Chapter 2. Within a few weeks Will graduated from single spoonfuls to whole toddler-size portions of several foods. Will is now eighteen months old, and Rachel has a hearty eater who enjoys his mom's cooking.

Three smart strategies are especially useful in dealing with toddler instincts:

1. INCREASE YOUR CHILD'S FOOD REPERTOIRE USING VARIETY AND REPETITION

Most one-year-olds will usually be happy to eat anything you put in front of them, if they are hungry and you don't overencourage them. Introduce foods you want your child to like at a good pace (one new food every three to four days). At first he may eat only a spoonful or two before wanting something he is more used to. Some foods may not even be touched, but just seeing them on his tray can help him become comfortable enough to try them another time.

Once a food has been accepted, maintaining its familiarity is also important. If your child learns to like, say, rice pilaf and then doesn't have it again for three months, he may well have forgotten what it is, and you will have to start all over again.

While maintaining familiarity, you also need to prevent the boredom that leads to food refusals. Most children (like their parents) have an instinctive liking for variety, and any food your child eats every day, with the exception of staples such as milk and bread, will soon seem tiresome. Nonstaple foods are best offered every three to fourteen days, depending on how popular they are (the more popular, the more often they can be given). So, for example, lunch for your toddler might include milk and bread every day, with a hard-boiled egg and pear one day, sliced turkey and banana the next day, and peanut butter and jelly and apple slices the day after. The following day you could repeat a hard-boiled egg or offer something new again. If your child is one of the few who becomes conservative early and starts to want the same foods every day, turn to Chapter 11 for advice on maintaining a varied menu.

Different preparations and presentations also provide variety. Potatoes can be mashed, or boiled and cut into pieces, or put into potato salad. Pasta comes as spaghetti, flat noodles, spirals, alphabets, and elbows. A turkey sandwich can be made with white, oatmeal, rye, or whole-wheat bread, and with or without cheese, onion, lettuce, and tomato slices. Raw veggies can be cut up and dipped, made into salad, or stuffed into a pita pocket, and are quite different from cooked.

Another way to get variety without extra effort is to give your toddler each meal item separately. For example, bread and butter separate from turkey and tomato slices may be preferred over a single mixed sandwich, because it gives him more different things to try. One toddler we know likes to eat chicken noodle soup as three courses—chicken pieces, noodles, and broth—and in fact eats more total food this way than when they are all in the bowl together.

If you find that a once-popular food is being rejected, take it off the menu for two to three weeks. Chances are it will be accepted again when you next offer it.

Once exception to the variety-familiarity strategy is for seasonal fruits and vegetables. You may want to let your child have them daily if they are popular. Locally grown cherries (pitted and cut into small pieces to prevent choking), for example, are often available for only a few weeks in early summer. By the time your child is thoroughly bored with cherries, the season will be almost over. Next year he will have forgotten how boring cherries got and will probably attack them again with enthusiasm.

2. TAKE A BACKSEAT

As your child's instincts prompt her to take charge of her own eating, she is also testing her relationship with you. It is all too easy to set up conflicts that will turn into genuine control battles around the age of two. Like the small scientist that she becomes by about twenty-one months, she is starting to explore her control over food and over you through daily "experiments" in which you are the unwitting research subject. Why does she drop food on the floor? To watch it fall—and see if you pick it up. Why does she squash blueberries on the tray? To see what they look like after squashing, and also to see what you think about it. Although her instinct to test you peaks after her second birthday, now is the time to learn appropriate ways to deal with this behavior.

- *Let her feed herself as much as she wants to.* You can continue to offer spoonfuls in between her own efforts, as long as she's willing to let you, but increasingly she will want to take over, and you should let her. She will probably take to using a cup and spoon—more or less efficiently. Self-feeding is a developmental experience children seem to really enjoy. Your part of the deal is to forgo table manners to some extent for the time being. If your child eats with her mouth open, dribbles (especially during painful teething), and sometimes bangs her spoon and shouts, this is all normal and expected, as is a certain amount of food play. Some food will also get into her hair and clothes just because she can't help it yet. Newspaper under the high chair can catch any food that accidentally goes overboard. But if she's deliberately smearing food everywhere, you'll know. A few meals where you take the bowl away briefly and tell her nicely not to put dinner in her hair will establish that food is not a toy. Once she has learned this rule, you can make playing the signal that it is time to stop the meal. She has plenty of things to play with, and you don't need to feel guilty about restricting the use of just one of them.

- *Let her eat as much or as little as she wants at each meal.* Never encourage, bribe, or threaten your child to get her to eat more than she wants or to "just finish the last two spoonfuls." Calorie needs are low during this year, and trying to sneak spoonfuls into her unwilling mouth by forcing it open or offering a toy at the same time, or playing "airplane" after she has stopped opening her mouth for regular bites, are all examples of common habits that will be taken— rightly—to mean you want her to eat that particular food. The result—if your child is at all typical—is that she may quickly go off it, and will be more likely to start being fussy about what she tries in the future. It's the formidable discounting principle at work.

- *Don't make a big deal out of refusals and don't take them personally.* Provided that your toddler never realizes you care, she won't be encouraged to try refusing just because it makes you react! Chances are she is just being cautious if she refuses a new recipe. Offer one plain alternative, such as cereal and milk, or bread and cheese, and make that the rule. Leave the refused item on her tray for the rest of the meal and let her see you eat and enjoy your portion.

    If she refuses a food, such as chicken casserole, that she usually likes, let it pass. Maybe she is not hungry, or hasn't eaten it in a while and doesn't find it familiar, or simply doesn't feel like it today because she ate it three days ago. Be consistent and offer one plain alternative, but don't rush to do so. She may voluntarily start to eat the chicken after she has enjoyed saying no. If you are low-key and give the impression that the choice is hers, she may eat it later in the meal, or the next time it's on the table. Remember, she instinctively wants to eat the same foods as you, as long as she feels in control. You don't have to worry that allowing her to have a simple alternative will make her gravitate to the plain food. It just lets her know that you are on her side in the matter of choice and gives her the security to be more adventurous, with an alternative to fall back on.

3. SET A GOOD EXAMPLE

Table manners are hard to teach but easy to demonstrate. As hand-to-mouth coordination improves, and with your help as a role model, you'll find your child turns into a reasonably neat eater somewhere between three and five years without much effort on your part.

FLUORIDE FACTS

Fluoride is thought to strengthen teeth by three mechanisms: it gets incorporated into the developing crystalline structure of the enamel and makes it less soluble to bacterial acids; its presence in saliva inhibits loss of minerals; and it inhibits the growth of acid-forming bacteria. Fluoride strengthens teeth more effectively now than at any other time of life—it's yet another example of the power of early nutrients.

More than half of American water supplies are now fluoridated—and as a result Americans now have only half the cavities and missing teeth of previous years. But too much fluoride causes the unsightly tooth mottling known as *dental fluorosis*.

The new 1998 Daily Recommended Intake (DRI) recommendation for fluoride is 0.7 milligrams for ages one to three. The maximum upper limit is 1.3 milligrams daily.

Your child will need a supplement if she doesn't drink 8 ounces of fluoridated water daily. Some foods and drinks do contain fluoride but not in sufficient quantities to meet the DRI. If your family drinks tap water, ask your town's water department if your supply is fluoridated to the usual level of 1.0 milligrams per liter. (Home water filters don't usually remove fluoride.) If you use bottled water, be aware that the fluoride content of bottled water is very variable, ranging from negligible quantities to more than 1 milligram per liter, even in brands that don't advertise a fluoride content. If your water source contains less than 0.3 milligrams per liter of fluoride, your pediatrician can prescribe a supplement to make up the difference.

For best absorption, fluoride supplements should be taken at night with a little water only. If milk is drunk at the same time, only about 30 percent of the fluoride is absorbed.

Major-brand toothpastes contain a lot of fluoride. This is generally healthful because of the local hardening effect of fluoride on tooth enamel, but young children often swallow some or all at every brushing, and this can lead to fluorosis. This is the reason that most dentists recommend either using just a tiny dab of toothpaste or even holding off using it at all until two years. You can also talk to your dentist about his recommendations on fluoridated versus unfluoridated toothpaste at this age.

COMMON PROBLEMS AND
FREQUENTLY ASKED QUESTIONS

Rebecca, just one year old, was recently weaned from breast-feeding and will not drink more than a few sips of milk or eat more than one small piece of cheese and one or two spoonfuls of yogurt at any given meal. Her mother had correctly avoided these foods until recently to reduce her daughter's risk of allergies, but now she is worried that Rebecca is not getting the high-calcium foods she needs for strong bones and teeth.

The main thing here is not to panic. The single spoonfuls of these foods that Rebecca now eats will turn into whole portions within a very few weeks if her mother continues to offer them without pushing them. Leaving these foods on the high-chair tray during mealtimes and offering different types of cheeses (for example, both cheddar and mozzarella) and both plain yogurt and yogurt mixed with favorite fruit pieces should produce good results, as will patience at mealtimes and making sure that Rebecca is hungry before meals containing milk and other dairy products. Warming the milk to body temperature (whether she has a bottle or has already gotten used to a cup) is another thing to try; this will be more similar to the breast milk she is familiar with.

Alexa, fifteen months, is willing to give up her bottle, but she won't drink a daily total of at least 16 ounces of milk when it is given in a cup. Her pediatrician advises stopping the bottle by fifteen months, but her mother doesn't know whether that or maintaining her child's milk consumption is more important.

If it comes to the choice, milk consumption should always come before giving up a bottle. No child of six still uses a bottle, so extended bottle use is a self-limiting problem that disappears when peer pressure sets in. However, very extended bottle-feeding can make it hard for a child to enjoy milk any other way when the bottle is removed.

By using gradual techniques, most fourteen- to seventeen-month-old children are willing to switch over from a bottle to a cup, but a few simply don't like drinking that much milk if they can't cuddle up and take it by sucking. For them, first try a cup with an built-in plastic straw (which most children can and will use happily by this age) and be careful to keep the temperature of the milk the same as it was in the bottle. If Alexa still won't drink enough milk this way, using one morning or evening bottle a day to keep the total adequate is a good compromise.

Sarah's parents are worried about their seventeen-month-old daughter. She has barely gained weight for four months, and has also had a lot of diarrhea.

At this age, a pause in weight gain lasting a few months is not in itself a major cause for worry, provided that weight was normal to start with. Children do grow in spurts. When coupled with frequent diarrhea, however, the picture changes. Sarah's parents should consult their pediatrician for an evaluation of her diet and other factors. Several dietary factors might be important, including a natural fruit sugar called sorbitol, present in many juices, that Sarah may be sensitive to. (Teething was once thought to causes loose stools, but this is now known to be incorrect.) If the diarrhea is traced to sorbitol, eliminating the problem juice will fix the symptoms. Decreasing carbohydrate intake and increasing fat and fiber is also frequently effective in stopping loose stools.

James, fourteen months, was on the 50th centiles of weight and height at birth but has been falling off steadily and is now on the tenth centiles. His parents, both of below-average height, are concerned that he may be suffering from "failure to thrive."

Many parents naturally worry when their children seem to grow slowly in relation to "normal" growth patterns, but with both weight and height on the same centile, no history of diarrhea or feeding problems, and two parents of less than average height, James is probably a small but healthy toddler. Birth weight reflects many factors and in fact is *less* influenced by the baby's genetic blueprint than by maternal hormones and placenta function, and by the mother's diet and physical activity during pregnancy (a good diet and moderate activity promote fetal growth). After birth, genetic inheritance takes a larger role and usually causes children to gradually move into their natural range. James' parents should be aware that their small son will probably need fewer calories than larger children and that trying to feed him more will only cause feeding problems and perhaps excessive fat gain. Finally, James should have a daily complete multivitamin/mineral supplement appropriate for his age, to ensure that zinc deficiency, for example, is not contributing to his slow height gain.

———————— ❖ ————————

CHAPTER 11

Twenty-one Months to Three Years

Feeding Your Terrific "Terrible Two"

On Jason's second birthday his parents congratulated themselves on having such a well-behaved son. No temper tantrums for them! When they went for Jason's routine two-year assessment, their pediatrician's sympathetic inquiries about "terrible two" behavior seemed like a validation that they were doing a great job. A week later they were wondering what had happened. Literally overnight Jason had started creating huge battles about everything, including mealtimes and what he would and wouldn't eat.

If your child is nearing his second birthday, you've probably already seen the beginnings of his declaration of independence. Maybe it's his constant no, even when there is nothing to argue about, or the way he deliberately ignores your requests not to climb the bookcase. Although he still needs your support for everything from physical care to emotional fulfillment, his increased physical and mental capabilities coupled with his instincts to grow up and "do it himself" are starting to crystallize in a whole new pattern of assertive behavior. He's determined to challenge every rule you make and do it all himself—while diligently copying what you do!

Your child is also coping with a dawning awareness of the need to be cautious and live within the boundaries of what he knows is familiar and safe. In some cases this may be exacerbated by unavoidable but stressful events such as the birth of a new baby, a move, or family problems.

WHAT IF YOU HAVE PREMATURE HEART DISEASE IN YOUR FAMILY?

The antecedents of heart disease begin early in childhood and can be prevented by a healthy diet. If you or your partner has risk factors for premature heart disease (elevated LDL cholesterol, triglycerides, or blood pressure), or one or more grandparents had a heart attack or angina before age fifty, there are four steps you can take from two years on to start programming a lower risk of heart disease in your child.

1. **Keep saturated fat, trans fatty acids, and cholesterol low.** Starting early in childhood, saturated fat increases blood LDL cholesterol, which (like dietary cholesterol and trans fatty acids) encourages the plaque formation in arteries that leads to heart disease. Using low-fat, including skim milk and low-fat cheeses, is one way of reducing saturated fat and dietary cholesterol. Serving lean, rather than fatty, cuts of meat is also important.

   Aim to keep your child's total fat intake at about 30 percent of calories from fat to ensure adequate growth, even as you reduce her saturated fat intake. Use liquid vegetable oils such as canola, corn, and olive in your cooking. These oils contain monounsaturated fatty acids, which some scientists believe minimize heart disease risks even more effectively than the polyunsaturated fatty acids found in oils such as sunflower and safflower.

However, all two-year-olds experience some degree of increased conservatism and pickiness—it's the necessary counterbalance to their growing urge to be independent.

In daily life this conservative instinct manifests itself as demands for his "blankie" or special toy, and consistent routines for everything from getting dressed to going to bed. The same conservative instinct is seen at the table, too, in your child's increasing dislike of the unfamiliar and—frequently—loud demands for the same foods every day. It can drive you crazy and set the stage for future problems if you don't know how to deal with it. It can also make you unnecessarily give up lots of the family foods that you used to love.

But, as with many things, there is a good reason for this conservatism. As

2. **Prevent excess weight gain.** Being overweight is an important risk factor for heart disease. Chapter 15 tells you how to start normalizing a childhood weight problem.

3. **Avoid high salt intake.** About 60 percent of people susceptible to hypertension are "salt-sensitive"—meaning their blood pressure increases if they eat a high-salt diet. A certain amount of salt is essential for normal metabolism, but most Americans eat two to three times as much as they need. You won't be able to tell if your child is salt-sensitive, but since our perception of saltiness depends on how much of it we eat, you can keep your child's salt intake low and be confident she can still enjoy her food. Keep the salt shaker off the table, choose low-salt products in the supermarket, and either omit salt from the foods you cook or use a quarter to half the amounts suggested in recipes.

4. **Offer your child the recommended amounts of fruits and vegetables.** In addition to the disease-preventing phytochemicals they contain, fruits and vegetables are rich in "soluble fiber" (so called because it dissolves in water). Soluble fiber is thought to decrease blood pressure by slowing the body's production of the hormone insulin, which is one of the metabolic controllers of blood pressure.

we suggested in Chapter 2, we think that what you are seeing is a successful evolutionary strategy at work. Imagine the two-year-olds of times long past, youngest of a clan of hunter-gatherers and just now able and determined to run around without constant supervision. An instinct to watch others before trying new foods, and then cautiously try a small taste before having a whole meal, would help determine which wild foods were good to eat without serious risk. Being cautious makes perfect sense in the context of some tens of thousands of years ago, a mere blip in the evolutionary timetable.

OPPORTUNITIES AND GOALS FOR FEEDING FROM TWENTY-ONE MONTHS TO THREE YEARS

Between twenty-one months and three years your child's nutritional needs edge closer to your own. At this important juncture he is also laying down the last subconscious memories that will guide his future feelings. Foods that he enjoys eating before about two and a half years will become the instinctive basis for his future preferences. Your patient efforts now will have a lifelong payoff.

- *With brain cell development largely complete, at two years your child is ready to move to a diet closer in its fat content to your own, with both lower total fat and lower saturated fat for long-term cardiovascular health.* Switching from whole milk to 2 percent milk is the easiest way to accomplish this change. To ensure maximum bone and tooth strength in the future, maintain his calcium intake with 16 to 24 ounces of milk, yogurt, or the equivalent in other calcium sources daily. Make the transition to 2 percent milk from whole milk gradually, mixing the two kinds over two weeks or more, with increasing proportions of 2 percent milk, so that he does not start refusing this important food. The main (and relatively uncommon) exception to a diet containing plenty of dairy foods is for a child with a milk protein intolerance (see Chapter 16).

- *Prevent anemia and resulting developmental impairment by offering iron-rich foods and a multivitamin/mineral supplement.* A standard complete children's multivitamin/mineral supplement with 50 to 150 percent of the childhood RDAs for most vitamins and minerals can be purchased over the counter in pharmacies and supermarkets, in a chewable form that most two-year-olds love.

- *Help your child maintain or build a liking for fruits and vegetables.* To protect against future weight problems, cancer, and heart disease, use smart strategies designed for the "terrible twos" to ensure enjoyment of $^3/_4$ to $1^1/_4$ cups of mixed fruits and vegetables daily during this conservative year.

- *Complete your child's daily nutrient intakes with a healthy balance of foods.* Your toddler will benefit from a daily 1- to 3-ounce serving of lean meat, poultry, eggs, or fish, and/or $^1/_2$ cup fortified cereal, and about 400 to 800 calories' worth of other good foods such as cereals, breads, and legumes, as his appetite demands. Total calorie needs continue to increase slowly in proportion to your child's weight, so offering a nutrient-rich diet is important to ensure enough essential nutrients without excess calories.

● *Be vigilant about maintaining good eating patterns.* Food habits established now can be hard to break later, so prevention and elimination of fussiness, food jags, and cravings for unhealthy foods are important goals for this year.

● *Food allergies that developed in your child's first year have often disappeared by now.* If your child was allergic to cow's milk or formula, a controlled reintroduction of milk and dairy products under your pediatrician's supervision may allow you to add these valuable foods back into his diet (see Chapter 16).

WHAT TO FEED YOUR CHILD

You will notice that fruit and vegetables are usually suggested for at least two meals per day in the menus on page 190. Children of this age do not often voluntarily eat a whole cup of fruit or vegetable at one sitting. Frequent exposure to a wide variety of tasty items is what gets the ³/₄ to 1¹/₄ cups of fruits and veggies consumed and enjoyed, especially if they are sometimes combined with dipping sauces for interest. Although 4 ounces of juice can reasonably substitute for ¹/₂ cup of fruits and vegetables daily, more than this on a routine basis is still not a good idea at this age.

Because the fiber needs of two- to three-year-olds are much lower than those of adults, they continue to need less high-fiber products now than you do, provided enough fruits and vegetables (which also supply fiber) are eaten. Some kids do like high-fiber foods (especially the ones that are not low-calorie), but if yours is not one, you don't need to worry. Casual regular exposure is more important now than trying to get large portions consumed.

Choking can still be a hazard, meaning that everything from hot dogs (nitrite-free only) and peanut butter to prunes, grapes, and cherries needs to be reduced to child-sized bites. Cutting fruits and vegetables into thin vertical strips instead of cross-sections or rounds makes these foods safer. To maximize the chance that the food gets chewed and swallowed safely, it's also important to make your toddler eat while seated and under supervision.

SAMPLE MEALS FOR A CHILD AGE TWENTY-ONE MONTHS TO THREE YEARS

Day 1	Day 2	Day 3	Day 4
BREAKFAST			
1 scrambled egg 1/2 slice oatmeal toast 8 oz 2% milk	1/3 cup fortified cereal 10 oz 2% milk 1/4 cup grapes	1/2 bagel 1 tbsp peanut butter 8 oz 2% milk	1/3 cup fortified cereal 10 oz 2% milk 2 grapefruit segments
MORNING SNACK			
6 oz 2% milk 1 plain cookie	6 oz 2% milk 1/4 cup pretzels	4 oz orange juice 1 graham cracker	6 oz 2% milk 3 crackers 2 tsp cream cheese
LUNCH			
1/2 peanut butter and jelly sandwich on white bread 1/4 orange Water	1/4 cup cottage cheese 1/2 English muffin 1/4 cup peaches Water	1/2 turkey and cheese sandwich on whole-wheat bread 1/2 banana 8 oz 2% milk	1/2 cup noodles with butter and cheese 1/4 apple Water
AFTERNOON SNACK			
4 oz low-fat fruit yogurt Water	3 dried figs Water	1/4 cup raw vegetables 2 tbsp cheese dip Water	1/4 cup mixed carrots and peppers 2 tbsp cheese spread Water
DINNER			
1/2 cup pasta 1/4 cup tomato sauce 1 tbsp grated cheese 1/4 cup mixed salad with oil and vinegar 1/4 cup blueberries Water	2 baked chicken nuggets with BBQ sauce 2 oz baked potato 1/4 cup broccoli with sauce 1/4 cup watermelon Water	1 oz baked cod 2 oz baked yam 1/4 cup string beans 1/4 cup cantaloupe Water	2 oz hamburger on a piece of roll 1/4 cup mixed salad with dressing 1/4 cup frozen yogurt Water

WHAT ABOUT COOKIES AND SNACK FOODS?

On-the-go two-year-olds need morning and afternoon snacks to keep their energy up. So what about cookies, chips, and other foods that are such an easy option? Plain cookies and some commercial snack foods are okay in moderation, as long as you rotate them with high-nutrient foods such as yogurt, fresh fruit, and dried fruit. There are also cookies, chips, and crackers in health food stores that are not high in salt, saturated fat or partially hydrogenated fat.

Many of your own favorite recipes can be modified to make them healthier, though you may have to go through a few trials to get the new proportions right. For example, you can often substitute oil for butter or, if this doesn't work, try half butter and half oil. Similarly, white flour can be completely or partly replaced with wheat flour or oat flour (with some wheat germ thrown in for good measure), and salt can be reduced to a quarter of the amount suggested. Many recipes are overly sweet, and you can often make them taste better by cutting out a quarter of the sugar. We developed the recipes on page 193 for our own families.

EATING OUT

By the time your child is twenty-one months old you can let her eat virtually anything on a restaurant menu. Don't bring any foods from home, and suggest some reasonable things for her to choose from. Even if she eats only milk, fruit, and bread and butter, they won't be exactly what she eats at home, giving her extra experience of variety in a pleasurable circumstance. If your child finds it hard to wait for food, ask your server to be as quick as possible, or see if there is something you can do with them until the order comes. Mel finds the fire station across the street from his favorite restaurant an invaluable resource when he takes his boys out for breakfast on the weekend!

SMART STRATEGIES FOR KEEPING A BASICALLY GOOD EATER ON TRACK

Melissa started refusing food that she normally liked soon after turning two. "No!" she would shout when told it was dinnertime. We suggested Melissa's parents focus on three things to keep this offer of a confrontation from turning into a pattern of genuine food refusals: patience, an ability to

*read their daughter's real food needs from her behavior, and a stock of
smart strategies for different difficult situations. By requiring Melissa (who
was clearly hungry) to join the rest of the family at dinner but telling her
she didn't have to eat anything, her mother ensured that Melissa felt in control of her eating, and she ended up consuming normal meals.*

Now that your child is two, you'll especially need backseat management
and patience to keep eating on the right track. In many ways, feeding a
two-year-old is analogous to toilet-training her. Progress has to be initiated by her and is never consistent; setbacks are part of the normal course.
This section deals with strategies for basically good eaters, and the next
section gives additional help for common difficult problems.

1. KEEP CONTROL BATTLES FROM BECOMING FOOD BATTLES

Testing your limits is what two-year-olds are designed to do, but since battles over food can be more difficult than battles about almost anything else
at this age, it is worth some effort to avoid them.

- *Don't assume all food refusals are caused by orneriness.* Some food refusals at this age stem from resistance, but others are for good reasons:
  lack of hunger (many children need fewer calories than their parents
  think), lack of familiarity, or simply because the food itself doesn't
  taste good to the child.

- *Work with your child's eating patterns.* Control conflicts often start at
  this age when parents try to get their child to eat vegetables before
  higher-calorie items such as pasta. Two-year-olds instinctively go for
  the high-calorie foods first when they are hungry. Don't try to subvert
  this normal behavior. Any attempt on your part to micromanage will
  rightly be seen as interference. After eating calories, children often
  move on to vegetables and other foods, provided they have enough
  time at the table. If your child finds it hard to sit still long enough,
  have some cut-up veggies available before dinner starts. They may get
  consumed immediately, just because your child is genuinely hungry.

- *Offer appropriate portion sizes.* Many parents, concerned about small
  appetites at this age (unnecessarily, since growth is *supposed* to be

HEALTHY SNACKS

WHOLE-WHEAT SESAME CRACKERS

2 cups wheat-blend flour (available in most supermarkets) or 1½ cups whole-wheat flour plus ½ cup white flour
1 tsp baking soda
½ tsp salt
½ cup corn or canola oil
¼ cup buttermilk powder
¾ cup sesame seeds (not dehulled)
¾ cup water

Mix flour, baking soda, and salt together, and mix in oil until you get a crumbly mixture. Stir in buttermilk powder and sesame seeds. Then add enough of the water to make a firm pastry that sticks together without being sticky. In two batches, roll out the paste to a sheet about 9 by 12 inches, using a little extra flour to prevent sticking. Cut into 1½-inch squares and place on cookie sheet, with each cracker a little separated from the others. Bake for about 20 to 25 minutes at 325°F until light brown and very crispy (you can bake both batches at the same time). Store in a plastic bag or airtight container to retain freshness. Makes about 80 crackers.

CHOCOLATE OR VANILLA COOKIES

1½ cups flour (minus 4 tablespoons if you are adding chocolate powder)
4 tablespoons cocoa (optional)
1½ cups oat flour (see page 175)
3 tbsp toasted wheat germ
6 tbsp canola or corn oil
4 tbsp butter
⅔ cup plus 2 tbsp sugar
2 tsp vanilla
¼ cup light corn syrup
1 tsp baking soda

Mix all ingredients together by hand or in a food processor until dough forms a single ball. Remove and knead by hand for 1 minute until smooth. Form into two long rolls, each about 1½ inches in diameter. Cut ¼-inch slices and place on cookie sheet at least 1 inch apart. Bake 7 minutes at 400°F until just starting to color. You can freeze one of the rolls for another occasion; defrost before slicing. Makes 60 cookies.

slow), overload their child's plate. The sight of all that food can have unpredictable effects. Some children eat less in the face of such large parental expectations. Others overeat simply because the food is there. Large portions coupled with excess variety (for example, more than two or three high-calorie foods at lunch and dinner) can easily lead to unnecessary weight gain.

- *Don't use rewards, encouragement, bribes, or punishments to get your child to eat.* Now that your child can understand everything you say, it is tempting to encourage her to "finish your plate" (since you know she'll be hungry later) or "eat one more bite of zucchini and you can have ice cream." Just a few attempts along these lines can virtually guarantee an entrenched dislike of the foods you are trying to encourage.

  If your child refuses zucchini (or whatever), feign indifference and keep bringing it back at one- to two-week intervals, especially when there is time for a leisurely meal. If it doesn't get eaten today, it quite likely will be accepted next week or the week after, when she has decided she likes it. Make it clear that she doesn't *have* to eat the zucchini, while at the same time showing her that *you* enjoy it. Though counterintuitive, this works. First, your child feels in control of what goes in her mouth (very necessary). And because you haven't overencouraged her, she's not suspicious of the food. Finally, her conservatism and resistance are defused by her desire to imitate you.

  Some two-year-olds loudly declare, "Yucky," after eating most of a portion. Don't try to argue with your child's logic. Research studies have shown that our perception of food palatability really does decline during the course of a meal—it's what encourages us to eat a varied diet. Provided you treat it as if it's no big deal, chances are the food she rejected with such vigor will be enjoyed again the next time you serve it.

- *Remember that out of sight is out of mind at this age.* Instead of leaving the pizza or cookies on the dinner table, remove them after everyone's been served, but keep a bowl of fruit within easy reach.

- *Have a consistent policy for responding to food refusals and requests.* For refusals, a four-step approach works well over time: First, make it your rule that everyone stays at the table through the main course; second, leave refused foods within reach so your child can try them later in the meal after she has forgotten she said no; third, offer one plain alternative (cereal and milk, bread and cheese, fruit) with little or no comment; and fourth, let your child see you enjoy some of the food she refused.

Making the alternative plain is important. If dinner is lemon chicken with Chinese vegetables and the alternative is the same cornflakes and milk she had for breakfast, your child may decide that chicken and snow peas are better than she first thought. But if she knows you will reluctantly come through with an ice cream sundae covered with sprinkles, or even a different main course, you can anticipate regular refusals now and in the future.

Once your child is old enough to ask for specific foods, you need another game plan. First, decide whether a food request is being prompted by hunger. If she asks for chips in the supermarket, it may simply be snack time and she'll be content with plain crackers.

There will come a point, though, when you need to say no. A neutral explanation works best; otherwise the refused food will become more attractive. If you can say "No, the cookies are all gone" or "No, we never eat candy in the morning" rather than "I know you like cookies but you have had enough for today," you will give your child an answer that doesn't work against you next time—or the time after that.

- *Never allow temper tantrums about food to succeed.* If your child has a tantrum in the supermarket because she wants something you don't want her to have, stop and carry her out. You can always come back later, with or without your child, but if you give in, it will be years before you can shop in peace.

- *Learn to recognize hunger signals.* Although most two-year-olds are quite capable of telling you if they are hungry, often they don't. You need to read their behavior. Whining for a cookie in the late afternoon, getting fussy shortly before lunchtime, or sitting pale and still when thirty minutes earlier he was playing a wild game usually means that your child got hungry early today. A small low-calorie snack such as a few carrot sticks, crackers, or apple slices and raisins will keep him in good humor until mealtime.

Likewise, food signals during meals will tell you how full he is. Most two-year-olds start off eating at a great rate when they are hungry. Big spoonfuls, crammed in at a rapid pace, are completely normal. Halfway through the meal, your child is eating at a more leisurely pace, stopping to talk and look around. Toward the end of the meal, spoonfuls will go in very slowly, at perhaps a quarter of the rate they did at the beginning, and he'll be ready to take an interest in whether cheese can really be mixed with milk if squashed flat. Either the meal will grind to a complete halt or your child will realize that the last mouthful was a mistake—and back out it comes.

Use these signals as your guide. If you finish your main course at dinner and your child is still shoveling in food at a great pace, just relax and wait until he seems done. You can then offer some crackers and fruit for a second course, heading off whines for cookies later in the evening. Conversely, if your child refuses a usually popular hamburger and then picks at the requested cereal and milk, you can be reasonably confident that he is not hungry and should be left in peace.

2. CONTINUE TO USE THE RULE OF FIFTEEN AND PRACTICE VARIETY AND REPETITION TO INTRODUCE NEW FOODS

For conservative two-year-olds, intervals of about three to fourteen days are the best for building a real preference for foods they seem to have some interest in. For less popular items, make it two to three weeks between tries. Remember to keep portions of familiar foods small when introducing a new food.

We're often asked whether parents should make a rule that every food must at least be tasted. Our recommendation is no. Tasting rules are hard to enforce, lead to arguments, and in the long run don't work.

But by all means help her to understand what is nice about the new food—a crispy crust you can give her a special piece of, or a tasty sauce she might like a spoonful of all by itself. If you do it casually, as a "food opportunity" instead of a requirement, she may give it a try rather than being put off. Low-key positive propaganda by the other parent (for example, complimenting you on how good the broccoli or fish is) can also be very helpful.

3. USE GARDENING, COOKING, AND OTHER FOOD-RELATED ACTIVITIES TO FAMILIARIZE YOUR CHILD WITH THE FOODS YOU WANT HER TO LIKE

At age two Emily did not eat tomatoes. All that changed the next summer, when cherry tomatoes were grown in pots in the backyard. Emily helped water them as they turned from green to red, and she came to love eating them straight from the vine.

Like the primitive agriculturalist your child instinctively resembles, he may enjoy planting seeds in your garden or a window box, watching them grow, and watering the plants. He will probably be ready to harvest them even before the fruits and vegetables are really ripe. Don't expect him to do more than nibble at first (those conservative instincts again); familiarity will lead to larger portions. Cherry tomatoes are one of the easiest vegetables to grow (and are especially popular), but don't ignore less obvious choices such as lettuce, arugula, peas, green beans, peppers, and even herbs such as mint, parsley, and basil. Just don't let on that you *want* him to eat the results—or you may find that your work backfires.

The supermarket can also be your ally—instead of a potential nightmare. Help your child name all the different-shaped fruits and vegetables; he'll enjoy learning how they grow and tasting them once you get them home. This kind of introduction also works for fish from the fish counter and cheese in the dairy section.

If you enjoy cooking, there are many things your child can safely do in the kitchen now. Helping mix the batter for muffins or pancakes, tearing lettuce for salad, and making salad dressings and dips are good projects for two-year-olds. Tasting during cooking, by the way, is a case where we happily break our own rule about indiscriminate snacking between meals. If your child dips lettuce leaves in the dressing he has just made, he's already eaten his salad and learned to enjoy it!

4. A WORD ABOUT MAKING MISTAKES AND RECOVERING FROM THEM

Even if you are generally careful about offering the right foods in the right way, sometimes you will slip up. We know from experience how quickly a two-year-old will pick up on your mistakes as his own window of opportunity! Maybe you consciously avoid overencouragement of vegetables, but one night after he has been sick your patience snaps and you tell him he ought to eat them because they are good for him. Chances are you will see refusals of the same item in the next few days. Then perhaps one night you are exhausted and decide to eat chocolate cookies in front of the TV, and the next night he is asking for cookies again.

RECIPES FOR MAKING WITH A SMALL HELPER

CREAMY PARMESAN DRESSING AND DIP

3 tbsp low-fat sour cream
5 tbsp plain yogurt
I tbsp low-fat mayonnaise
I tbsp corn, olive, or sunflower oil
I tbsp vinegar
I tbsp sugar
I tsp finely chopped onion
$1/4$ cup grated Parmesan cheese
I tsp chopped parsley (optional)

Whisk or blend ingredients together. Keeps three to five days in the refrigerator. Great for serving with cut-up raw veggies.

KATHLEEN'S PUMPKIN MUFFINS

A graduate student of mine devised this moist and delicious recipe one fall when her parents (who are farmers) had so many pumpkins that they didn't know what to do with them all. It also works well with the canned variety at other times of the year.

2 cups white or whole wheat flour
$3/4$ cup sugar
3 tsp baking powder
$1/2$ tsp cinnamon
I cup cooked, pureed pumpkin
2 tbsp canola or corn oil
I egg
I scant cup milk
2 tbsp rolled oats

Mix together all dry ingredients except oats. Beat egg and mix with oil, pumpkin, and milk. The batter should be soft. Pour into a greased $9 \times 6 \times 2$-inch pan, sprinkle with oats, and bake 50–60 minutes or until the top is springy and a skewer comes out clean. Cool in pan and cut into squares before storing in your refrigerator or freezer.

In these cases, go right back to your usually careful behavior. You can tell your child, "Candy is only for sometimes," or "That's fine. You don't have to eat salad if you don't want to—give it to me and I will eat it," and the problem will likely sort itself out in a short while. Two-year-olds are wonderful for all kinds of reasons, not least of which is the fact that their short memory spans give you room to learn from your mistakes before the more challenging times ahead.

HANDLING FOOD JAGS AND EXTREME FUSSINESS

Food jags are quite common at this age. Your child insists on the same thing at every meal for several weeks—and then suddenly refuses to eat it at all and goes onto something different. If you don't nip this behavior in the bud, you may end cooking twice for every meal or eating macaroni and cheese more than you want (not to mention your concern that her diet is completely lacking in antioxidants, iron, or whatever). So if your child has been insisting on the same lunch or dinner item for more than a week, don't turn it into a battle, but just make "off" days when a similar option is available ("We don't have any macaroni and cheese today. Would you like a grilled cheese sandwich with cherry tomatoes instead?"). If she says no, the plain alternative is cereal and milk or bread and cheese. No child will hold out against more interesting alternatives, kindly presented, for long—and you will prevent the overfamiliarity that makes food jags turn into food refusals.

Some two-, three-, and even four-year-olds don't go on food jags but will eat only a very few foods, sometimes even demanding the same brand or recipe every time. Once you've made sure you are not fueling the problem with too much encouragement to eat other foods, get beyond it by establishing a "bridge of familiarity" to similar foods. This way your child never feels threatened by the strangeness of the new things you want her to enjoy.

Start by making a list of foods she likes—you may be pleasantly surprised that there are more than you thought. Each favorite food will be the "bridge" to one that hasn't yet been accepted.

If she likes white-bread peanut butter and jelly sandwiches, you might offer peanut butter and jelly on fresh oatmeal bread instead—and from there move to peanut butter and sliced ripe banana. If pasta with butter and cheddar cheese is a favorite, try noodles, polenta, gnocchi, or couscous, perhaps with a little grated Parmesan cheese and olive oil. If she likes orange slices, offer tangerines (making sure you remove the seeds). Baked chicken nuggets with barbecue sauce might be replaced by crispy fried fish with barbecue sauce.

When you are offering very similar foods to your child, don't give in and provide the original favorite if your child doesn't rush to try the new one. Eat the new food yourself. Tell her it is very similar to the one she normally enjoys, but that she doesn't have to eat it. If you make sure she remains at the table until you finish your main course, she will very likely make a meal of it after all, especially if you provide some minor distraction such as music or something interesting to talk about.

As you gradually introduce more related foods, you are not only expanding your child's repertoire but also making her more comfortable about trusting what's new. Introduction should get progressively easier, enabling you to create a varied diet by repeating individual foods only once every three to fourteen days.

WHAT ABOUT FOOD TRICKS?

Sometimes, when a toddler is going through a particularly difficult period, it is tempting to get the right nutrients in with strategies such as cutting sandwiches in fancy shapes, making raisin-face pancakes containing grated zucchini, or adding milk powder to the mashed potatoes. We think this is a slippery slope you don't need to go down. If you enjoy food as art, that's fine. The Japanese aesthetic of shaping vegetables as flowers and arranging foods in a precise pattern comes to mind, and we know one mother who makes whimsical pancake shapes just for fun. But as a desperation measure, it can work against you. Even trying to cut sandwiches into different shapes every day of the week will backfire if your child decides that she will eat only the shape you didn't make today. Highly decorated foods simply raise your child's expectations for food as entertainment and make it harder to win acceptance of the plain fruits and vegetables you want your child to like. Simply focus on making healthy food that tastes great, and let your child learn to enjoy that taste combined with the pleasure of shared family meals.

COPING WITH CONSTIPATION

Tom, a healthy boy of twenty-eight months, has started having problems with his bowel movements. Two or three times a day he will stand in the corner, crying and crossing his legs, for ten or fifteen minutes. When his mother saw blood on the outside of his stool, she finally took him to his doctor, who performed a rectal examination and diagnosed constipation with an anal tear. Along prescribing a stool softener to help the tear heal, Tom's doctor recommended increased dietary fiber to prevent future problems. But Tom already eats whole-grain cereal for breakfast and sandwiches made with whole-wheat bread. What should his mother feed him?

Children who are eating the amounts of different foods recommended earlier in this chapter will almost never suffer from constipation because they are taking in plenty of fiber—the one nutrient that prevents constipation in the first place, and treats it if a problem arises. But constipation is quite common between two and four years, and can be especially noticeable around the time of toilet training, when easy bowel movements are essential for progress.

In his gastroenterology clinic, Mel finds that *too much milk* is one of the common causes of constipation. During this period, when new foods are viewed with suspicion, many parents fall back on plenty of milk and juice for trouble-free feeding, and their conservative two-year-olds are often perfectly happy to go along with such a plan. Intakes of 35 ounces a day of milk and 8 ounces of juice are not uncommon, and at these high levels many children need few additional calories to make up their total daily requirement. Even if those calories, like Tom's, come from whole-grain cereal and whole-wheat bread, there is simply not enough solid food to make up the daily fiber requirement.

In these cases, limiting milk to 16 ounces per day to encourage consumption of more solid foods, offering plenty of water for thirst, and providing a variety of vegetables and fruits (bananas excluded) will help increase fiber intake to a level where bowel movements become easy again. High-fiber snacks such as whole-wheat sesame crackers (page 193) can also provide a fiber boost in a pleasurable way, and prunes are a high-fiber treat that is popular with many two-year-olds.

Be aware, however, that too much fiber can cause gastrointestinal bloating and discomfort—especially if you switch very abruptly from a low-fiber diet to a high-fiber one, and can also impair mineral absorption. For this reason, avoid large amounts of very high-fiber products (such as more than two or three prunes daily, or more than ¼ cup of very high-fiber cereal).

If changing what your child eats does not completely fix a constipation

ADDING UP THE CALCIUM FOR A CHILD WHO WON'T DRINK MILK

If your child doesn't drink 16 to 24 ounces of milk daily, you are probably concerned about calcium. Take heart! In the first place, the 16- to 24-ounce recommendation actually provides *more* calcium than your child's recommended allowance of 500 mg. In fact, about 12 ounces of milk plus the calcium contained in your child's multivitamin/mineral supplement will supply most of her calcium needs, and the rest of her diet will supply the balance because most foods contain at least some calcium. (And though milk contains many essential nutrients and is an all-around good food, those nutrients are present in other good foods, too.)

If your child won't drink milk at all, use the list below to see how much calcium she is already getting on a typical day and to improve her diet if necessary. Provided you can add up 400 milligrams on most days of the week, and her multivitamin/mineral supplement contains at least 50 milligrams, you can assume that the remaining 50 milligrams are coming from the other foods she is eating.

FOOD	MILLIGRAMS OF CALCIUM
3 ounces calcium-fortified orange juice	100
1/2 ounce hard cheese such as cheddar or mozzarella	100
1/4 ounce Parmesan cheese	100 (note that Parmesan has twice as much calcium, ounce for ounce, as cheddar)
1/4 cup yogurt (plain, fruit, frozen)	80–100
1/2 waffle (calcium comes from the milk, eggs, and raising agent)	90
1/3 cup macaroni and cheese	80
1/2 packet plain instant oatmeal	80 (even more if you add milk)
1/3 cup ice milk	70
1 slice processed cheese	60
1/3 cup cream soup made with milk	60
1/3 cup spinach or collard greens	60
1/4 cup broccoli	50
2 dried figs	50
1/4 cup cooked beans	30

I egg yolk (whites don't contain calcium)	28
I ounce tofu	27
I slice bread	25
¼ cup orange segments	15
¼ cup carrots	15
¼ cup peas	10

If your child really isn't getting enough calcium, use a calcium supplement for the rest (you only need to do this calculation once for a typical day, not every day). The supplement can be chewable or liquid, in the form of either calcium carbonate (sometimes called oyster calcium) or calcium citrate—both are absorbed about as well as milk calcium. Adult antacids (the kind made with calcium, not magnesium or sodium) are a widely available chewable source, and your child can crunch up small broken pieces equal to the amount she needs. Look in a health food store if you want a liquid calcium supplement, making sure that any supplement you buy contains *only* calcium.

problem, your pediatrician can prescribe mineral oil for a few days to help return your child's bowel movements to normal. Enemas and suppositories should be avoided, however, to avoid sensitizing your child to psychological concerns related to his bottom and the act of defecation.

COMMON PROBLEMS AND FREQUENTLY ASKED QUESTIONS

Dylan, two and a half years old, weighed 8 pounds at birth and grew well; he was on the 50th centile for weight and height until he was one year old. Since then his growth rate has slowed, until he is now on the 25th centile for height and the 10th centile for weight. His parents, who are both of normal weight and height, say he eats like a bird and are at a loss for what, if anything, they should do.

Some pediatricians suspect that growth failure and nutritional stunting are a serious emerging problem among affluent, nutrition-conscious families. Any child who stops growing needs to be examined by a pediatrician, because there are a number of possible explanations and only a detailed evaluation will get to the root of the problem.

If no metabolic explanations are found for Dylan's growth failure, food may be the explanation. About 15 percent of children examined for failure to thrive are thought to suffer from accidental malnutrition. Often this is because the child has been given meals that are too low in fat and calories to allow for normal childhood growth. High-calorie foods such as whole milk (up to 24 ounces), other full-fat dairy products, meat, and refined starches and grains, all given in a form the child enjoys, will be part of the short-term solution while catch-up growth is established. In addition, a multivitamin/mineral supplement is necessary to ensure that he gets enough micronutrients. Once weight and height are headed back in the right direction, a focus on feeding Dylan meals and snacks with a normal fat content for his age will be important to prevent a relapse and to allow his body composition to continue to normalize.

When she was two Natalie loved broccoli, but by the time she was two and a half she consistently refused to eat it. Her mother loves broccoli and wants to know how to get her to like it again.

Children typically get put off food by being overencouraged to eat it. How you deal with it depends on the age of the child. Quite likely Natalie refused broccoli one day simply because it wasn't as good as usual or because she was not hungry and then was overencouraged to eat it, which stopped her from liking it. It is also possible that she had been given it too often and started rejecting it simply because she got bored. The solution at Natalie's tender age of short memories is to take a low-key approach, not pushing the broccoli but letting Natalie see that her parents enjoy it even if she doesn't want to eat it today. Natalie's mother can also experiment with some different ways to make broccoli—raw or cooked with a different sauce, perhaps in a cream soup or quiche—and try to put it on the table only every two weeks, at times when Natalie is hungry. It is worth remembering, too, that lots of other foods have similar nutritional value, including spinach, cabbage, and cauliflower.

Christy, age two, has started having mild diarrhea most days, especially in the late afternoon and evening. However, she is cheerful and continuing to grow well. Her mother wonders if this is something she needs to see her pediatrician about.

Diarrhea that doesn't resolve in three to seven days definitely needs a call (and possibly a trip) to the pediatrician. The most likely candidates at all ages are viral or bacterial infections. However, persistent diarrhea is sufficiently common at this age that it has been given the name "toddler diarrhea" or "chronic nonspecific diarrhea of childhood." Children with toddler diarrhea show no signs of malabsorption and continue to gain weight normally. This diagnosis is made only after excluding other causes of chronic diarrhea, including malabsorption syndromes (celiac disease, cystic fibrosis, *Giardia* infection), and lactose and other food intolerances. The symptoms of toddler diarrhea resolve spontaneously by three to four years, and have no adverse long-term effects.

All treatments are diet-based, and frequently effective measures include reducing fruit juice, adding fat, and cutting out cold foods (which stimulate colon motility). Increasing fiber can also help in some cases, though in others it has the opposite effect. Although many children with toddler diarrhea later become lactose intolerant, removing milk now doesn't help, and can make achieving a balanced diet harder.

Danny started refusing milk shortly after his second birthday. His mother knows that milk is important but doesn't know how to get Danny to start liking it again.

As with Natalie and her broccoli, Danny was probably put off milk when he accidentally found out that his parents want him to drink it. The easiest way to get Danny to drink milk again is to be patient and keep putting it in front of him at mealtimes. (You might also try a different type of milk, such as skim instead of low-fat.) Especially if you set a good example by drinking it yourself and don't give him water with his meal for a while (though make sure to offer him water afterward), he will get thirsty and want to drink it. This is a different strategy than the one for broccoli, because milk is a bland drink, and kids usually learn to drink it out of habit and thirst rather than because it is especially interesting.

It is also worth checking that Danny's cup is not difficult to drink out of, that the milk is the temperature he likes, and that there is no bad odor. Danny's mom should avoid rushing to give flavored milk instead of plain milk, as the extra calories are something that he doesn't need now or in the future.

CHAPTER 12

⸭

Three to Six Years

Moving into the Outside World

Kaela, four, was taken to a restaurant where she saw an older girl drinking an orange soda. She asked for one, too, and it arrived at the table along with fresh orange juice for her dad, who offered it to her to taste. Although the orange soda was attractive because a "big girl" was drinking one, taste and a low-key approach won out, and after a few sips she asked for orange juice instead. A casual emphasis on being a good role model and providing your child with healthy food that tastes at least as good as the competition will help keep the strong peer influences at this age from spoiling your good work.

Most three-year-olds seem like a species apart from the terrible twos they were just a year earlier. Compliance (usually) and communication par excellence are the hallmarks of this age, enabling you to see into the subtleties of how your child resembles you and your partner and yet is his own person, too. Past the stage where early subconscious feelings are formed, your child is now busy forming the first conscious memories that will last a lifetime. Irascible behavior and control battles are temporarily set aside, heralding a wonderful time for you both. More subtle changes are also taking place that profoundly affect all aspects of your child's behavior, including his behavior with food.

MEET YOUR PRESCHOOLER, THE SOCIAL ANIMAL

Your child is now becoming an active member of the human family, and increasingly wants to interact and cooperate with people outside her immediate family.

In this, she is expressing our uniquely human evolutionary heritage. Although other social animals such as chimpanzees and wolves also spend their lives in groups, these groups are composed almost exclusively of extended-family members. Animals outside the family pack are at best distant strangers. We, in contrast, interact and cooperate with completely unrelated work colleagues, neighbors, and even people we don't know at all.

Evolutionary biologists believe that these social bonds between genetically unrelated individuals contribute to our enormous success as a species. They make it possible to become a specialist (be it in child care, medicine, or carpentry) and to trade that skill for the different skills of other people. And because it is more efficient to specialize in one task than in many, there is time for things such as art, music, and invention. Collectively we accomplish more than if we socialized and traded only within our own family.

In the times of our distant ancestors, families with a natural inclination to cooperate, specialize, and learn from others would have been more successful than less gregarious ones—and became the lineage from which we all descend. Seen in this light, it is clear why our children are influenced by the eating behavior of children and adults they meet: Their instincts are propelling them to do so.

In the same way that your child may take on the games and slang expressions of her peer group, so she will also start to absorb their food habits, both good and bad. This does not mean that you will lose your own influence over what your child eats. As her parents, you are in the inner circle, and she continues to spend much of her time intently trying to mimic everything you do. Just as she may want to dress like you and discipline her stuffed animals the way you discipline her, so her food likes and dislikes are modeled on your own. Our smart strategies for this period focus on making the most of your influence.

OPPORTUNITIES AND GOALS
FOR FEEDING FROM THREE TO SIX YEARS

By the time your child is ready for kindergarten, he can enjoy eating the full spectrum of foods that will support his health for a lifetime. Beginning at age three:

- *Move your child to a diet with lower, adult levels of fat and saturated fat.* Switching from 2 percent milk to 1 percent or skim milk is one easy way to accomplish this change. Which type of milk is right for your child will depend on the fat content of your family meals and snacks and whether you have a family history of premature heart disease.

● *Continue to plan daily menus containing 16 to 24 ounces of milk (or other foods to ensure calcium intake) and 1 to 1½ cups mixed fruits and vegetables.*

● *Protect against anemia by offering iron-fortified cereals and lean meats.* A child's daily chewable complete multivitamin/mineral supplement (providing 50 to 150 percent of the RDA for most essential nutrients) can be used if your child doesn't eat these foods. It is not essential for other nutrients now if your child eats a consistently good diet, but it is harmless and offers good insurance against a shortfall in one or more important nutrients.

● *Complete your child's nutritional needs with a healthy balance of foods.* A child this age needs about 700 to 1,100 calories' worth of other good foods such as cereals, breads, and legumes, as his appetite demands, and water for thirst.

WHAT TO FEED YOUR CHILD

From the time he was a small baby, Ricky used to watch his father eat bran flakes for breakfast. At around age three, bran flakes suddenly became Ricky's favorite breakfast, too! Like many children, Ricky learned to like higher-fiber cereals at just the time when his body was ready for them.

Nobody knows exactly why, but many parents find that their child will now enjoy regular portions of the whole grains he ignored earlier. At three years your child's body is more mature in some important ways (for example, most brain cells are fully formed), and it may simply be that high-fiber products now taste better. If one cereal or bread doesn't work, try another! One of Mel's boys likes only high-fiber cereals that don't contain nuts—something that took a while to identify. If your child is attached to white bread but will occasionally eat whole wheat, try buying less tasty brands of white (maybe the ones with potato or extra fiber) and make delicious homemade oatmeal bread as an alternative (page 214). The new

SAMPLE MEALS FOR A CHILD THREE TO SIX YEARS OLD

Day 1	Day 2	Day 3	Day 4
BREAKFAST			

1-egg omelet
¼ slice toast
 	
8 oz 1% milk
	⅓ cup fortified
	    whole-grain cereal
	Piece melon
	10 oz 1% milk
		⅓ cup oatmeal
		    with 2 tbsp
		    raisins, 1 tsp
		    sugar, and 1 tbsp
		    half-and-half
		8 oz 1% milk
			1 waffle
			2 tbsp maple syrup
			¼ cup strawberries
			8 oz 1% milk

MORNING SNACK			
6 oz 1% milk ⅓ cup homemade popcorn	4 oz orange juice 2 graham crackers	6 oz 1% milk ¼ avocado, sliced	4 oz orange juice 15 corn chips ¼ cup salsa
LUNCH			

⅓ cup ravioli
1 tbsp grated
    cheese
¼ cup carrots
2 tbsp hummus
¼ cup grapes
Water
	⅓ cup bean soup
	Small roll-up with
	    chicken, cheese,
	    and salad
	½ apple
	Water
		½ cup macaroni
		    and cheese
		1 plum
		Water
			2 tbsp peanut
			    butter and 1 tbsp
			    jelly on whole-
			    wheat bread
			½ orange
			¼ banana
			Water

AFTERNOON SNACK			

1 oz plain cake
1 low-fat mozzarella
    cheese stick
Water
	6 oz low-fat fruit
	    yogurt
	Water
		1 slice pumper-
		    nickel with
		    butter and
		    jam
		Water
			6 oz low-fat fruit
			    yogurt
			Water

DINNER			

2 oz roast chicken
⅓ cup scalloped
    potatoes
¼ cup cabbage
¼ cup pineapple
Water
	2 oz salmon
	⅓ cup mashed potato
	¼ cup peas
	1 kiwi
	Water
		½ cup rice
		⅓ cup chili con
		    carne with grated
		    cheese and sour
		    cream
		1 ear corn, buttered
		½ apple
		¼ cup frozen
		    yogurt
		Water
			¾ cup pasta
			¼ cup tomato
			    sauce
			2 tbsp grated
			    cheese
			¼ cup mixed
			    salad with oil
			    and vinegar
			¼ cup blueberries
			6 oz 1% milk

OBESITY DURING THE PRESCHOOL YEARS

Three to six years is a time when children are more vulnerable to excess weight gain than previously (one in seven are overweight by age six). Although you should never, of course, restrict your child's food against the possibility of a problem, do keep a firm rein on high-fat snacks and sweets to prevent the increase in fat calories that is usual at this age—and paradoxically so, since fat requirements actually decrease. Maintaining your child's vegetable and fruit consumption will also help prevent a budding problem, as will offering whole-grain rather than refined cereals, breads, and pasta, and giving water for thirst instead of high-calorie juices and sodas. Turn to Chapter 15 for help normalizing an existing weight problem.

"mild" brands of whole-wheat flour can also be used to make bread that looks like whole wheat but tastes more like white.

An increase in the amount of fruits and vegetables provides the gradual increase in vitamins and minerals your child needs to keep pace with increasing calorie needs. If you continue to serve fruits and vegetables at least three times per day, chances are your child will automatically increase her intake with no other help from you. If she does not, try increasing the number of choices you offer while reducing the variety of other foods. The variety principle is still on your side.

Calorie intakes are very variable now, with perfectly normal children eating as little as 900 or as much as 1,800 calories per day. Average daily intakes do increase by 150 to 200 calories each year during this period, but the actual amount will depend on growth rate and how physically active your child becomes.

FOOD ON THE ROAD

Vacations with a three- to six-year-old can be wonderful fun, although maybe not as relaxing as vacations of old! *Always* make sure to take food with you—a hungry child will be pretty wearing, and airports and highway rest stops may offer only fast-food outlets.

One sandwich that packs well is turkey and cheese; another easy-to-carry one is peanut butter with jelly, cream cheese, banana, or honey. A bag of baby carrots, a cut-up red pepper, and washed lettuce leaves provide healthful variety. Low-salt crackers, graham crackers, and fruit that can be

ROLL-UPS

Given a tortilla or other kind of wrap and a few tasty fillings, your three-, four-, or five-year-old may relish foods he might disdain if served another way. And because they are so much fun to make and eat, roll-ups make a good lunch option for noontime birthday parties at this age. Here are just a few types we have found popular with three- to six-year-olds.

Salad roll-ups. White or whole-wheat pita bread is a good base, sliced in half to give a kid-sized portion. Most supermarkets also offer large square sandwich wraps, and some Middle Eastern specialty stores sell soft home-made Lavash made fresh daily. Or use lettuce leaves themselves as an interesting alternative. Serve with a selection of the following: thinly sliced turkey, hummus, peanut butter, grated hard cheese, crumbled feta cheese or cream cheese, finely shredded lettuce, thin tomato and onion slices, strips of red pepper and cucumber, and vinaigrette dressing on the side or for dipping.

Roll-ups with cooked fillings. Almost any hot meal can be turned into a roll-up. All kinds of wraps work well. Good fillings include creamed spinach with grated Parmesan cheese, warm sliced chicken with a little mashed potatoes and vegetables, and Chinese stir-fried vegetables (page 169) with small slices of omelet or sauteed tofu.

Mexican burritos. Although white-flour tortillas are sold in almost every supermarket, try to find the tastier whole-wheat or corn kind sold in health food stores. Serve with a selection of the following: grilled chicken or steak cut into thin strips, refried or whole cooked beans, rice, sour cream, guacamole, mild salsa, shredded lettuce, tomato and onion, and grated cheese.

eaten out of hand are good, too. Oranges, apples, plums, and cherries are tasty fruit selections (grapes and peaches, though delicious, often get squashed in transit). If your child likes his apples cut in slices, you can prevent browning by soaking the slices for fifteen minutes in water containing the juice of a quarter lemon. Homemade cookies, snacks, and Fruit Newtons containing some fiber are other healthy options worth trying, as is cold home-cooked pizza (page 214).

While you are on vacation, you may find yourself eating in restaurants much more than normal. To prevent disruptive behavior, take along some

WHAT ABOUT STRONGLY FLAVORED AND SPICY FOODS?

Your child can eat anything you do now, including the strongly flavored and spicier recipes that you may have held back on earlier. Children living in countries where spicy food is the norm typically learn to love it only after age two or three. Most Indian families, for instance, feed their children only bland food until three years.

As with any other new food type, most children need regular—but not too frequent—exposure to spicy foods for popularity to grow, and a low-key atmosphere. They often take to Chinese food easily, and generally popular items include mixed vegetables, lemon chicken, garlic shrimp, lo mein, scallion pancakes, and crispy fried tofu (sometimes called bean curd) with vegetables. One boy we know learned to like broccoli with black bean sauce before he would eat it any other way. Restaurant and take-out Chinese food is often loaded with oil and is very high in sodium. But healthy stir-fries are quite easy to prepare at home. Simply use less oil than recommended in the recipes and substitute low-sodium soy sauce for the regular kind.

For very spicy foods, such as chili con carne or Indian curry, try making your usual recipe with only a quarter of the usual amounts of spices at first, gradually increasing the amounts each time you prepare them. Especially if you encourage your child to try making up his own plate—with condiments such as grated cheese, onions, and sour cream for chili con carne, and raita and chutney for Indian food—you may find that acceptance is quicker than you might imagine.

crayons and paper for drawing projects, and ask your server to bring some bread as soon as you are seated. When the bread arrives, you can quickly order your food, including some appetizer items such as soup to keep your child in a good humor. For extended stays away from home, we have found that the best parts of a restaurant menu to graze from can be the appetizers, soups, and side dishes. That's where you may find such staples as cottage cheese or favorite vegetables in small helpings. With the enormous portion sizes offered by many restaurants today (look around to see how much you will get), you may also find that two adult entrees will serve two adults and one or two small kids with plenty left over for seconds. Kids can also, of course, have a kids' meal if one is offered, but the choices are usually less healthy than many items on the adult menu.

SMART STRATEGIES: MAINTAINING GREAT EATING HABITS—OR ESTABLISHING THEM

Lauren, four years old, often says she isn't hungry at dinnertime because she is too busy playing. Fortunately, her mother has held to the rule that Lauren has to sit at the table while others have their main course, even if she doesn't want to eat. This easy rule works its magic repeatedly, with Lauren realizing she is hungry after all.

Many of the strategies you have worked with up to now will continue to be important as your child moves through his preschool years. However, as in the past, no one strategy will work all the time, and now that your child is older and savvier, simple subterfuge is less successful than previously. Few self-respecting five-year-olds will turn around and eat something you left on the table after they told you repeatedly it was yucky two minutes ago, in contrast to their more innocent selves at age two and a half. Likewise, a fixed aversion to everything green will not disappear if you simply cook broccoli at regular intervals.

Your preschooler can be helped especially with the following smart strategies:

1. USE ACTIVITIES AND GAMES TO ENCOURAGE INTEREST IN HEALTHY FOODS

Preschoolers learn by *doing*. Mixing, tasting, and watching the transformation that cooking brings to food are compelling activities for many children at this age, and new healthy foods can become firm favorites if you allow your child to help prepare them.

Encourage sons to cook as much as daughters—boys enjoy cooking just as much, especially if they see their dad in the kitchen sometimes. One young man we know liked nothing better when he was about four than to use a spoon as a steam shovel in the biscuit flour.

Do allow tasting even if it means that hunger is less at mealtimes. And be sure to instruct your child about not touching stoves and sharp knives.

RECIPES TO MAKE WITH YOUR SMALL HELPER

OATMEAL BREAD

Children who disdain whole-wheat bread may love a warm oatmeal roll spread with peanut butter or honey. And because oatmeal has as much fiber and essential minerals as whole wheat, this is also a good introduction to whole grains.

Preparation time: 10 minutes
Rising and baking time: 3–4 hours

> *For a 1¹/₂ pound loaf:*
> 2 teaspoons yeast
> 2 cups white flour
> ¹/₂ cup whole-wheat flour
> 1¹/₃ cups instant or quick-cooking oats
> 2 tablespoons sugar
> 2 tablespoons molasses (omit for rolls and pizza dough)
> 1 teaspoon salt
> 1¹/₄ cups water (be prepared to add 1 or 2 tablespoons more depending on your make of bread machine and whether the weather is dry)

For a bread machine: Mix all ingredients in their usual order for your bread machine, and set for a light crust and whole-wheat kneading if you have the options.

For hand kneading: Mix all ingredients in a food processor and blend for 2 minutes, or knead by hand for 5 minutes. The dough should be soft, just this side of actually sticky. Cover and allow to rise for 1–2 hours, until at least doubled in size. Knead again for 2–3 minutes and shape into a round. Place on cookie sheet, cover, and rise until doubled in size again, about 1 hour, or divide into 10–12 portions and let your child make rolls. Preheat oven to 425°F. When bread dough is ready, bake for 5 minutes before reducing heat to 350°F. Bake until bread is pale golden and sounds hollow when tapped underneath (35–45 minutes for a loaf, 8–12 minutes for rolls).

ANYTIME PIZZA

Most pizza places slather their pizzas with so much cheese that the grease runs off when you pick up a slice. Pizza in Italy is not like this, and yours doesn't have to be either. This recipe got a top rating from our kid testers, one of whom rated it "better than strawberry Twizzlers"—high praise indeed!

Preparation and cooking time: 25 minutes

> 1/2 recipe oatmeal bread dough
> Spray olive or corn oil
> 1/2 cup tomato sauce (fresh or canned)
> 2 tablespoons grated Parmesan cheese
> 3 ounces sharp cheddar cheese, grated
> Toppings (pick as many as you like): finely chopped onion, thinly sliced mushrooms, thinly sliced green pepper, finely diced pineapple, cooked ground turkey shaped into meatballs

Preheat oven to 450°F. Prepare dough according to recipe. Allow to rise for 1/2–1 hour to make the dough pliable, and then stretch out to completely fit a 15-inch-diameter pizza tray, or make small individual rounds for each family member. Spray stretched-out dough lightly with oil and cover for 1/2 hour if you have time (this step is not essential). Spread tomato sauce evenly all over. Sprinkle first with Parmesan cheese and then with cheddar cheese. Sprinkle on toppings. Bake for 12–15 minutes until cheese is bubbling and starting to brown all over.

WATERMELON COOLER

On a really hot summer day, almost nothing will seem as refreshing as this vitamin-packed watermelon drink from Malaysia.

Preparation time: 2 minutes

> *Per thirsty adult or child:*
> 1 cup seedless watermelon cut into chunks, flesh only
> 1/2 cup ice cubes
> 2 teaspoons sugar or to taste

Get your child to cut up the watermelon with a blunt knife and throw everything in a blender. Blend until completely smooth. Serve outside with a straw for best enjoyment!

Physical abilities usually exceed an awareness of safety issues at this age, so vigilance is important.

The more your child knows about vegetables, the more she will be willing to try them, so continue to involve her in gardening and shopping. The fact that carrots, beets, and potatoes grow under the ground and have very different kinds of roots will be interesting now—as will the fact that carrots, lettuce, and other greens are a rabbit's favorite food.

Many three- to six-year-olds spend hours every day involved in pretend activities that seem to be vitally important to their psychological development. If you ask your child to make a pretend meal for you featuring a chicken sandwich with mayonnaise, lettuce, and cucumber, she may request a real one in a day or two. Likewise, suggesting that she "cook" a soup with beans and vegetables can make tomorrow's lunch more likely to succeed. Good cooking props are important, because if your plastic or paper food extends only from cakes to hot dogs, you may encourage preferences you don't want. Since even the best sets of plastic food may include some less-than-desirable items, you may want to make a few "disappear."

2. HARNESS GOOD OUTSIDE INFLUENCES

Watch for books and videos that send good messages about food—some for a particular dish. Think of "Goldilocks and the Three Bears" as an ad for oatmeal! You can also embellish on traditional tales. One grandmother we know used to tell her family that the vegetable soup she made on special occasions was the one Little Red Riding Hood and her family had for dinner after getting rid of the wolf.

These messages can counterbalance those you don't want absorbed, which unfortunately are everywhere. Every time a picture-book rabbit eats only cake for dinner or the child in the story makes a face over a plate of broccoli, your job is made a bit harder.

Book Suggestions

Anansi and the Moss Covered Rock. Eric A. Kimmel. Holiday House, 1990. A greedy spider steals all the fruit and vegetables belonging to his jungle friends.

Stellaluna. Janell Cannon. Harcourt Brace, 1993. Story of a baby bat who loves mangoes.

Mufaro's Beautiful Daughters. John Steptoe. Lothrop, 1987. An African tale

about kindness in which yams and sunflower seeds are given and received with pleasure.

Green Eggs and Ham. Dr. Seuss. Random House, 1960. Childhood classic
suggesting that adventurous eating is worth a try.

Bread and Jam for Frances. Russell Hoban. HarperCollins, 1964. A fussy little badger learns that the same food day in and day out is not as much
fun as she thought, and a friend has creative ideas about lunch.

Chicken Soup with Rice. Maurice Sendak. HarperCollins, 1962. Wonderful
and educational, this well-known tale may convert even a confirmed
soup-hater.

Movie Suggestions

The Wishing Bear (A Winnie-the-Pooh Story). Disney. Rabbit tries to protect his vegetables from the voracious bugs.

It Takes Two. Warner Bros. Suspicion over something new (sloppy joes) is
won over by taste.

Small friends with good eating habits are pure gold. If your daughter's
friend loves spinach pasta or hummus with pita bread and strips of
red pepper, think about asking to have it served when she eats lunch
at her friend's house. On the other hand, if your son eats salad, broccoli,
and peas even though they're not particular favorites, keep them off
the menu if an influential friend who hates green vegetables stays for
lunch.

Supermarkets, farmers markets, and restaurants can also be allies. If
your supermarket leaves samples of fruit, crackers, and so on around to
taste, or maybe even does cooking demonstrations, let your child try what
is offered. She will feel all the more adventurous for seeing other kids and
adults tasting, too. And if your child normally refuses fish but loves eating
out, take her to a seafood restaurant. The combination of a special place to
eat and seeing other customers enjoying their meal can have remarkably
rapid results.

Finally, even animals can be great food models. Preschoolers take note of
what every animal eats, including your pet hamster or the sheep at a local
farm. Offer your child a carrot or piece of lettuce while she is watching a
rabbit enjoying the same, or a piece of whole-wheat bread while the goats
are greedily pushing to be first, and she may join them.

3. LIMIT QUESTIONABLE OUTSIDE INFLUENCES

My daughter at four enjoyed pizza with all kinds of vegetable toppings until the day she watched the movie *Home Alone*. All it took was the scene in which eight-year-old Macaulay Culkin refuses to eat any kind of pizza except "plain cheese." That weekend she asked if she could have plain cheese pizza for dinner, and it took nearly six months and a good deal of patience on my part before any other kind would do.

Likewise, if your child comes home and tells you she wants some jelly beans like her friend Alison, or refuses to eat dinner because she had chocolate pudding at four o'clock at Eric's house, you will be seeing the side of food influences you have tried to avoid.

Here are a few strategies we have found helpful:

- Use your absolute power over what food comes into the house to ensure that at least two-thirds of what your child eats is under your direct control. Provided that you do this, and you give her a children's complete multivitamin/mineral supplement, she will get the nutrients she needs even if some of her meals are not what you would wish.

- Don't make a big deal out of unhealthy foods when your child eats them outside your house, and don't fall into the trap of actively discouraging them while actively encouraging healthier choices. This also applies to foods you don't want your child to like for other reasons (for example, meat in families of strict vegetarians). When you provide tasty alternatives and don't overreact to undesirable choices, she will never become fixated on them. At the same time, when you do eat out with your child, a little passive discouragement of unhealthy choices doesn't hurt. Giving your child a big meal at home before going to the mall or to see a movie, for example, minimizes the attractiveness of all the candy, ice cream, and other undesirable foods she will see there.

- Don't succumb to keeping foods you don't want in the house. Just because Justin eats fruit rolls (which, nutritionally speaking, resemble candy) every afternoon for a snack doesn't mean you have to keep them in *your* house. If you have a clear division between home food and other food, your child will enjoy each in its different setting. It is actually surprising how place-specific most children are in their food

TELEVISION AND FOOD

TV advertising is such a negative and powerful food influence that you may simply want to consider restricting your child's viewing to PBS and other noncommercial channels. In any case, if you make a rule that you never buy any item in the supermarket just because your child saw it on TV, you will help him make the distinction between TV food and home food—and you won't get badly pestered when you go shopping together. Once your child reaches five or six years you can have some fun reality-testing the ads. Kids catch on pretty quickly to overinflated claims, and you may be surprised at your child's shrewdness if you ask whether she really thinks the cereal can talk.

Keeping the TV off during meals will save you many irritations. Research studies have shown that children who watch too much TV are at greater risk of becoming overweight. Your child will also be a more adventurous eater when she doesn't have the distraction of watching a screen at the same time.

requests. Even if you fall into the habit of letting your child have a bag of chips after her weekly swimming trip, she likely won't even think of them at other times if you don't keep them around.

- If your child tries to mimic her friend—for example, by wanting a peanut butter and jelly sandwich for lunch *every single day*—nip it in the bud by making the ingredients disappear for a few days. It is easier to prevent habits from forming than to stop them once they become entrenched.

4. TAILOR THE DISCOUNTING PRINCIPLE TO YOUR CHILD'S DEVELOPMENT

As at earlier ages, overencouragement, bribes, threats, and punishment about particular foods and eating in general are actively counterproductive.

Now, however, you can exploit the discounting principle in more sophisticated ways. You want your child to love beans and be lukewarm on commercial pudding? Try offering a trip to Uncle Bill's garden to pick beans if he hurries up and finishes his snack. This is not as ridiculous as it

HOLIDAY FOOD

Many parents and grandparents are disappointed when a child refuses the special foods they make.

Part of the problem is all the excitement—food may simply not get onto the radar screen of a wired three-year-old playing with cousins or family friends he sees only a few times a year. Lack of familiarity may play a role, too; items rejected at three years may become popular at four or five as your child's memory span increases. My daughter at age four refused to touch pecan pie at Thanksgiving but was ready to give it a try at Christmas after watching our enjoyment four weeks earlier. Avoid urging your child to eat—even to please an elderly relative.

Aren't many traditional holiday foods unhealthy? Yes, but it really doesn't matter as long as they're in the house for only a day or two. And, of course, festive foods don't all have to be sugary or rich. You can offer special vegetables such as asparagus and wild-greens salad, or a beautifully arranged bowl of blueberries, raspberries, and pineapple, along with your traditional holiday dishes.

might sound—we know a child who learned to prefer green beans precisely because her parents offered this choice. Or you might occasionally try telling your child in a joking way *not* to eat the mushrooms and carrots you gave him for dinner—and see how quickly they disappear!

PRESCHOOL

Even if your child has been in day care, starting preschool may seem like a big deal to both of you, only one step removed from kindergarten. With respect to food, preschool is, in fact, a big deal and may have a significant influence on what your child eats.

Most preschools provide reasonably healthy snacks, and so the only school meal you really have to think about is lunch. The best way to make certain that your child is exposed to good lunch foods is to ask your school to provide a suggestion list for parents, if there isn't one already. This will help ensure that everyone brings in healthy food and you don't get pestered for less healthy items your child's classmates bring with them.

Standard but healthy items usually work best, because peer pressure can make your child feel that foods nobody else brings are yucky—even if he was previously happy to eat them at home.

How do you decide what to prepare for your child on any given day? Some people recommend preparing several different items with much more total food than your child will eat, so that he can pick and choose. We think this is the wrong approach for three reasons. First, research studies have shown that excess variety encourages overeating. Second, it encourages fussiness by building the expectation that there should be many different foods at each meal. Third, you spend money on lots of food that gets thrown out.

The better approach is to prepare one sandwich or hot item, one fruit, one vegetable, and one drink that you know your child likes. The amount of food can be about 25 percent more than you would normally expect your child to eat—but not too much more. Large portions, like excess variety, encourage overeating in kids who are susceptible to weight gain. For the sandwich or hot item, tell your child two or three options the night before, and let him pick. This way you encourage responsibility about eating and food choices, and also ensure that he enjoys his lunch.

As well as helping guide food choices, preschools can also make new foods seem interesting. When preschoolers help to make snacks such as instant wheat pizza (English wheat muffins topped with tomato sauce and a modest amount of cheese), oatmeal cookies, pumpkin muffins, and vegetable plates with a dip, they are not only learning new physical skills but are also becoming familiar with foods they may not have at home.

If your preschool encourages parent participation, consider a cooking project or maybe taking in foods that come with an educational message. For example, holidays can be celebrated with international foods drawn from the backgrounds of children in the class, and seasons of the year can be illustrated with growing and harvesting (apples and squash in fall, lettuce and peas in spring).

TALKING ABOUT NUTRITION AND HEALTH

We are often asked whether children should be told about food and health at this age. Should parents, for example, explain that milk makes bones and teeth strong, or that green leafy vegetables can help keep colds away?

Offering some limited information is a good idea starting at age four to

LUNCH SUGGESTIONS FOR PRESCHOOLERS

SANDWICHES, ROLLS, ROLL-UPS, AND PITA POCKETS WITH DIFFERENT FILLINGS

Cheese, including cottage cheese
Peanut butter and jelly
Egg salad
Tuna
Honey
Turkey or chicken
Sauteed or steamed tofu
Falafel (mixes available in health food stores)
Salad items such as lettuce, tomato, cucumber, celery, and red pepper

ALTERNATIVE COLD ITEMS

Crackers, including graham
Bread, bagels
Cheese sticks
Hard-boiled egg
Hummus or cheese dip with cut-up vegetables
Fruit yogurt, with or without cereal to mix in
Vegetable sushi, whole-wheat sesame crackers (see recipe page 193), or
    empanadas

ALTERNATIVE HOT ITEMS (SENT HOT IN A THERMOS, OR COLD FOR HEATING UP)

Soup with bread or crackers
Ravioli and cheese
Pasta with sauce
Rice with vegetables

SIDE DISHES

Fresh cut-up vegetables such as carrot sticks, cherry tomatoes, and slices of
    red pepper
Fruits, including grapes, blueberries, strawberries, apple slices, orange
    segments, and banana

SOMETHING TO DRINK

Water
Juice
Cold milk in a thermos

Avoid sending candy, soda, chips, sugary desserts, and other less healthy choices
that you and other parents may want to keep off the children's menu.

five years if your child seems interested. If you have one of the body books with a picture of a stomach leading to an intestine and so forth, he may enjoy a simple explanation of how the food he eats get mixed up in the stomach with special stomach juices that turn the food into liquid, and all the essential chemicals are then taken into his blood to travel through his body from his fingers and toes up to his head. Excretion can also be brought into the story, as the parts of food left after the body has taken everything it needs.

If your child finds this information interesting, you might go on to say that food is used for growing, giving him energy to run around (like putting gas in the car) and keeping him healthy and strong. If he enjoys this, too, he may even be ready to know that foods such as candy and soda don't contain any good chemicals, and this is why it is not a good idea to eat too much of them. Your child will respond better to having a short list of foods that should not be eaten regularly rather than a long shopping list of things he ought to like.

Leave aside for now the fact that different foods have different nutrients, because if you focus too much on different foods, you may be opening the door for unhealthy food obsessions that you want to avoid.

YOUR CHILD'S BODY IMAGE

Sometime between the ages of four and six, your child, especially if she is a girl, may become aware of how her body stacks up against those of other children she knows. Maybe she will come home from a play date one day and say, "Mom, my tummy sticks out," or "Daddy, am I fat?" At the same time, she may be playing imaginative games in which there is a "fat beast" or will tell you that she doesn't want to play with Alexandra because "she's too fat."

When your child starts to think that bodies matter and that some may be nicer than others, your response is critically important. Children who develop feelings of inferiority about their body now risk developing an eating disorder in the future.

What you need to know is that your child does not have a truly objective sense of her body yet, but is working through ideas she is gleaning from peers, books, TV, movies, and her own initial observations. You are still her most respected source of information and can give her the confidence that will insulate her from budding inferior feelings about her body.

However fat or thin your child really is, however much her tummy sticks out compared to other kids', what she needs to hear from you is that she has a very nice little body that you really love. If she genuinely is overweight, you might also say that some children grow fast early but that it evens out as they get older, and that in any case being a nice person—which she certainly is—is the most important thing. If any other adult makes your child feel fat for any reason, ask them to stop immediately.

Remember also that all your good work can be undone if your child hears you obsessing about your own weight or thighs, or overhears you talking about a neighborhood kid who is getting really fat.

COMMON PROBLEMS AND FREQUENTLY ASKED QUESTIONS

> *Tina, four years old, enjoys a generally healthy diet but will eat almost nothing for dinner after playing at her friend Sophie's house. The reason is that Sophie (whose family eats dinner rather late) has a snack of pudding around five o'clock, and when Tina joins her it is enough to put a stop to dinner at six. Tina's mother would like to handle the situation without upsetting Sophie's mother.*

How often does Tina play with Sophie? If it is only occasionally, one solution is to delay dinner fifteen minutes and offer Tina less pasta, rice, or potatoes than usual so she can focus on meat, vegetables, and fruit. If Tina plays with Sophie regularly, perhaps more of the play dates can be moved to Tina's house, where food can be better controlled, or the time of snacking changed. Alternatively, Tina's mother can ask Sophie's mother to give Tina only a quarter portion of pudding, telling her that otherwise Tina will not be hungry for dinner.

> *Patrick, now nearly six, is extremely fussy about food—so fussy, in fact, that his mother has created a set of "emergency rations" that go everywhere with him, so that he won't starve when he is visiting friends. She would dearly love him to eat a wider variety of foods.*

Problems like these are much easier to nip in the bud than to eliminate once established, but a two-pronged solution usually works, given patience and some time. First, Patrick can be told that now he is so grown-up that he is ready to be more independent about food. The "emergency rations" should be renamed his "lunch box" and reserved exclusively for school lunches. If he gets hungry at other times, he will be less fussy when the next meal or snack comes around. Second, Patrick's parents should use smart strategies to increase his food repertoire when he is at home. While these changes are given two to three months to work, Patrick should take a children's multivitamin/mineral supplement. Deficiencies of some micronutrients, such as zinc, have been linked to loss of appetite, and this can create a vicious cycle in picky eaters.

Dillon, aged four, still needs a sippy cup, and actually refuses milk if it is offered in a glass. How can his mother get him to give up his "sippy" without also losing an important food?

There is no urgent reason for Dillon to switch over now. (Many children use sippy cups until 5 years or older.) Waiting a few months may make the problem go away by itself. If it doesn't, plastic straws can ease the transition. Dillon's mother can explain that the change is necessary and that these straws will be Dillon's new "sippy." Because the sucking action is so similar, Dillon will probably get used to straws within a few days, and can use them indefinitely if he wants.

John is a healthy, active boy of four who began having hard stools two months ago. He recently began refusing to go to the bathroom and has had fecal soiling in his pants.

John probably has a typical case of impacted stool, and excess stool in the colon is now beginning to leak out around the hard mass. A pediatrician or pediatric gastroenterologist can provide guidance to help John eliminate the hard stool and encourage John's bowel habits to return to normal.

Impacted stools often start as constipation caused either by a lack of fiber or by a lack of fluid (the latter being especially common in summer months). Once a child finds it difficult to go to the bathroom, he tries to hold off as long as possible and this can lead to the downward spiral cumulating in impacted stool. Offering extra fluid, especially fruit juices, can resolve a budding problem in its early stages by softening the stools, as can additional high-fiber breads and cereals if normal fiber intake is low.

> *Irene, mother of three children ages one to six years, likes to serve desserts but wants to keep them under control. She has noticed that whenever ice cream is on the menu, her kids skimp on their main course and often leave vegetables untouched.*

Saving ice cream and other sweet treats for occasional use is definitely the easiest way to keep a dessert habit from derailing a healthy diet. Some parenting books actually suggest serving dessert at the beginning of the meal to get it over and done with. We don't think this is a good idea, as it encourages abnormal eating patterns and reinforces the child's belief that desserts are the best kind of food. Also, dessert helps satisfy your child's variety instinct whether served at the beginning or end of a meal; either pattern reduces his interest in vegetables and fruits.

If Irene really wants to serve regular desserts at home, we recommend:

- Don't make a big deal of desserts when they are served.
- Decide on one or two types (for example, chocolate or vanilla ice cream) and don't ever offer anything else for dessert; familiarity will lead to boredom.
- Give very small portions. For ice cream, the side of a spoon can be used to make thin slivers, which can then be piled up in a bowl to look like a pleasing amount.
- Make a "no seconds" rule and stick to it.

Combined, these strategies will help prevent dessert from seeming like the best part of the meal, and will also demonstrate the restrained behavior over sweet foods that helps children regulate their own intake when they are older and more in control of what they eat.

LOOKING FORWARD

As your child grows up she will become an increasingly active member of the community you live in, with play dates, after-school activities, and sleepovers part of her normal life. This whirlwind of new activity threatens to disrupt family closeness, but it needn't. Shared meals can become one of the regular family activities that you can use to actually strengthen family ties. The simple pleasure of having everyone gathered at the table for a wholesome sit-down meal will not only continue to reinforce the good nutritional habits you have instilled, but can become a time for helping each other in ways that only families can. And as you watch your child's bright face over the dinner table, you will be reminded that growing a healthy child is not only one of the biggest responsibilities of parenthood, it is one of life's greatest joys, too.

PART FOUR

Food Solutions for Common Problems

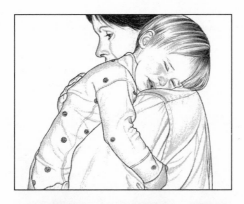

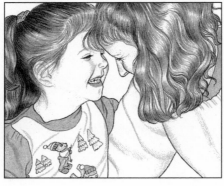

CHAPTER 13

✦

Feeding Your Sick Child

Diarrhea, Vomiting, and Other Common Illnesses

Peter, fifteen months, has a temperature of 103°F and is vomiting. His father called the pediatrician after Peter vomited twice in one hour and had watery diarrhea, and was told to give Pedialyte. The trouble is, Peter can't keep any down. Even 2 ounces comes straight back up. What should his parents try now?

Some babies get sick in the first few months. Others avoid illnesses early on, only to catch virus after virus later when they join a play group. Whenever it happens, the first time can seem very shocking. Your priceless child suddenly seems so vulnerable, and the pediatrician is too far away for real comfort.

Fortunately, there is help right at hand for many illnesses—in the shape of food and fluids! In fact, food and fluids can often provide the most effective relief and treatment for common problems.

Because feeding your child during illnesses involves using some foods different from what you usually eat, it is good to know what to expect and to store some of these items in your cupboard. With this in mind, we hope you are reading this chapter *before* your child gets sick, or at least have a partner available to rush to the store if necessary.

DIARRHEA, VOMITING, AND FEVER

Most bouts of diarrhea, either as a single symptom or combined with vomiting and fever, are viral in origin and cannot be cured with medicine. Antibiotics are rarely prescribed even when the diarrhea is bacterial, because gastrointestinal upsets are almost all self-limiting and antibiotics can sometimes prolong both the symptoms and the time patients carry the organism. Over-the-counter antidiarrhea medicines should also be avoided—they merely hide the symptoms (by bottling the fluid up inside your child's intestine) rather than treating them, and can give you a false sense of security.

Food and fluids are your most effective aids when it comes to helping your child recover. Research has shown that good feeding strategies can actually reduce symptoms and speed recovery, as well as prevent dangerous dehydration. And preventing dehydration is tremendously important: It is a leading cause of hospital visits in children under five years (accounting for more than 10 percent of admissions), and is fatal in 0.2 percent of cases. Home-based feeding plans can keep your child safe—*and* prevent sleepless nights in your local emergency room.

When your child begins to have diarrhea or starts vomiting, the first thing you need to know is that more fluids should go in than come out through the obvious routes. This is especially important when your child has a fever, because fever increases evaporative water loss that you can't see. Because dehydration reduces stomach motility (the normal stomach movements that shunt food along into the intestine), maintaining fluid balance also minimizes vomiting. As described below, how much and what kinds of fluids to give your child depends on his weight and the severity of the illness.

The second thing you need to be aware of is that it is important to reestablish normal feeding as soon as possible. Until recently parents were often advised to withhold food for one or two days after an attack of diarrhea, to allow a period of "intestinal recovery." Research has shown, however, that reestablishing normal feeding as soon as your child is willing to eat actually reduces the severity and duration of diarrhea episodes, and also prevents the nutritional depletion that comes with prolonged fasting. This is true even if your child continues to have diarrhea, because there is a net nutrient benefit to feeding even if some of the food is lost.

Here is what to do:

Infrequent diarrhea (once per four hours or longer), even if it is very watery, should not require major dietary changes provided your child is otherwise fine and doesn't have vomiting or fever. Simply continue feeding your child his normal diet. The digestive enzyme lactase (which breaks down milk sugar, or lactose, into absorbable subunits) sometimes gets reduced during diarrhea, theoretically making it harder to digest cow's milk and formula (breast milk is more easily digested). However, studies have shown that most infants with mild or moderate diarrhea have enough remaining lactase to obtain some—if not all—of the usual nutrients from a regular diet. Having said this, some solid foods and liquids are more easily tolerated than others, and are listed on pages 237 and 238.

The amount of usual foods and drinks during infrequent diarrhea will depend on what your baby or child is willing to take. However, since intakes at meals and snacks often drop to half or less of normal, you may need to keep fluids up in another way to prevent gradual dehydration. Oral electrolyte solutions such as Pedialyte or Infalyte are the best choice and can be offered by bottle, teaspoon, syringe, or cup every hour, or more frequently if desired. Amounts can be dictated by your child's thirst, but you should check that he urinates at least every three hours; if he is urinating this often and the urine is light-colored, he is not dehydrated.

More severe diarrhea (watery stools every one to three hours), or any diarrhea coupled with repeated vomiting or a fever over 100°F, requires more stringent measures to prevent dehydration and keep some nutrients going in.

- Try feeding your child appropriate foods for her age, but if they induce vomiting or if she refuses them, wait half an hour and then try again.
- Switch over to an oral electrolyte solution if your child can't keep anything down, or refuses to try, and aim to feed enough to ensure your child urinates at least every three hours (this may mean about ¹/₂ ounce per 5 pounds of body weight per hour). Use a teaspoon or syringe to give tiny amounts every five minutes. If vomiting is severe, give 1 teaspoon of oral electrolyte solution every two minutes. Giving small amounts frequently during the worst of the illness will usually be tolerated better than larger amounts given less often, and so prevents vomiting and dehydration better. As vomiting diminishes, you can gradually increase the volume per feed and lengthen the time interval between feeds. Don't stop the oral electrolyte solution if your child continues to vomit or have diarrhea—studies have shown that the amount lost in vomit or diarrhea is less than the amount consumed.
- If your child doesn't urinate every three hours, increase fluid intake to 1 teaspoon every one to two minutes for four hours to restore lost fluids.
- Try offering a small amount of appropriate foods every few hours, so that you return to normal feedings as soon as your child is able to tolerate them.

DEHYDRATION AND OTHER DANGEROUS SIGNS

Because dehydration is such a risk, your pediatrician should be notified within twenty-four hours even for infrequent diarrhea, and within twelve hours for severe cases. In addition, if your child exhibits any of these signs of dehydration, call your pediatrician immediately:

No tears if crying

Poor skin elasticity (returns slowly to normal if pinched)

Dry mouth

Eyes sunken

In babies under 9–12 months, fontanel (soft spot on head) hard and sunken

Other symptoms that you should tell your pediatrician about immediately include:

Diarrhea combined with repeated vomiting or fever greater than 100°F

Seven or more episodes of diarrhea in twenty-four hours, or hourly diarrhea for five hours

Change in mental status (lethargy, unusual sleepiness, apathy)

Pus or blood in the stool

Rapid breathing or heart rate

Severe abdominal pain

GOOD FLUIDS TO PREVENT DEHYDRATION AND SPEED RECOVERY

There has been much confusion over what kinds of fluids are appropriate during diarrhea and vomiting. For young babies with infrequent diarrhea without vomiting, continuation of the usual milk (breast milk or formula) works best in about 90 percent of infants. Even in severe diarrhea, about 80 percent of infants who are not also vomiting can tolerate their usual formula. If you are breast-feeding, you should continue to nurse your baby, no

ORAL ELECTROLYTE SOLUTIONS: WHY ARE THEY SO EFFECTIVE?

I was an early witness to the remarkable powers of oral electrolyte solution in the late 1970s, when one of the early field trials of dehydration prevention was conducted in the African village where I was working. The results were astonishing. Babies with vomiting and diarrhea could keep down oral electrolyte solution, even though milk, water, and everything else came straight back up; young children recovered their hydration within hours, and with it some energy and alertness; and before a day or two had passed, the diarrhea was gone, even though previously diarrhea lasted for several days to a week in that community.

In fact, the precise formulation of commercial oral electrolyte solutions makes them as good as a magic potion. What they do is exploit scientific knowledge of the way water, sodium, and glucose are absorbed through the gastrointestinal wall during infections. Normally the walls of the intestine secrete an enormous amount of fluid (about 15 pints per day) into food as it is being digested, and this fluid plus the broken-down nutrients are later absorbed into the bloodstream by a variety of different mechanisms. During gastrointestinal infections, most absorptive mechanisms become temporarily nonfunctional, resulting in the accumulation of a large volume of fluid in the intestine, which then leads to watery diarrhea.

One absorptive mechanism remains, however: the glucose-sodium co-transport system. This mechanism allows pairs of glucose and sodium molecules to cross the intestine wall together, and water is able to tag along provided that the solution is dilute enough. So the combination of glucose and sodium in a weak solution is actually what activates water absorption when children drink oral electrolyte preparations. Fluids without both sodium and glucose, such as fruit juices and soda, and solutions that are too concentrated (such as sports drinks) don't work because they don't activate the special carrier mechanism. Commercial glucose electrolyte solutions also contain valuable potassium, to replace that lost during diarrhea, and bicarbonate to buffer excess acid production, making them generally more effective than homemade preparations.

matter how severe the diarrhea gets. Studies now show that lactose-free formulas, once recommended for diarrhea, confer no particular benefit above regular formulas at this time. If your baby refuses formula or vomits it all back again, try diluting it 50 percent with water before giving up on milk. Often a more dilute formula is tolerated even if a full-strength one causes problems.

If additional fluids are needed, or if your baby vomits after food or formula, commercial oral electrolyte solutions (called oral maintenance solutions) will do the best job at preventing dehydration and speeding recovery. Pedialyte and Infalyte come in several flavors, as both liquid drinks and frozen pops. Electrolyte packets, which can be dissolved in water at home, are also available but are a less preferable option unless you can be sure to get the dilution exactly right.

A recent study reported that Pedialyte and Infalyte are equally effective, on average, in preventing dehydration. They do, however, have a rather different composition, with Pedialyte containing more glucose, and Infalyte containing more carbohydrate as "rice syrup solids" (which is easily converted into glucose but has slightly different metabolic effects). Because of this, you may find that one brand works well for your child even if another doesn't. As for liquid versus frozen, studies have shown that they are equally effective at preventing dehydration, although the ice pops may be a bit more popular (an important factor in determining how much your child will take).

But although oral electrolyte solutions are highly effective, some parents find their children refuse to drink them because of their poor taste. A small percentage of children (my own child included, alas) find the taste so horrible that it actually makes them retch. Manufacturers are working to improve the taste of their products, so in the future this may become less of an issue. In the meantime, homemade preparations (see page 237) are not as ideal in the abstract but can provide a safety net if they are the only oral electrolyte solution that your child will take.

Caution: Soda, fruit drinks, full-strength fruit juice, and sports drinks are often recommended during diarrhea and vomiting but can actually make symptoms *worse*. They do this because their high sugar content pulls water into the stomach and intestine, resulting in increased intestinal volume. Their high sugar content may also exceed the capacity of your child's sick intestine to digest sugar, leading to a further worsening of symptoms. For this reason, you should avoid these drinks until your child is fully recovered, although fruit juice diluted 50 percent with water can be given in the late stages of recovery.

HOMEMADE ORAL ELECTROLYTE SOLUTION, AND A SOLID-FOOD EQUIVALENT

Use one of these recipes when your child really won't tolerate a commercial one, or when you get caught short and need a substitute for a few hours. Do not use either of these if your child is under two years, or for longer than twenty-four hours in an older child, without consulting your pediatrician, because the balance of nutrients is less optimal than commercial alternatives. Also, be very careful to use exact quantities—the wrong balance of water and nutrients can worsen symptoms, and can be positively dangerous if the solution ends up too concentrated.

1. Mix together $\frac{1}{2}$ tsp salt, 8 tsp sugar, and 32 ounces (1 quart) of clean, sterile water (boil tap water for 5 minutes and cool before using). Store refrigerated and use within twenty-four hours.

2. If your child prefers something solid and has a mild or moderate sickness, allow 10 saltine crackers per 8 ounces dilute apple juice (3 ounces juice, 5 ounces clean, sterile water).

GOOD FOODS DURING INFREQUENT DIARRHEA AND DURING RECOVERY FROM SEVERE DIARRHEA

Early refeeding with solid foods can actually speed recovery in severe cases of diarrhea. Focus on starchy foods such as rice, potatoes, pasta, and bananas (depending on what is appropriate for your child's age) because starches are better tolerated than many other foods. Although the BRATT diet (bananas, rice, applesauce, toast, and tea) is no longer recommended because it doesn't contain all the essential nutrients, the individual BRATT foods (though not the tea) continue to be valuable for children convalescing from diarrhea. Eggs and yogurt are also well tolerated by most children and provide protein, vitamins, and minerals. Avoid very sweet foods because they may exceed the capacity of the recovering intestine to digest sugar.

COLDS AND OTHER ILLNESSES
THAT PRIMARILY REDUCE APPETITE

For colds and other illnesses that primarily reduce appetite (many babies and children will eat only a quarter to half of their usual calories when they have a stuffy nose), it is good to focus on nutrient-dense items that have calories and protein as well as plenty of fluids. For children over one year, items such as baked custard, scrambled eggs, and creamy rice pudding are all good choices, provided they are familiar and usually popular. You may even want to give your child these foods periodically when he is *not* sick so that you can use them when you need to. Don't worry too much about fruits and vegetables for now unless your child will enjoy them for refreshment (for example, watermelon, applesauce, and cooked strawberries can be nice)—a few days without these usually important items won't matter in terms of his overall health.

To keep fluids high during colds, you can ignore your usual ceiling on fruit juice and offer apple or grape juice, up to 8 ounces pure juice daily diluted with water, and extra water for thirst if requested. Juice frozen in ice-pop molds is often a hit with toddlers and older children, especially if you make "rainbow pops" by filling each container a third full of one juice, allowing it to freeze, and adding another and then another. Soup and hot lemon (a little fresh lemon juice mixed with warm water and honey to sweeten) are other options worth trying if your child usually likes them. Some children find milk hard to tolerate when they lose their appetite unless it is mixed with cereal (as in the case of rice pudding).

A word of warning: Although making an effort to prepare nice things will help prevent a complete cessation of eating, don't go too far. A mother we know tried so hard one time when her daughter was really sick that she offered things that were normally prohibited—including bacon, chips, and candy. Her daughter did eat a lot while she was sick, but subsequently became so fussy that it took weeks before eating was back on a healthy track. Some degree of appetite loss is normal during sickness, and you don't need to go to extreme lengths to keep calorie intake completely normal.

FREQUENTLY ASKED QUESTIONS

Jesse, three years old, has been starting to sniffle. His mother suspects he is catching a cold and is wondering whether vitamin C, zinc, or an herbal supplement will help prevent it.

Scientists continue to bicker about vitamin C and the common cold, but the emerging consensus is that it has no effect in most people. The few people who experience good results probably had vitamin C deficiency to start with—in which case the supplement was really correcting a deficiency rather than boosting an already adequate intake.

Concerning zinc, several recent studies have reported that zinc gluconate initiated within one to two days of the onset of a cold can decrease the severity and duration of symptoms. However, as we pointed out in Chapter 3, the RDA for zinc is actually pretty hard to meet without a multivitamin/mineral supplement, and the improvements may again have been in people with insufficient intake from their usual diet. A recent double-blind placebo-controlled study of zinc and the common cold in 249 schoolchildren consuming five 10-milligram lozenges of zinc gluconate per day found no measurable benefit and an *increase* in adverse symptoms (nausea, throat discomfort, and bad taste). Long-term zinc supplementation can also decrease absorption of copper (zinc and copper are absorbed by similar mechanisms), potentially causing symptoms of copper deficiency such as degeneration of the nervous system and anemia.

Echinacea is also sometimes suggested as an herbal supplement that can prevent colds. However, the evidence isn't good. Although echinacea has been shown to have beneficial effects on the immune system in laboratory experiments, there is little data supporting its use in humans. One recent trial of echinacea in 300 volunteers found no protective effect against respiratory infections. Moreover, there are potential problems, such as severe allergic reactions in some individuals and the possibility of toxic metabolic effects during regular use, that suggest echinacea shouldn't be used lightly.

For these reasons, Jesse's usual multivitamin/mineral supplement (suggested for all ages up to six years) and a good diet for additional nutrients will probably provide the best insurance against unduly prolonged or frequent colds. Megadoses of vitamins, which have sometimes been suggested for cold prevention, are dangerous for children and should never be used.

Two-year-old Michael started having loose stools three days ago, which progressed to watery diarrhea six to ten times per day and a fever of about 102°F. At first he was able to eat normally, but in the last twenty-four hours he has vomited all solid food and is now refusing to eat or drink anything, including oral electrolyte solution. His urine is dark, his mouth is dry, and his mom is afraid he is dehydrated.

Dark urine and a dry mouth are signs that Michael needs fluid and could develop serious dehydration if he doesn't get it. His parents should tell their pediatrician of the symptoms and start getting Michael to take fluid immediately. Teaspoons of oral electrolyte solution every one to two minutes for four hours should accomplish this. Small, frequent spoonfuls are easier for a child to tolerate than large amounts, and it is likely Michael will accept small sips and retain some fluid this way. If he resists liquids, frozen pops made from oral electrolyte solution may be more acceptable. As he starts to pass light-colored urine again (showing a normalization of body fluid), his vomiting, diarrhea, and fever may start to improve. Even if they don't, the oral electrolyte solution should be continued at a rate to maintain adequate urine output, and solid foods should be offered every few hours so that he begins to eat again as soon as he is able.

Marsha, age seventeen months, has had diarrhea off and on for almost two weeks. Her mother has been giving her lots of fluids, including water and apple juice, but the diarrhea keeps recurring. What's going on?

It is possible that Marsha's diarrhea started with a gastrointestinal virus and has actually been prolonged by excess fruit juice (which contains a natural sugar, called sorbitol, that can cause loose, watery stools in some children). Marsha's parents should restrict fruit juice to 4 ounces per day and offer her normal foods to give her intestines a better chance to recover. If her symptoms do not disappear within two or three days, Marsha should be taken to her pediatrician for evaluation.

Amelia, twenty months, has her first bad cold. Her mother has heard that dairy foods increase mucus production and should be avoided to minimize her cold symptoms. Is it true?

Children between one and four years of age typically catch several colds per year, and restricting milk intake has sometimes been suggested as a way to reduce mucus.

However, a recent large study of volunteers experimentally infected with the cold virus found no relationship at all between mucus and milk intake. Amelia's mother can continue to give her daughter milk with a clear conscience, confident that the mucus is caused by a cold virus and not by anything she drinks.

CHAPTER 14

✧

Food, Sleep, and Your Baby

Jane and Michael, parents of thirteen-month-old Matthew, were desperate—and desperately tired. They had not slept through the night since Matthew was born. On a typical night Matthew woke and cried to be fed every one to two hours! It wasn't because he was growing poorly or needed little sleep, and all conventional treatments for sleep problems had failed. Then Jane and Michael learned about recent research suggesting that milk allergy might be a possible cause of poor sleep in some cases. Within a week of removing cow's milk from Matthew's diet, he started sleeping thirteen hours a night with no awakenings. Jane and Michael are now the joyful parents of a happy and lively toddler and are firm believers in the fact that, contrary to widespread opinion, food has profound effects on our children's health and well-being at all levels, including even sleep.

There are many professional skeptics who discount the interconnectedness of eating and sleeping. Pediatricians and parenting books often tell parents that babies do not wake up according to how well or poorly they are fed. But the widespread belief that the right food can help your child—and you—get a good night's sleep persists. Why is this?

It's partly because many factors affect how well or badly infants and young children sleep. Food is only one factor, and other problems can be easier to identify and solve. But it may also be because research on sleep and food is usually conducted either by nutritionists or by sleep experts—not both. The outcome often is studies that are imperfectly planned, and the results can be inconclusive.

We are among a growing number of researchers who believe that food and sleeping *are* connected and that changing how you feed your child can sometimes help solve an apparently intractable sleep problem. This is not to say that food is the only answer to sleep problems. It is one of several factors that parents should consider if the more obvious and usual explanations don't lead to a solution.

ENCOURAGING YOUR BABY TO SLEEP THROUGH THE NIGHT

There comes a point in the life of most new parents when they desperately need some unbroken sleep, and getting a baby who is a poor sleeper on track can seem like an impossible task. Often this point comes when your baby is three or four months old and you are back at work and yet still have to get up twice a night for feedings. Like you, Mel and I have been there and know that it can make life miserable for a while.

Sleep experts tell us that most babies are capable of sleeping through the night by four months, but many older babies—breast-fed and formula-fed alike—get into the habit of relying on one or more middle-of-the-night snacks to keep them going. What can you do to help yourselves break out of this cycle?

If your baby is less than two months old, you should not be restricting nighttime feeding—it is simply too early. What you can do, though, is make sure to clearly distinguish night from day in how you handle the feedings. Between one and three months babies start to develop the cicadian rhythms that determine sleep patterns—which means that dim lights, quiet voices, and no playing at nighttime encourage an early return to unbroken nights as soon as your baby is metabolically ready.

If your baby is between two and four months, provided that he was not premature and is healthy and normal, he is ready for just one middle-of-the-night feed (though there will always be exceptions). By the middle of the night, we mean the time between the 10 P.M. or midnight feed and the first morning feed at around 5 or 6. If he regularly wakes twice or more between these times, studies have shown that you can shift him onto a better pattern without skimping on the food he needs for growth, and without compromising your milk production if you are nursing. Here's how.

1. Check with your pediatrician that your baby is ready for a sleep modification program. It's important to not start prematurely.

2. Wake your baby and make sure he has a good feed between 10 P.M. and midnight, before you go to bed. If you are breast-feeding and tend to run out of milk late in the day (a not uncommon pattern), consider expressing some of your milk in the morning and using it for an early evening feed. This will have the dual effect of increasing your milk supply overall and also providing you with a spare feed. However, even if you use this supplemental milk, make sure that your very last feed each night is by breast. If your breasts get overfull at night, it will tend to decrease your milk supply.

3. When your baby wakes at, say, 1 A.M., don't immediately feed him if he is just whimpering. This is very important, because it breaks his association between waking up at night and expecting milk. Instead, go to him, comfort him, and do alternative caretaking activities such as diapering. Delay feeding for ten or fifteen minutes unless he is really awake and crying to be fed. Gradually try to lengthen the delay until he is fed only once in the middle of the night. Research has shown that you can expect positive results within one to two weeks.

4. If you are breast-feeding, remember to make up for fewer nighttime feedings by nursing longer when you do feed, to keep your milk supply up.

5. By the time your baby is four to five months old, you can try the same approach to get her to sleep through the whole night. By this time most babies are physiologically ready to manage without food for seven to eight hours or even longer, so you don't have to worry that you are being cruel. When your baby wakes up, delay feeding her for a while and try to put her back to sleep after doing alternative caretaking activities. If you have difficulties stopping the feeding, try giving an ounce of water instead of breast milk or formula. If your baby gets used to not receiving any calories during the night, her metabolism will slow down and there will be fewer hormonal changes encouraging her to wake up. One night shortly after you have committed yourself to this approach, *you* will wake up at 3 A.M. but your baby will sleep through. Then you will know that you have made it to another of life's milestones.

6. After your baby starts on her first solid food, between four and six months, try offering her 1 to 2 tablespoons of rice cereal (mixed with breast milk or formula) with dinner. Most doctors say that dinner-time cereal doesn't make babies sleep through the night, but our ex-perience is that it works for some children. As with so many aspects of parenting, trial and error is important when it comes to working out what is best for your own baby. Don't, incidentally, add the ce-real to your baby's bottle rather than giving it by spoon—it won't be any more effective, and your baby will lose out on valuable practice eating solid food.

GETTING YOUR BABY TO SLEEP

Ann gave up nursing at three months, when she went back to work. Almost immediately she noticed a change in her daughter's sleep habits. "She used to fall asleep so easily. Even when we wanted her to stay awake, her body was so determined to sleep that there was nothing I could do," Ann recalled rather wistfully. "Now everything has changed. It takes forever, and we both get cranky, wishing for the days when she just drifted off in my arms."

Babies who are fed formula often take a while to fall asleep. This can be frustrating for tired parents who want the day to finish so they can go to bed themselves. If you watch your formula-fed baby, it often looks as though she is trying to go to sleep but simply isn't sleepy yet. Breast-fed ba-bies, on the other hand, typically can't wait to drop off. If allowed, they often fall asleep while they are still nursing.

Scientists have traced this phenomenon—called "sleep latency"—to the amino acids in breast milk and formula. Although formulas are similar to breast milk in many ways, they are certainly not identical, and one of the ways they differ is in amino acids, the building blocks that make up proteins. The amino acid tryptophan seems to be one of the keys to sleep latency. Tryptophan is the dietary precursor of the brain neurotransmitter serotonin, which is involved in helping us go to sleep. Absolute amounts of tryptophan are actually less important than a tryptophan score, denoting the amount relative to similar amino acids that compete for the same transport mechanism into the brain.

Formula-fed babies tend to have low relative levels of tryptophan in their blood, causing them to fall asleep more slowly than breast-fed babies by an average of ten to fifteen minutes for each sleep. Not all formulas have the same amount of tryptophan; if your baby seems to have a problem falling asleep, you can consider switching to the one in your formula group that has the highest tryptophan score.

Remember that dietary supplements, other than the infant multivitamins/minerals, should *never* be given to babies. Even though tryptophan acts like a kind of sleeping drug (and was used as such by adults until it was taken off the over-the-counter market), you should never give it or related substances to your child. Similarly, if you are breast-feeding, you shouldn't take a supplement to help yourself sleep. Any substance you ingest has the potential to pass into your breast milk and so into your baby's body.

When breast-fed babies have trouble falling asleep, the foods their mothers eat may contribute to the problem. Caffeine is the first suspect. Caffeine's effects are obvious—it causes the same jitteriness and sleeplessness in your baby (via your breast milk) that it does in adults who are not habituated to it—but its sources can be less so. Some sodas and teas, in particular, contain almost as much caffeine as coffee. The other common problem in a nursing mother's diet may be—surprisingly—cow's milk.

TRYPTOPHAN SCORES	
REGULAR FORMULAS	
Enfamil	4.6
Good Start	7.2
Similac	4.6
SOY FORMULAS	
Alsoy	4.4
Isomil	5.8
Prosobee	4.5
HYDROLYSATES	
Alimentum	6.7
Nutramigen	4.7
Pregestimil	4.7
FOLLOW-UP	
Enfamil Next Step	4.3
Enfamil Next Step with soy	4.5
Follow-Up	4.4

COW'S-MILK SENSITIVITY AS A CAUSE OF CHRONIC SLEEP PROBLEMS

A sensitivity to cow's milk or other food will most often manifest itself with diarrhea, abdominal pain, eczema, or wheezing. Research has shown, however, that occasionally none of these signs is apparent, and instead very poor sleeping habits are seen.

A recent research study followed 146 children under five who had chronic sleep problems that could not be traced to any particular cause. One in nine were completely cured within seven days of total removal of cow's milk from their diet. Instead of sleeping an average of only five and a half hours a night, their sleep jumped up to a much more normal thirteen hours. Needless to say, their parents were overjoyed. Their joy did not prevent them from further helping science, however. All but one of the families agreed to try their child on cow's milk again, to confirm the result, and every child went right back to sleeping as badly as before. Other studies have also shown that not only does the total amount of sleep improve in cow's-milk-sensitive children when they are taken off the milk; their quality of sleep is also much better, with many fewer nighttime awakenings.

The children in those studies were old enough—past one year—to be consuming cow's milk as part of their own diet. But for breast-fed and formula-fed babies under one, the effects can theoretically be the same. In some nursing mothers, cow's-milk proteins can pass directly into the bloodstream without first being broken down into amino acids, and then pass intact into breast milk.

Be aware that food is a possible cause of your child's sleeplessness only if he has not slept well since at least six weeks of age. If he learned to sleep through the night at four months and started waking again at nine months, separation anxiety is a more likely cause. However, if your baby is older than eight months and has had persistent sleep problems that you haven't been able to solve in other ways, consider milk sensitivity and involve your pediatrician to help you address the problem.

The first step in testing whether cow's milk is the problem is to remove all dairy foods and cow's-milk products from your baby's diet for ten days, including cow's milk, regular formula, yogurt, cheese, and all foods containing these items. Substitute a hydrolysate or elemental formula such as Nutramigen, Alimentum, Pregestimil, or Neocate for regular formula, to make sure that your baby gets all his essential nutrients. If you are breastfeeding, remove all cow's-milk products from your own diet and be sure to eat other foods for protein and take a calcium supplement. Turn to page 202 for information on nondairy sources of calcium.

When you remove dairy products and regular formula from your child's diet, or begin avoiding dairy products yourself if you are nursing, don't expect immediate results. When a food intolerance has been present for a while, it takes time for all the symptoms to go away. You may, however, expect improvement within seven to ten days if your child is one of the 11 percent with undiagnosable sleep problems that improve with removal of cow's milk.

If you find that eliminating cow's milk and dairy products does not help your child's sleep problem, you can assume that cow's-milk sensitivity is probably not the cause and switch back to what you were feeding before.

If your child does show improvement, you should break out the champagne, and while you are having your celebration, read more about allergies and food intolerances in Chapter 16. Food allergies are triggered as easily by small amounts of the offending food as by large amounts, and care needs to be taken to eliminate all foods containing cow's milk to prevent a recurrence. Happily, most early childhood food allergies disappear by two to three years. Meanwhile, because milk, cheese, and yogurt contain many essential nutrients, you should talk to your pediatrician about a referral to a dietitian for help in replacing them with other foods.

A WELL-RESTED BABY IS EASIER TO FEED

The interconnectedness of eating and sleeping works in the other direction, too: Poor sleeping habits can affect what your child eats. There is no good research on this issue, but as parents, both Mel and I have seen how good nutritional habits are obliterated by a bad night's sleep.

My daughter, now six, is usually a great kid about food. She eats good meals, does not need to snack too much, and is eager to try most new things we cook at home. This rosy picture is transformed after a few bad nights: She will pick at her meals, demand snacks at odd times, and want cookies, chips, and other unhealthy foods that she normally ignores.

Chronic sleep problems, which occur in about 25 percent of infants and young children, cause even more difficulty. For this reason, we think of the interconnectedness of eating and sleeping as a circle of influence: A well-fed child sleeps well, and a well-rested child eats well. But a circle of influence can also turn into a vicious cycle—when a food problem makes for bad sleeping habits, or poor sleeping habits encourage a poor diet, and each problem feeds on the other. If this happens, knowing how to break the cycle makes getting back on track possible.

Dr. Richard Ferber, a sleep expert at Children's Hospital in Boston, is one good source of suggestions that can help break bad sleep patterns or prevent them from occurring. Three points Dr. Ferber considers especially important:

1. *Know your child's sleep needs.* The typical amount (nighttime plus naps combined) is fifteen hours at two months, decreasing gradually to twelve to thirteen hours at one to two years. Some children will sleep more than this and some less, but most will need within an hour of the average amount.

2. *Develop consistent routines around bedtime and sleeping.* Different routines work for different people, but having standard times for taking a bath, getting into bed, and reading stories (for older children) is very helpful. Established routines for middle-of-the-night problems (which will always happen occasionally, even in good sleepers) should be kindly without being rewarding enough to encourage repetition.

3. *Let your child learn to fall asleep by herself in her own bed.* Being too active in helping your child go to sleep—rocking her or cuddling her and then putting her to bed after she has started sleeping—encourages your child to need you in the night. Avoid these habits and you will avoid the middle-of-the-night awakenings that go along with them.

Whether it's a food problem creating a bad sleep pattern, or a nonfood problem that then makes your sleep-deprived child a poor eater, the circle of influence can be interrupted. And when it finally is, you'll probably wake up once or twice during the night anyway. Go back to sleep. You've earned it.

Additional Reading

Solve Your Child's Sleep Problems. Richard Ferber, M.D. Simon & Schuster, 1985.
Touchpoints. T. Berry Brazelton, M.D. Perseus Books, 1992.

CHAPTER 15

———◈———

Problems with Weight

The Spectrum from Obesity to Anorexia and Bulimia

Three-year-old Karen is on the 50th centile for height but the 90th centile for weight, and seems to have gotten a little fatter every time she visits her pediatrician. Her mother is also somewhat overweight at 5 feet 5 inches and 160 pounds. Should she do something now about her daughter's weight? Is Karen genetically programmed to be overweight? Or will she simply outgrow her "baby fat?"

Problems with body weight are at such epidemic proportions in the United States that virtually every family is touched by them. Recent weight statistics made headlines in newspapers all around the country because they showed that average body weight has increased progressively over the last thirty years. More than half of all adults are now overweight. In fact, more adults and children are overweight today than ever before in our history.

What these shocking statistics tell us is that most weight problems are *not* caused by unusual genetic defects. A small minority of people do seem to be afflicted by genetic mutations that promote obesity, but American adults had the same gene pool thirty years ago and weighed an average of 10 pounds less. This does not, of course, imply that we are individually to blame for greed and slothfulness. Rather, we are members of a culture that actually makes it hard not to gain excess weight—and this problem has been exacerbated by misinformation about what we can do to help ourselves.

The good news is that by exploiting new research showing how to reduce calorie intake without promoting hunger, you can now do a lot to help your child and your whole family. Even if your family history suggests that your child has a genetic predisposition to obesity, the effects of this predisposition can be minimized.

And minimizing excess weight is important, because obesity is not just a cosmetic issue. Like overweight adults, overweight children often suffer from symptoms of premature heart disease, bone and joint problems, physical limitations, and depression. Recent statistics also suggest that very overweight children are also at risk of diseases such as adult-onset (type 2) diabetes, which was previously thought to occur only after age forty.

Even as obesity is on the rise, clinically diagnosable eating disorders are increasingly common. According to one recent study, an estimated 20 percent of adults and adolescents—especially, but not only, women and girls—have bulimia at some point in their lives, with its bingeing and purging behavior, or anorexia nervosa and its attendant severe weight loss. Because of our society's obsessive equating of thin with beautiful, and with creating thin bodies at almost any cost, every child who is part of our culture is at risk.

The problems of overweight and eating disorders seem diametrically opposed, yet paradoxically they often have their roots in similar childhood situations. And, as you will see in this chapter, both are easier to prevent and treat by early intervention than to resolve once they have been established for several years.

DOES YOUR CHILD WEIGH TOO MUCH?

If you think your child may be overweight or at risk of developing a weight problem, and he is one year or older, your first step should be a call to your pediatrician. Do, by the way, make this call when your child is not with you. One mother we know still remembers with horror the day when she was six years old and overheard her pediatrician telling her mother she was getting too heavy.

The second step is for your pediatrician to measure your child's weight and height. You can then use your pediatrician's charts, or the ones on pages 318–330 to see whether your child's weight is greater than it should be, taking into consideration how tall he is. Weight-for-height charts are generally more useful than separate charts for weight and height, because you don't have to compare two different graphs to see whether your child has a problem.

If your child is anywhere between the 25th and 90th centiles of weight for height, he is not overweight. If he is on or over the 90th centile of weight for height and one year or older, he is heavier than desirable, and

BEFORE YOU START

If you think your child may be overweight, or heading in that direction, there are several effective steps you can take right now. First, however, there are three things to avoid:

1. Do not start any form of treatment before twelve months of age. Uneven growth spurts before one year can make a child appear overweight when there is actually nothing wrong at all.

2. Do not put your child of six years or less on a "diet"—that is, by giving her less total food than she wants to eat. Instead, give her healthy meals and make sure she gets plenty of exercise to help her maintain height growth while reducing weight gain. In this way she will "grow down" to a better weight without your ever having to deny her food when she is hungry.

3. Do not tell your child of six or less that she is overweight or too fat, or even tell her you are trying to help her lose weight by changing what she eats. You can normalize her weight without her ever being aware of what is going on, and she will do better and be happier because of it. In the meantime, if she confronts you with the idea that she is too fat, or hears another adult telling her she shouldn't eat so much, explain that you love her just the way she is and that some people are big and others are small—and that it really doesn't matter.

now is a good time to think about moving him onto a lower centile, with your pediatrician's help. A child who is close to the 90th centile is not yet overweight but can be watched for possible future problems. (A child who is under the 10th centile of weight for height is underweight and should be evaluated by a pediatrician for possible causes.)

Your family history is a factor here, too. If your child is overweight or heading in that direction but neither you nor your child's other parent has a weight problem, it is a good idea to wait twelve months or until your child is three years old (whichever comes sooner) to see if the problem corrects itself naturally. It quite probably will, because "lean genes" definitely help protect against long-term weight gain. If, however, your child is overweight and you (or his other parent) struggle with your own weight, being more proactive is the right strategy.

WHY SOME CHILDREN BECOME OVERWEIGHT

We each have a unique genetic weight range within which our body weight tends to stay. For one person that range might be 110 to 140 pounds, for another 200 to 260 pounds. What exactly we weigh within our own genetic range depends on what we eat and how active we are. A few lucky people, because of their unusual lean genes, can maintain a healthy weight whatever they eat or do. For the rest of us, environmental factors converge with our genetic blueprint to make us overweight or not, depending on how we lead our lives. This convergence between normal genes and lifestyle is the root of most twentieth-century weight problems.

How do we know this? Probably the best evidence comes from recent research comparing the body composition of ethnic groups living in different locations. Japanese-Americans, for example, are typically heavier than their counterparts in Japan by an average of 15 to 20 pounds, a difference that can be related directly to the different lifestyles and dietary practices in the two countries.

The same observation has been made even in groups that appear to have a severe genetic susceptibility to obesity. The Pima Indians of Arizona and Mexico are a case in point. Virtually 100 percent of Pimas living on reservations and exposed to a modern American lifestyle are obese, while adult Pimas following the traditional life of their ancestors are lean and healthy, and average 60 pounds lighter! Such an extreme genetic susceptibility is rare, but the same pattern applies to most of us on a less dramatic scale.

What this research tells us is that by reversing some of the modern aspects of our lifestyle, it is possible to keep our own weight—and our children's—at the lower end of our personal genetic range. This is not an effortless change for parents, who need to learn new recipes and plan new family activities (children are so adaptable they usually find it easy), but it gets less difficult over time as the changes become routine.

Another factor in long-term weight problems is that excess weight can become self-perpetuating. This is an unfortunate instance of metabolic programming working in a negative way. Once we move into the top end of our genetic weight range and become overweight, our bodies start to take on the metabolism of a fatter body.

Why does this happen? Scientists don't yet have all the answers, but there are a number of pieces of the puzzle in place. Perhaps most important, body fat used to be thought of simply as the warehouse for surplus calories. We now know that this is not correct at all, and that fat tissue actively synthesizes hormones and enzymes that have many important metabolic effects.

For example, as a child becomes overweight, he actually grows more fat cells than a lean child. These excess fat cells secrete several hormones, including estrogen and leptin, that in turn influence metabolic rate and hunger.

The action of the enzyme *lipoprotein lipase* is another example of how becoming fat can change a child's metabolism. Sitting on the surface of fat cells, this enzyme has the job of drawing fat from digested foods into the cells for storage. More fat cells mean more lipoprotein lipase, working to store still more fat. The body's fat, in effect, takes on a life of its own.

Once weight has increased, our bodies also tend to be better at fighting back against caloric restriction than they were at fighting the original caloric excess. It is one of the genetic legacies of our hunting-gathering ancestors, who were more likely to suffer from food shortage than food excess, and were less likely to survive if they lost weight easily. The result is that the status quo tends to be maintained, and it is harder to drop weight after a prolonged period of overweight than it is to prevent weight gain in the first place.

For these reasons, it is easier to fix weight problems in childhood than later. Nipping your child's weight problem in the bud, *before* it gets entrenched, can be the best way to help him attain a normal adult weight.

It is important to remember, too, that you don't have to radically reduce your child's weight to see significant health benefits. Even bringing weight for height down from the 95th to just below the 90th centile may yield big long-term results in terms of health risks and adverse psychological consequences.

HOW TO NORMALIZE A WEIGHT PROBLEM

If your child is now over the 90th centile of weight for height, it will take several months to a year to effect the change you want. Your aim is for her to slow her rate of weight gain while she grows taller, rather than to actually lose weight. You can think of this as "growing down the centiles." Time is on your side, and there is no need to rush the following eight steps:

1. WORK WITH YOUR PEDIATRICIAN AND HAVE REALISTIC GOALS

Working with your child's pediatrician is essential to prevent problems, and setting a reasonable goal for your child will help you work within the limits of her genetic potential. If both you and your child's other parent are a normal weight for height, then you can reasonably expect that your child can grow down to the 50th or 60th centile for weight for height. If you are both overweight, the 75th or 80th centile may be a more achievable goal. In this case, your child may never be quite as lean as some other children, but you will have scored a major victory for her future health and well-being.

2. DO A REALITY CHECK

You may think that you are already feeding your child healthy foods and that what she eats is not part of the equation, but research has shown that most overweight children and adults eat more high-calorie, low-fiber foods than their lean counterparts. In this respect, our perceptions about what we eat are rather like our perceptions about exercise. I, for example, think of myself as a person who exercises four days a week, but if I keep a daily record of when I do exercise, it often turns out to be less—sometimes a lot less!

Begin this step by recording everything your child eats and drinks for three days (including one weekend day). As you record what your child eats, don't give her different foods from normal, or try to change how much she eats. The aim is to see what her baseline is. This gives you a starting point for the changes you need to make and tells you what specific habits may need correcting.

If your child eats some food away from home, ask your child-care provider to record the information without your child's knowing about it. Explain that you don't think anyone is at fault or to blame, and that you want your child to eat as usual so you can better understand how to improve her weight.

Once you have your food record, you can look at what your child has eaten and when she has eaten it. Here are ten factors that can contribute to a child's weight problem and which the program described below will help eliminate.

1. Eating fewer vegetables and fruits daily than recommended for her age

2. Eating daily desserts

"REALITY CHECK" FOOD RECORD FOR AN OVERWEIGHT THREE-YEAR-OLD

DATE: JULY 24

TIME	FOOD	APPROXIMATE AMOUNT
7:00 A.M.	Whole milk	8 oz
	Cheerios	$\frac{1}{2}$ cup
	Buttermilk waffle with syrup	$\frac{1}{4}$ waffle
10:00 A.M.	Chocolate chip cookies	2 cookies
	Apple juice	8 oz
Noon	Peanut butter and jelly sandwich	2 slices white bread with 2 tbsp each peanut butter and jelly
	Canned peach slices	$\frac{1}{2}$ cup
	Whole milk	8 oz
3:00 P.M.	Microwave popcorn	$\frac{1}{2}$ cup
	Whole milk	8 oz
4:00 P.M.	Small packet gummi bears	1 oz
5:30 P.M.	Chicken nuggets	3 pieces
	Ketchup	3 tbsp
	French fries	$\frac{1}{2}$ cup
	Frozen yogurt	1 cup
	Apple juice	8 oz
7:00 P.M.	Whole milk	8 oz
	Oreo cookies	2 cookies

Note how many of the ten factors on pages 254–256 are contributing to this child's weight problem.

3. Drinking more than 6 ounces of juice daily, or *any* regular soda or juice drinks (such as fruit punch) or sports drinks

4. Drinking whole milk rather than 1 percent or skim, or more than 24 ounces of any kind of milk daily

5. Eating more than two small cookies or one small bag of chips daily

6. Eating more than one fast food, take-out food, or restaurant meal every three days

7. Eating more than one deep-fried entree or vegetable (for example, fried chicken, fried fish, or french fries) every three days

8. Eating only white bread, rather than some white and some whole wheat, if she is older than three years

9. Eating candy more than once a week

10. Regularly eating more than three meals and two snacks daily if she is older than eighteen months

3. FOCUS ON GOOD FOOD CHOICES

Making sure that your child gets to choose how much he eats—*but from a carefully controlled list of foods and drinks*—will go a long way toward ensuring he achieves a normal weight without feeling deprived. Keeping less desirable foods out of the house is by far the best way of making sure they don't get consumed.

In the past, there has been a great deal of misinformation about what foods and drinks help keep weight under control—whether for adults or for children. Fortunately, very recent research is making it easier to give recommendations that genuinely help regulate calorie intake.

For children, foods that help reduce calorie intake are (1) lower in caloric density (in other words, they have relatively few calories per ounce of food) and moderate or low in fat; and (2) are lower in glycemic index (releasing glucose into the bloodstream more slowly).

Foods with a lower caloric density and lower glycemic index actually reduce hunger and your child's desire to eat. They do this by causing a delayed rate of absorption, giving your child the right feelings of satisfaction at the end of each meal and preventing the return of hunger before it is time to eat again.

This is not to say that you should only feed your child low-glycemic-index, low-caloric-density foods. Moderation is very important, to prevent the severe calorie restriction that will cause nutritional deficiencies and even stunting in children. So you don't need to ban cereals, bread, and other foods with a moderate to high glycemic index and moderate caloric density in favor of broiled fish and spinach. Simply avoiding foods with an extremely high glycemic index and high caloric density will reduce overeating.

Many of the good foods with a low or moderate glycemic index and caloric density are ones your child is already familiar with:

- *Vegetables, fruits, and beans.* Most vegetables and fruits (except potatoes, yams, and bananas) and all beans have a low glycemic index, and usually a low caloric density, too. And although cooked vegetables and fruits are great, raw fruits and vegetable salads are even better. The firm texture slows down digestion—and delays the return of hunger.

- *Lean meats, poultry, seafood, and low-fat dairy products.* High-protein foods such as these are good because they have a low caloric density and glycemic index. However, don't serve more than the normal amount for your child's age; too much of any one food group can unbalance the diet and cause deficiencies of one or more essential nutrients.

- *Whole-grain breads and cereals.* The "soluble" fiber in whole-grain oat, barley, and rye cereals lowers the glycemic index by forming a gel in the stomach and slowing the rate at which food empties into the intestine (where absorption takes place). The "insoluble" fiber in whole wheat is valuable too, because it reduces caloric density and increases the sensation of fullness, making whole-wheat products far preferable to their refined, rapidly digested cousins even though they don't have a big impact on glycemic index. Whole-grain cereals made up of actual pieces of cereal grains (such as Irish oatmeal) are even better than processed cereals made from whole grains, because the intact cereal kernels further slow digestion and so decrease hunger.

- *Plain carbohydrates.* Carbohydrates such as rice, potatoes, and white bread are generally considered to have a high glycemic index (pasta less so, especially if cooked al dente). For adult dieters, therefore, carbohydrates should generally be restricted. However, for slightly reducing calorie intake in children growing down the centiles they are not bad foods, because they have a lower caloric density than al-

CALORIC DENSITY AND FAT

Research studies from my own laboratory and others around the world are showing that foods with lower caloric density (in other words, foods with fewer calories per ounce) are one of the important keys to healthy weight. This is because our bodies tend to be better at sensing the bulk of food we have eaten during a meal than how many calories we have had. The result is that we feel more satisfied and eat fewer total calories when foods with fewer calories per ounce dominate the menu.

Fat, of course, contains plenty of calories (9 calories per gram, or 250 per ounce), and so most high-fat foods have a high caloric density. Cookies, cakes, fried entrees, and french fries are just a few examples of foods that are usually loaded with fat and high in caloric density. However, fat and caloric density don't always go hand in hand. Green beans cooked with a little olive oil and garlic, for example, might provide as much as 70 percent of calories from fat but still contain only 12 calories per ounce. Fat-free cookies, on the other hand, often have 100 calories per ounce. In this example, a 4-ounce helping of green beans would provide fewer calories than $1/2$ ounce of low-fat cookies, and would do much more to stop hunger and overeating.

WHAT ABOUT COMMERCIAL LOW-FAT AND NO-FAT PRODUCTS?

Unfortunately, because of the recent focus on fat rather than caloric density, food manufacturers have been encouraged to create whole lines of products that are low in fat but have a caloric density that is as high as—or higher than—the regular product. Extra sugar and other carbohydrates have simply been added to replace some or all of the fat, and these low-fat, low-fiber, but high-calorie products encourage overeating just as much as traditional recipes. It's a good example of how overly simplistic nutrition messages (in this case, "Reduce fat") can actually create problems. We hope that in the future, nutrition labels will carry information on caloric density, or will at least standardize portion sizes better so that different foods can be compared directly. In the meantime, reading nutrition labels for both calories *and* serving size will help you make choices that are truly healthy for your family.

ternatives such as french fries or rice pilaf cooked with lots of butter or oil. The moderate caloric density of plain starches is a plus that can help moderate overeating.

On the other hand:

- *Serve oils and fats in moderation.* They don't affect blood glucose and insulin, so they effectively have a glycemic index of zero, but with 9 calories per gram, they have the highest caloric density of any single food. We recommend the same 30 percent of calories from fat that we recommend for children without a weight problem—but packaged in foods with fewer calories per ounce. Again, moderation is the key. Spreads such as butter, margarine, and cream cheese are easy to moderate without its being obvious. Be aware, too, that liquid oils are no better than solid fats when it comes to weight gain—in fact, ounce for ounce, butter actually has slightly fewer calories than oil because it also contains a little water and protein.

- *Strictly limit cakes, cookies, chips, and other high-carbohydrate, high-fat treats.* The combination of fat with sugar and/or starch creates a powerful combination of high glycemic index and high caloric density. Such foods not only are easy to overeat: they also encourage a rapid return of hunger. When you do serve these items, make sure never to give your child the impression that *you* think they are tastier than other, healthier foods. This way you will avoid making them seem better than they really are.

You can almost always turn less-than-desirable items that your child overeats into good foods that he doesn't, by cooking them yourself. Homemade pizza with an oatmeal, whole-wheat, or sourdough crust, less cheese, and a few vegetables is still tasty pizza but provides only half the calories and a good deal more fiber than take-out pizza. Macaroni and cheese, hamburgers, and even cookies can be turned into healthy foods your child can enjoy but not overeat.

Will your child like these versions as much as, say, pizza from your local pizzeria? Quite likely yes, but whatever the answer, one thing you can be sure of is that he will find them more filling and won't eat as much—and you will have achieved your goal of a voluntary calorie reduction! It's critical, incidentally, to make sure that the whole family eats the new foods,

WHAT IS THE GLYCEMIC INDEX?

The glycemic index is a measure of how quickly carbohydrate-containing foods are digested to release glucose into the bloodstream. Rapidly digested carbohydrates have a high glycemic index, while slowly digested carbohydrates have a low glycemic index.

Although several recent diet books have based their recommendations on the glycemic index, there have never been any good research data to support the claims—until now. A research study from my own laboratory has provided the first direct evidence that foods with a low or moderately low glycemic index actually decrease hunger and overeating in overweight children. When provided with a breakfast and lunch having a moderate or low glycemic index, the children in our study were less hungry and ate fewer calories in the afternoon compared to when they were given a breakfast and lunch with the same amount of calories but a high glycemic index.

The difference in hunger and overeating was traced to the metabolic effects of the glycemic index. The foods with a high glycemic index caused massive spikes in blood glucose and the hormone insulin, followed by a precipitous fall in blood glucose to below fasting levels. And because low blood glucose is one of the signals that tell the brain that food is needed, the subjects became extremely hungry. Foods with a low or moderately low glycemic index, in contrast, moderated glucose and insulin levels, and in consequence reduced hunger and the desire to eat.

Most vegetables, fruits, and beans, especially the ones containing plenty of fiber, have a low glycemic index (because fiber decreases the glycemic index by slowing digestion). In addition, raw fruits and vegetables tend to have a lower glycemic index than cooked ones, and whole cereal grains have a lower glycemic index than flour made from those grains. In both cases, this is because the firmer texture slows digestion. Foods such as meat and fish also have a low glycemic index because they mainly contain protein, which doesn't affect blood glucose and insulin.

not just your overweight child. Otherwise he will feel punished and unloved, and the whole plan will backfire.

And remember that you certainly don't need to feel guilty about depriving your child of foods he loves. Children are remarkably resilient, and given a little time your child will learn to enjoy the new foods you serve. Provided you show him how much you love him in other ways, he probably won't care that some old favorites are off the menu. And as you change the foods your child eats, you will also have the satisfaction of knowing that you are helping him avoid the lifelong struggles with food and eating that afflict so many adults today.

Bear in mind that variety is the spice of life, but not when it comes to carbohydrates, desserts, high-caloric beverages, and condiments. As discussed in Chapter 2, variety is an important factor determining calorie intake. This works for your child when the variety instinct helps him seek out fruits and vegetables, but it can work against him, too. New research from my own laboratory is showing that too great a variety of high-calorie foods encourages overeating, whereas a smaller variety of the same foods encourages moderation.

When you offer your child a plentiful variety of fresh fruits and vegetables and high-fiber cereals while offering a smaller number of high-calorie options, you encourage him to eat the one or more cups of fresh fruits and vegetables daily that minimize his desire for other (higher-calorie) items. This is easier to say than to do, of course, because it often involves rethinking shopping lists and popular family menus, as well as sacrificing some foods that you enjoy yourself. But be reassured: As we mentioned before, it is much harder for you than for your child (he likely won't notice that anything unusual is happening), and it gets easier over time as the new patterns become familiar.

For best results offer at least three, and preferably more, different fruits or vegetables daily (for example, one with breakfast, one with lunch, and two with dinner). *Don't,* incidentally, focus on fruits to the exclusion of vegetables. Vegetables are more protective against obesity than any other food group, because they are particularly low in both glycemic index and caloric density.

Desserts are very important in the context of variety, because we eat them even after we have had a good main course and are no longer hungry. For this reason, simply abandoning sweets and desserts is the best plan if you can bear it. If you just can't, consider offering a controlled amount of something sweet at snack time instead. A small piece of plain cake, a little frozen yogurt, or a plain cookie along with some pieces of fruit, in place of juice and crackers, is perfectly okay provided that the portion size is right. This way your child can enjoy something sweet without its interfering with his calorie regulation at lunch and dinner.

MEAL AND SNACK SUGGESTIONS FOR A CHILD GROWING DOWN THE PERCENTILES

Instead of these	Try these alternatives with lower caloric density and/or lower glycemic index
BREAKFAST	
Refined cereals with whole or 2 percent milk	Whole-grain cereals with at least 2 grams fiber per $1/2$ cup, served with skim or 1 percent milk or plain low-fat yogurt
White bread, toast with butter	Whole-wheat or oatmeal bread, lightly buttered
Bagel with cream cheese	Whole-grain bagel with a little lite cream cheese or a thin smear of regular cream cheese
Pancakes or waffles with syrup	Whole-grain or oatmeal pancakes or waffles with fruit sauce or a small amount of lite syrup and no butter
Muffins (including commercial low-fat varieties)	Whole-wheat or oatmeal muffins with fruit pieces
LUNCH	
White-bread sandwiches with high-calorie fillings such as peanut butter and jelly or tuna with mayonnaise	Any sandwich on whole-wheat, oatmeal, or rye bread; white-bread sandwiches if filling is lean (e.g., turkey and lettuce with one thin slice of cheese and no mayonnaise, tuna salad made with lite mayonnaise or yogurt and shredded carrots)
Macaroni and cheese	Homemade macaroni and cheese with a lower fat content and whole-wheat pasta
Pasta with alfredo sauce	Pasta with tomato sauce and Parmesan cheese
DINNER	
Pizza	Oatmeal- or whole-wheat-crust pizza with less cheese and more vegetables
Fried or fast-food chicken nuggets	Baked chicken nuggets
Sausages, hot dogs, fried entrees	Lean entrees with meat, fish, poultry, and beans
Cheeseburger, fast-food hamburgers	Homemade lean hamburgers (90 percent lean meat) with whole-wheat rolls, lettuce and tomato or ketchup and relish, no mayonnaise

French fries, onion rings	Baked potato or potato mashed with milk, and plenty of raw and cooked vegetables of all kinds
Desserts such as ice cream, cake, cookies, cheesecake, muffins, brownies	Fresh fruit, fresh fruit salad with no added sugar
SNACKS	
Regular cookies, chips, pretzels, crackers, popcorn with butter, candy, chocolate, granola bars, puddings	Higher-fiber, lower-caloric-density cookies, plain low-fat yogurt mixed with fresh fruit, breakfast cereals with fiber, fruit and vegetable sticks, air-popped popcorn, whole-grain bread lightly spread with hummus or reduced-fat cottage cheese, reduced-fat hard cheese, low-fat chips served with no-fat salsa
DRINKS	
Whole milk, chocolate milk, juice, juice drinks, and sodas	16–24 ounces unflavored 1 percent or skim milk (less if yogurt and cheese are also eaten), a maximum of 4 ounces juice, and water for thirst

Drinks have calories, too, so controlling what your child drinks is as important as stocking your pantry with the right foods. Water, skim or 1 percent milk (up to 16 to 24 ounces daily), and juice (up to 4 ounces daily, diluted with water if your child prefers) are all good, with water for additional thirst. More milk or juice means excess calories. Avoid regular sodas, fruit drinks, and flavored milks altogether to save unnecessary calories. Total sugar consumption is now at the all-time high, and more than half of this sugar comes from soda and juice drinks.

Be patient and keep at it. You will quite likely find that starting to offer your child foods from the "try these" list will automatically encourage him to eat fewer calories than he would if he ate mostly from the "instead of this" list. If he does not immediately take to the new foods you are offering, you will need to switch gradually over a period of a few weeks or months, using psychological strategies such as the bridge of familiarity and the rule of fifteen to gain acceptance.

With gradual changes, you can introduce quite a number of new and healthier foods without your child's being very aware that anything has happened. If an older child does notice something and wants to know why you are not cooking the same things anymore, you can explain to him that you are changing the types of foods you keep in the house because you love your family and want everyone to grow up strong and healthy, and the new foods will do this better than what you used to eat. A simple explanation of this kind, without any mention of fatness, can help make a smooth transition.

Other smart strategies to speed acceptance of new foods are described in Chapter 2 and the chapters devoted to feeding children at specific ages.

4. AVOID FOOD RESTRICTIONS

Restricting the total amount of food your child is allowed to eat at mealtimes is not a good idea because, in addition to being hard to enforce, it can make your child more determined to eat as much as he wants. In older children it may also result in sneaking food. Again, the best way to head off overeating is to consistently offer only healthier versions of favorite foods, and let your child lead the way when it comes to deciding whether he wants to eat or not. This way he will learn to recognize the internal signals of hunger and satiety that will help promote good weight control in the future.

In the unlikely event that after changing the types of foods you put on the table you still feel that portion control is called for, offer smaller portions of particular foods rather than the whole meal. If you make a large amount of, say, chicken casserole, keep the casserole off the table and serve everyone with an appropriate amount so that they can have seconds without overeating. If your child finishes his casserole and asks for more while leaving the rest of the meal on his plate, you can give him a little more and say the rest has been put away for another day. Make sure to provide other healthy foods to fill up on, such as a salad with dressing, raw vegetable strips, or whole-wheat rolls and fruit, so he never has to leave the table hungry.

There may also be a number of daily meals where your child eats fixed amounts that you simply put in front of him (for example, cereal and milk at breakfast). In these cases, you can reduce amounts by just a little, 10 or 15 percent, and very likely he won't even notice. If he does and asks for more, you can give him a little extra or provide a lower-calorie alternative such as apple slices to fill up on.

One time when you *can* refuse to give your child food is when he wants to snack in front of the TV. Children are amazingly place-specific about food. If you never allow chips or other high-calorie munchies in front of the TV, you'll save arguments as well as calories. For an already established habit, change the house rules and give your child a plausible explanation—one mother we know told the children it was because she didn't want crumbs on the carpet. You can mention health reasons if you like, but don't talk specifically about weight.

5. LIMIT EATING OUT

Unfortunately, child-friendly restaurants are usually no help if you're trying to manage a weight problem. Some do have low-fat or heart-healthy choices, but if that just means a dried-up salad with tasteless fat-free dressing, or a stale roll instead of french fries, what child is going to eat them?

For this reason, limiting the number of times you eat out is the best solution. With only one or two meals a week out, you don't have to worry too much about what gets eaten, and can focus your attention on food coming into your own house.

If eating out more regularly is necessary, set a good example by what you yourself order, and pick items as carefully as you can, focusing on caloric density and fiber rather than fat. You can also try offering your child a piece of fruit or some raw veggies before you go out. This will not reduce meal size for all children, but in those for whom it does, it can be an effective way to control outside meals while simultaneously encouraging good food habits.

6. DON'T FEED EMOTIONAL HUNGER WITH FOOD

Many adults eat out of habit, boredom, or stress rather than because they are hungry—and inadvertently teach their children to do likewise. This is often a major cause of unnecessary weight gain. With forethought and strategies, you can teach your child how to eat when her body needs food, rather than simply out of habit.

- Serve an age-appropriate number of meals and snacks, and don't give your child any food except low-calorie snacks such as carrots and apple slices at other times. Children older than one year don't need more than three meals and two snacks daily as a general rule; more than this provides excess calories and is an unhealthy substitute for other activities.

- Make sure that your child sits down at the table with at least one parent for at least two meals every day. Take time to talk about the day and enjoy a few minutes of relaxation. Meals eaten on the run do not provide the emotional satisfaction that everyone needs, and can lead to excess snacking on unhealthy foods at other times.

- Take time to show your child that you love and value her at nonfood times as well as at meals, to reinforce the important message that she is a wonderful person and your love for her is unrelated to whether or not she eats.

- Never use any kind of unhealthy food as a bribe. A bowl of ice cream exchanged for a promise of good behavior at the supermarket after lunch will only make ice cream seem more attractive, and will encourage your child to overeat whenever she feels vulnerable or wants a treat. If you have already started down this slippery slope, you may be able to simply stop or at least reduce the occasions gradually over a period of a few weeks. A bribe with healthy food is an entirely different story. One girl we know learned to love mangoes when her mother started occasionally bringing them home after work as a "special treat."

- Never give your child food when she is not hungry. It might seem kind, but it's actually a form of cruelty because of the weight problems it fosters. Giving your child a fancy dessert after she has already had a good dinner, offering her a cookie just because she is upset, or giving her juice when she is simply thirsty and needs water are all ways to inadvertently teach a child to overeat.

- If you want to treat your child, offer to spend some special time with her. If she is older than about two, you can even let her pick what to do. Children value individual time with their parents more than a whole mountain of ice cream or candy.

7. ENCOURAGE PHYSICAL ACTIVITY

Physical activity is tremendously important for all children, but perhaps especially for those who are overweight.

- Exercise influences the way hormones and enzymes work in the body—with the important result that foods can be burned rather than stored.

- It increases the amount of fat circulating in the bloodstream. Only when fat is in the bloodstream can it be used as fuel throughout the body. If your child is inactive, the fat stays in the fat cells and can't be used.

- Exercise increases the amount of muscle in your child's body. This is also important because muscle is one of best tissues for using fat as a fuel. These effects of physical activity not only occur when your child exercises but also carry over to boost metabolism at other times, when he is relaxing.

You don't, by the way, need to worry that exercise will simply make him hungry and cause him to eat more than ever. Although exercise may increase your child's appetite, the calories of extra food consumed will not be as much as the extra calories being burned.

To make sure your child has plenty of opportunities for vigorous play:

- Start by limiting television and videos to ten hours a week or less. It's sedentary time—twenty-four hours a week of it for the typical American child—and (in the case of commercial TV) also encourages a desire for the high-calorie snacks, sweets, and overly refined cereals seen in advertisements.

- Encourage physical activity by playing active games with your child or setting up vigorous activities for your child and her small friends. Dancing, running, tag, ball games, swimming, active play groups, romping with friends or parents, bike rides, and energetic games of imagination such as staging a circus or Olympic games are all healthy ways to have active fun. The greater variety of active games you can think up, the more your child will like them.

- Aim for your child to be vigorously active for at least one hour a day and up to twice as much if possible. This doesn't need to be all at one time, but should ideally be in periods lasting at least ten to fifteen minutes each to maximize the metabolic effect of the exercise.

IN BRIEF: KEYS TO HELPING YOUR CHILD "GROW DOWN THE CENTILES"

1. *Involve your pediatrician and have realistic goals.* You will maximize success by working within your child's genetic potential and planning to make permanent changes that are sustainable for the whole family.
2. *Do a reality check.* Record what your child eats for three days.
3. *Focus on good food choices.* Offer your child a variety of healthy foods and drinks at regular meals and snacks, and keep undesirable items out of the house. Offering the right food is your most effective weapon against excess weight.
4. *Avoid food restrictions.* Attempting to restrict your child's total food intake to less than she wants will backfire. What your child needs to learn is how to self-regulate her intake of healthy foods.
5. *Limit eating out.* It's hard to find restaurants that make reduced-calorie food suitable for children.
6. *Don't feed emotional hunger with food.* It's a major—and unnecessary—cause of excess weight gain.
7. *Encourage physical activity.* It helps normalize your child's weight by burning excess calories and building muscle.
8. *Give a daily multivitamin/mineral supplement.* It will ensure adequate nutrition as you work with your child's eating habits.

8. GIVE A DAILY MULTIVITAMIN/MINERAL SUPPLEMENT

A multivitamin/mineral supplement appropriate for your child's age will ensure adequate intakes of essential nutrients such as zinc that are particularly important for sustaining continued height gain while weight levels off.

BE CASUAL ABOUT SUCCESS

When you realize that not only are your son's pants too short now, but he also needs a slimmer fit, it is very tempting to comment out loud and congratulate him—but don't do it. Just as you avoided involving him in the treatment, you should continue to treat the outcome as no big deal. Through your good efforts your child has managed to grow down the centiles without becoming sensitive about his weight. Like many other special things you do for your child, this is an example of how good parenting is its own reward.

EATING DISORDERS: EVERY CHILD IS AT RISK

Anne, a slim young woman of nineteen, has bulimia. Food obsesses her, and most days, after eating a big dinner with her family, she heads out to the store and buys a cake or a bag of cookies and a jar of peanut butter, which she smuggles home and eats secretly before vomiting it all up to prevent herself from getting fat. Anne is much too ashamed to seek help, and is devastated when her terrible secret is discovered. Her case history documents obsessions with food and body weight going back to age six, when she started secretly eating raw flour in the pantry. Her mother, herself a lifelong dieter, had told her she was getting fat and that she should not eat so much.

Eating disorders only appear to be much less common than obesity. They are a hidden problem, as Anne's story illustrates, and are fatal in up to 5 percent of cases. Every child is at risk, especially in our weight-conscious society.

Preoccupations with body weight and food are among the seeds of eating disorders. They are not the only factors, of course, but they do make an important contribution. Where do these preoccupations come from? In the case of our children, they come in part from watching us, their parents. Television, magazines, videos, popular music groups, and their peers are all important, too, but as parents, we play an important role because of our children's instincts to copy everything we do when they are young.

More than two-thirds of adults think they are overweight, and more than a third are dieting at any given time. If your child hears you talking about wanting to lose weight or sees you weighing yourself, she may want to do the same. And sometimes tragically, she does. Dieting obsessions are frequently seen in girls and boys as young as eight to eleven years old, and can start years earlier.

Here is what you can do to help prevent an eating disorder in the future:

- Do, at every age, work to help your child develop and maintain the food self-regulation skills that she needs to stay on the right track. Encouraging her to decide whether she is hungry or thirsty (or both) at snack time from age eighteen months on, reminding her that she doesn't have to finish all her dinner if she doesn't want to, and never offering food just because she is upset are just a few of the ways you can encourage her to listen to her internal signals about when she is hungry or full. More details on how to help your child's eating behavior are given in Chapter 2 and in the chapters on feeding children at different ages.

- Try to keep your own dieting or eating problems private from your child. If you do diet, choose a plan that lets you eat normal foods at mealtimes when you are home. Your child probably will not notice that you eat smaller portions than normal or that you are eating more vegetables and less pasta. She will, however, notice liquid replacement meals and other unusual diet foods.

- If another adult says inappropriate things—for example, telling your child to eat less, or talking about her body fat—ask him or her to stop immediately. Exert damage control by telling your child that everyone is different—some are big and some are small, and you think she has a very nice body that is just the size it is supposed to be right now.

- Use your role as gatekeeper of the household food to keep a plentiful variety of fruit, vegetables, whole grains, lean meats, and low-fat milk in the house rather than too many highly processed, low-fiber, high-fat, and high-sugar foods. To be protected against eating disorders, children with overweight tendencies need to learn self-regulation skills on healthy rather than unhealthy food choices. By giving your child the opportunity to learn to enjoy healthful foods, you make it easier for her to maintain a weight that is right for her without resorting to extreme measures.

COMMON PROBLEMS AND FREQUENTLY ASKED QUESTIONS

Two-year-old Jeffrey is overweight, and his parents have started giving him healthier foods. The trouble is, he won't eat them. Whole-wheat sandwiches go untouched, and fruit for dessert is disdained. His parents can't live with the idea that he might go to bed hungry, and so every night he ends up eating the foods they were trying to keep away from him.

Jeffrey's parents are quite likely dealing with the classic situation of a fussy two-year-old rather than the specific rejection of healthy foods. At around two most children get much more conservative about food, and new things are rejected in favor of old favorites. For this reason, Jeffrey's parents need to try some of the smart strategies described in Chapters 2 and 11. In the meantime, they should know that no child who is treated kindly and with respect will starve himself for more than a meal or two. A pediatrician should also be involved to monitor weight and height.

They should start by making a list of the foods Jeffrey likes and then picking from those the healthy choices, being careful to keep less healthy options out of the house. The already accepted foods can form the basis of the new menu. New foods that are introduced should be as similar to old ones as possible, to create a bridge of familiarity. Although some experts recommend that parents try to get their children to take at least one bite of each food, we find that saying the food is new and good but that they *don't* have to eat it is more effective!

Jeffrey's parents should also understand the value of patience and of offering him *opportunities* to eat rather than insisting. Remember that it often takes fifteen tries for a new food to be fully accepted. Knowing that even meals when new foods are not tasted can help contribute to long-term acceptance should help provide some of the patience that will be needed. In the meantime, a children's multivitamin/mineral supplement will provide essential nutrients and take away the worry that Jeffrey will become nutritionally deprived while learning to enjoy his new meals.

Susan, mother of two-year-old Tess and nine-month-old Matthew, feels helpless about the fact that both of her children are already over the 95th centile for weight even though their height is on the 50th centile. Tracing the problem to genetics (both she and her husband are not overweight, but have to struggle to stay that way), Susan tells us that she gives her children healthy food but that they are still gaining too much weight. Her own mother tells her it is baby fat and nothing to worry about, while her doctor has told her (correctly) that putting them on a diet should be off-limits, but has not given her any advice on what she should do instead.

A detailed case history from Susan documented two common problems. First of all, she thinks she is feeding her children a good diet, but they actually get quite a lot of high-calorie, high-glycemic-index, low-fiber foods, including take-out pizza, commercial-mix pancakes, and hot dogs. Switching to similar foods with fewer calories and more fiber and vegetables will help Susan to reduce her children's unnecessary overeating, as will making sure all involved adults are in the same place about what goes on the table. Second, Susan is giving her daughter juice throughout the day when she is thirsty. Substituting water (by gradually diluting the juice more and more with water over a few days) will ensure that Tess learns to enjoy drinking no-calorie water when she is thirsty, and will help reduce calories to a healthy level.

Peter is six months old and already has rolls and rolls of fat. He is always hungry and will eat anything. His parents would like to do something but feel helpless in the face of his insistent demands for food.

Although six months is too early to start any weight-correction program, Peter's parents can think about whether some simple changes are appropriate now. Sometimes infant-parent teams get on the wrong feeding track, and it becomes the parents' responsibility to move over to a better one. Because infants have so few ways to express their needs, and because some infants are less good than others at expressing their feelings, parents can get into the habit of solving all problems, not just hunger, with food. When this happens some infants will happily get used to having boredom, anxiety, thirst, and other problems solved with a bottle of milk, a breast-feeding, or a bowl of cereal. It may seem hard at first to substitute a game, walk, bottle of water, or cuddle for food, but this is what is needed, and a little persistence may bring results in a surprisingly short time.

Peter's parents should first keep a record of how much they feed Peter in a typical day. The average six-month-old needs only 30 to 35 ounces of milk, 2 ounces of strained fruit or juice, and 1 ounce of baby cereal per day, and Peter may be eating much more than this. If they are feeding amounts much above the recommendations, Peter's parents can try nonfood ways to solve their infant's problems first, gradually reducing the daily amount of milk to a more normal level. Giving only milk, incidentally, rather than a mixed diet, is not appropriate for a baby of Peter's age. He needs to get used to eating solid food during this time, when he is instinctively programmed to want it, and in any case many solid foods have fewer calories than milk. Making sure that Peter has the opportunity to try crawling and games that encourage movement is also important, because it will help burn calories and reduce the amount of weight he gains. If Peter continues to gain excess weight, he should be examined by a specialist with experience in the very rare syndromes of genetic obesity.

Amanda is a cheerful four-year-old girl who weighs herself when she goes to the bathroom. She also pretends to do "her exercises" so that she "doesn't get fat." Is this behavior normal, or something that her parents should try to change?

Weighing herself and making up games about being fat is definitely not normal. Amanda is copying somebody who has a weight problem (or is worried they do) and is letting Amanda in on it. If her parents are dieting, they should discuss their progress when Amanda is not around. If they think the problem comes from elsewhere, they should talk to the adults Amanda sees regularly. With the elimination of such adult behaviors to copy, Amanda will soon forget about them and find new games to play.

John is one year old and on the 90th centile of weight for height. Neither of his parents is overweight, and they wonder if they should do anything or not.

It is unusual, though less so than even ten years ago, to find two normal-weight parents and an overweight child. More often than not the child is simply growing unevenly and his weight will normalize over time. It is also possible, however, that his parents are not feeding him in the best way. For now, rather than actively trying to change the foods he is eating, they should be aware that a problem could develop and should get him measured for weight and height at eighteen and twenty-four months before embarking on any treatment program. They should also read Chapter 10 on what foods are normal at this age. Sometimes a simple change such as substituting water for juice above 4 ounces per day or reducing milk to 16 to 24 ounces daily is all that is needed.

Two-year-old Jason was overweight by the age of six months, and on their own initiative his parents introduced strict dietary measures. Jason actually lost weight, but has also moved from the 50th height centile down to the 25th. Is this connected with his weight loss, and if so, what should his parents do?

It is likely, although not certain, that Jason's loss of growth in height has been caused by his parents' being too strict about what foods they let him have. Children under six years of age should never be placed on a weight-loss diet because it can cause stunting and nutritional deficiencies. Jason's parents should introduce a wider range of foods into his diet, especially higher-fat but also healthy foods such as unhydrogenated peanut butter and entrees prepared with vegetable oil. They should also give Jason a children's multivitamin/mineral supplement, because it is possible that zinc deficiency is responsible rather than too few calories. If food is the problem, Jason's parents can expect to see a growth spurt in the next few months.

CHAPTER 16

———————— ✿ ————————

About Allergies, Food Intolerances, and Colic

Allie, now two, has been suffering from severe eczema and nagging bronchial wheezing since she was nine months old. The irritation from the eczema is so severe that Allie's pediatrician has told her parents to put cotton gloves on Allie's hands at night to keep her from scratching herself in her sleep. Several diagnostic tests have failed to identify a problem, but something is wrong. What is it?

A dverse reactions to foods may take many forms. While most people think of allergies in terms of the coldlike symptoms of hay fever, in fact food allergies and intolerances can also cause a wide range of other respiratory symptoms, as well as vomiting, diarrhea, gastrointestinal discomfort, skin rashes, and more.

In poor Allie's case, symptoms were eventually traced to foods eaten in infancy, when her body was not yet able to avoid becoming sensitized. With the right diagnosis and some remedial steps, further food reactions were headed off, but Allie's case underlines the fact that food allergies and intolerances can be difficult to pin down, even for pediatricians.

Many food reactions go undiagnosed, causing needless suffering for young children and their families. A program to weed out the causes of these reactions can be set up at home with the help of your pediatrician, but the better solution is to prevent them in the first place. For families without a particular susceptibility to allergies, three simple steps for routine prevention are outlined on pages 282–284. If you have a family history of allergies, additional preventive measures are described on pages 284–288.

If, on the other hand, your child is already showing symptoms you can't explain, you may want to read the whole chapter. Let's talk first about the signs that send parents to the doctor with the question "Could my child have allergies?"

RECOGNIZING ALLERGIES AND INTOLERANCES

The spectrum of allergic/intolerant reactions includes the following symptoms, which are increasingly being reported in infants and young children:

Most common symptoms

- Vomiting
- Excessive spitting up
- Diarrhea
- Colic
- Bloody stools
- Upper respiratory problems such as sneezing, nasal congestion, and runny nose
- Reactive airway problems such as wheezing, coughing, and asthma
- Skin rashes, including hives and eczema

Occasional and suggested but not proven symptoms

- Facial symptoms such as puffiness and dark circles under the eyes
- Severe sleeping difficulties (see Chapter 14)
- Failure to thrive (that is, poor growth and subsequent delayed development)
- Severe headaches or migraines
- Increased or decreased blood pressure
- Attention deficit hyperactivity disorder in older children (see Chapter 17)
- Ear infections

Food reactions can develop rapidly, within minutes or hours, or gradually, over days or weeks, and one symptom or several may be present. In controlled studies of children with proven food allergies, approximately 50 to 60 percent have diarrhea or vomiting (either chronic or intermittent), 50 to 70 percent have skin rashes (hives or eczema), and 20 to 30 percent have respiratory symptoms. However, if your child does develop some of these symptoms, your first assumption should be a viral or bacterial infection (especially if she also has a fever, which is not an allergy symptom), and you should consult your pediatrician accordingly. Food allergies should be considered only after seven to ten days of persistent symptoms.

If the symptoms don't disappear, your child's health care provider can help you decide whether they warrant further investigation. If the problem continues and you don't find an immediate cause, it's important to keep trying. Sometimes identifying whether foods are the problem—and if so, which ones—takes time and effort by everyone involved. Observant and involved parents can be the crucial element in solving the puzzle.

FOOD ALLERGIES AND FOOD INTOLERANCES ARE DIFFERENT

Most people don't realize that, strictly speaking, food allergies and food intolerances are different. However, because it can be difficult to determine whether a food reaction is an allergy or an intolerance, "food intolerance" has become a general term that can mean both.

Food allergies are caused by an immune-system reaction to foreign substances in the body, usually proteins. In about 5 to 10 percent of infants and children, some proteins not made by the human body cause an allergic reaction. They might be the proteins in cow or soy milk, egg whites, fish, peanuts, or some other food. The resulting symptoms—for example, vomiting, diarrhea, or eczema—are caused by the chemicals made by the immune system as it goes overboard trying to repel the alien proteins. Once an allergic sensitivity has been set up, just tiny amounts of the offending protein can trigger the immune reaction all over again.

Food allergies start in the first year of life in about 80 percent of cases. The most common food allergy is to the protein called ß-lactoglobulin, found in cow's milk, which affects 2 to 8 percent of all babies under one year. Infants up to four months of age are particularly susceptible to the development of a food allergy, because their intestinal tracts are immature and quite easily let significant amounts of partially undigested protein slip directly into the bloodstream. The source of the foreign protein is usually formula or solid foods, but can also be breast milk when the mother absorbs some undigested food proteins and passes them on to her baby.

FOOD CAUSES OF ALLERGIES AND INTOLERANCES

COMMON CAUSES

Cow's milk and products containing it

Egg whites

Peanuts and tree nuts (walnuts, pecans, cashews, pistachios, hazelnuts, and almonds)

Beans and bean products, including soybeans and soy milk

Fish and shellfish

LESS COMMON CAUSES

Wheat products such as bread and pasta

Citrus fruits, tomatoes, and strawberries

Chocolate

Chicken

Mushrooms

Food additives (such as tartrazine, sulfites, monosodium glutamate, benzoates)

Pesticide residues

Hormone residues in milk, beef, and chicken

If your family is bothered by allergies of any kind—ranging from dust or pollen to foods—your child will have an increased susceptibility to allergies in general, including food allergies. But this is not to say that he will definitely have allergies. You have an important role to play in whether your child's immune system gets activated to cause allergies during his early years.

Some infants from susceptible families will develop a food allergy despite everyone's best efforts. For those who do, it's necessary to track down the offending food or foods and eliminate them. This can be inconvenient and take time, but there is good news, too. Food allergies that develop during early infancy, unlike pollen and dust allergies that develop later, don't always last a lifetime. Milk, soy, and egg allergies, in particular, usually disappear by three years, and sometimes earlier.

Food intolerances differ from food allergies in several ways, though symptoms can be similar. An intolerance is a reaction to food that doesn't involve the immune system. With intolerances, it's often the case that small amounts of the problem food can be tolerated, while with allergies—because of their link to the immune system—even the smallest amount can trigger a reaction.

The bad side of intolerances is that the body almost never gets over them. There are many different kinds, and they are genetically linked: If both you and your spouse have the same intolerance, there is generally a 25 to 100 percent chance that your child will have it, too. Because of this link, intolerances come to stay, and sufferers—and their parents—have to find ways of permanently dealing with them.

The most common type of food intolerance is caused by the lack of an enzyme needed to metabolize a particular nutrient or substance in food. Lactose, or milk sugar (the carbohydrate in milk), may be the most widely known example. Lactose intolerance occurs in 70 to 80 percent of adults worldwide (relatively more in people of African and Asian descent, and less in Caucasians) and is caused by the lack of the digestive enzyme lactase, which is needed to break down lactose in the intestine before it is absorbed. Production of lactase can start diminishing early in childhood, and when this happens, the lactose stays in the intestine, rather than being absorbed, and is then metabolized by the intestinal bacteria to produce gases that lead to cramping, bloating, and pain. Lactose intolerance is uncommon before four years in otherwise healthy white children and before two years in nonwhite children.

Interestingly, biologists have shown that lactose intolerance was the original human condition. Prehistoric humans lost the ability to digest lactose in early childhood, but accidental gene mutations about ten thousand years ago gave some families the ability to keep producing lactase throughout life—and with it came the ability to drink large amounts of milk. This gene (which arose around the time when dairy farming was invented) was not especially needed by Africans and Asians, because they didn't practice dairy farming and lived primarily in warm climates where there was plentiful sunlight (needed for their skin to synthesize vitamin D) to allow maximum absorption of available calcium. However, the new gene *was* needed by white families living in the cold

SOME FOOD INTOLERANCES AND THEIR SYMPTOMS*

Problem Constituent	Foods It Is Found In	Symptoms in Sensitive Individuals
NATURAL FOOD COMPONENTS		
Phenylethylamine	Chocolate, aged cheeses	Migraine headaches
Tyramine	Aged cheese, French-style cheeses, yeast, tofu, sausages, bologna	Migraine headaches, red or white itchy skin patches, high blood pressure
Histamine	Fermented cheeses such as blue cheese, fermented foods (for example, sauerkraut), pork sausages (but not fresh pork), French-style and Swiss-style cheeses, canned tuna, anchovies, sardines, spinach, eggplant, yeast	Red skin patches, headaches, decreased blood pressure
Histamine-releasing agents	Shellfish, chocolate, strawberries, tomatoes, peanuts, pork, pineapple	Itching, red or white skin patches, eczema
Cyanide residue	Almonds, lima beans, cassava, and seeds of fruits such as apples, peaches, and plums	Weakness and blindness

northern climates, because vitamin D could only be synthesized by the skin during a few months every year when the sun was strong, and the extra calcium provided by milk counterbalanced the lack of vitamin D. The strong bones and protection against premature heart disease that calcium provided to families with the new gene would have caused the gene to be favored in natural selection. Nowadays vitamin D is added to food, so nobody has to rely entirely on sunlight for this essential nutrient, but our ancestors didn't have that advantage, and this one factor likely

Problem Constituent	Foods It Is Found In	Symptoms in Sensitive Individuals
FOOD ADDITIVES AND CONTAMINANTS		
Tartrazine or FD&C yellow no. 5	Yellow or yellow/orange-colored foods, soft drinks, medicine	Hives, rash, asthma
Benzoic acid or sodium benzoate	Soft drinks and some cheeses, salt-free margarines, and processed potato products	Hives, rash, asthma
Sulfites, metabisulfites, bisulfites, and sulfur dioxide	Shrimp, many processed foods, instant potatoes, dried fruits, acidic juices, and items in salad bars	Acute asthma, anaphylaxis, loss of consciousness
Monosodium glutamate	Chinese and Japanese dishes	Headache, weakness, sweating, chest pain, rapid heart rate, dizziness, and numbness of arms and legs

* Modified from *Krause's Food, Nutrition and Diet Therapy,* by L. Mahan and S. Escott-Stump. W. B. Saunders Co.

played a significant role in determining which families survived and which didn't.

The extent of lactase deficiency varies between individuals. One person might have to be very careful about all lactose in his diet, while another could drink perhaps two glasses of milk per day and be fine but would have trouble with three. Because of this, knowing the lactose content of different dairy foods can be very helpful in deciding what foods to offer your child and whether a lactase supplement (for example, Lactaid) is necessary at particular meals.

Lactose Content of Common Foods

FOOD	LACTOSE (GRAMS)
Milk, ice cream (1 cup)	10–14
Yogurt, frozen yogurt (1 cup)	5
Cottage cheese (1 cup)	5
Aged cheddar (1 oz)	0.5
Parmesan (1 oz)	Trace
Rice Dream and most cereal and soy beverages	0

Some other food intolerances occur because the body has an adverse reaction to a toxin or chemical in the food. The symptoms are often less dangerous than allergies—but not always, as shown in the table on pages 280–281.

ROUTINE PREVENTION OF FOOD ALLERGIES

Even if you come from a family without any particular susceptibility to allergies, it is worth taking basic precautions to prevent them in your child. The prevalence of allergies is increasing, for reasons that scientists don't yet understand. It may be simply that they are being diagnosed more frequently. It may also be that they are more common because not enough attention has been focused on prevention.

The following are good preventive measures for all parents, and are critically important for families with a history of allergies.

1. BREAST-FEED IF AT ALL POSSIBLE

Breast milk is the best insurance that your baby will receive primarily human proteins in his early months. Studies have shown that infants with no family history of allergies have about a 4 percent risk of developing allergies if they are fed formula, compared with a 2 to 3 percent risk if they are breast-fed. If breast-feeding is not the right option for you, substitute only formula for the entire first year. Because the proteins are broken down by heat treatment, cow's-milk-based formula reduces the risk of allergies compared to cow's milk itself.

In addition to protecting against allergies, breast-feeding may reduce the risk of juvenile-onset diabetes, an autoimmune disease in which the immune system destroys the beta cells within the pancreas that makes in-

CAUTION: PREVENT PEANUT ALLERGY

Peanut and tree nut allergies are less common than some other food allergies (affecting about one percent of children and adults) but can cause unusually severe symptoms—which can be life-threatening in some cases. They can also be precipitated by tiny amounts of the offending food (even mere skin contact in a few cases) and only rarely disappear once they develop. The first noticed reactions to nuts usually include one or more of the following: hives; wheezing; swelling of the throat, tongue, hands, or legs; repetitive coughing; and, less commonly, vomiting and diarrhea. About one in five first-time reactions is life-threatening and requires emergency treatment with injected epinephrine. These are called anaphylactic reactions.

Because of the very severe reactions caused by peanuts and tree nuts, particular care is needed to avoid inadvertently sensitizing your child by offering them before twelve months. In addition to avoiding obvious nut sources such as whole nuts and peanut butter, read food labels to exclude foods containing nuts. Common items that contain nuts are cookies, desserts, cakes, candy, ice cream, and Chinese, Southeast Asian, African, and Middle Eastern foods.

sulin. Although juvenile-onset diabetes (which affects two in every thousand children) has a strong genetic component and is thought to be promoted by viruses such as mumps and dietary factors such as nitrosamines (see page 10), one recent study suggested that fully 14 percent of juvenile diabetes cases may be attributable to a lack of breast-feeding. The reason for this protective effect of breast milk is not known for sure. However, the combination of the protective immune factors in breast milk and the lack of stimulation of the immune system by foreign proteins (such as in formula) probably prevents the early overactivation of the immune system that initiates beta-cell destruction.

2. STICK WITH BREAST MILK, FORMULA, AND PERHAPS A LITTLE WATER BEFORE FOUR MONTHS

Research has shown that giving solid foods earlier than four months increases the risk of allergies. One study showed a 30 percent prevalence of eczema at one year of age in infants who were introduced to four or more solids before four months, compared to a 4 percent prevalence in infants who were not introduced to solids until four months or later. Even small amounts of some foods can trigger an allergic reaction if given too early; a single lick of ice cream at two months can be all it takes. Occasionally it may be necessary to give solid foods early, when the risk of allergies is outweighed by some medical factor, but generally it is something to avoid.

3. BE CAUTIOUS ABOUT WHAT YOU FEED YOUR BABY BETWEEN FOUR AND TWELVE MONTHS

Rice cereal, considered to have less allergenic potential than other weaning foods, is a good first choice. If rice cereal is well tolerated, you can slowly introduce other safe foods on the "Good Solid Foods to Try" list (pages 140–141), being careful to not introduce each food before the recommended time to minimize the risk of food proteins directly entering the bloodstream.

ADDITIONAL STEPS FOR ALLERGY PREVENTION IN HIGH-RISK INFANTS

> *Mary nursed Daniel from birth. At five weeks Daniel developed colic and eczema. These symptoms continued until Daniel was eight weeks old, when Mary was advised to stop eating all dairy products. Daniel's colic and eczema cleared up completely within a week but came back promptly when she tried to eat dairy foods again.*

Daniel had a classic case of cow's-milk-protein allergy even though he was breast-fed. Contrary to common belief, food allergies and intolerances are not uncommon in breast-fed infants from high-risk families, unless extra precautions are taken. One study reported that breast-fed infants from families with allergies have a 20 to 30 percent risk of developing allergies, compared with a 49 percent risk for infants with a family history of allergies who were given formula.

If you or your partner has allergies or intolerances, you may already be putting pieces of the puzzle together, with some of those pieces being your symptoms or your child's. Many disorders run in families. Some of our research has dealt with adopted identical twins living in different families. During the course of these studies, Mel and I have continually been amazed at how strong an influence genetic inheritance plays in physiology, metabolism, and even personality. Susceptibility to food allergies and food intolerances is yet another trait where heredity is readily apparent.

There are some important things you can do to prevent food allergies in your child if your family is particularly susceptible. This good news comes with a caution, however, because you need to follow the directions carefully to maintain adequate nutrition for you and your baby.

1. CONSIDER MODIFYING WHAT YOU EAT DURING PREGNANCY AND NURSING

Recent research has shown that the adult intestinal tract is not as impermeable to food proteins as we used to think. Although the gastrointestinal tract was previously thought to digest food proteins into small particles of amino acids, we now know this does not always happen. In some people, a small number of partly undigested protein molecules actually gets directly into the bloodstream. From there they may pass directly to the baby—during pregnancy through the placenta, and during nursing through breast milk. One study identified cow's-milk proteins in the breast milk of about 50 percent of nursing mothers who drank milk. These food proteins can trigger allergic reactions in a sensitive baby in just the same way that they would if your baby actually ate them.

Some studies have shown that women who completely eliminate cow's milk and all dairy products, eggs, fish, and peanuts from their diet starting by the tenth week of pregnancy, and during lactation if they are nursing, substantially reduce the risk that their baby will develop allergies in the first year of life. One study showed a reduction from about 60 percent risk to about 15 percent for babies with two allergy-prone parents. On the other hand, other well-designed studies showed that changes in the mother's diet had no effect, perhaps because eliminating all high-risk foods is a challenge. Because food additives are also suspected of causing food reactions, an additive-free diet for the nursing mom until her baby is four to six months old may also help.

So if you have allergies in your family, should you give up high-risk foods during pregnancy and nursing? It can be a good option—but only if you can be sure to eat a balanced diet without milk, other dairy products, eggs, fish, peanuts, and soy products. Most people find this takes a lot of effort. If you're planning to try it, you should get a referral to a dietitian, who will review nutrient intake and probably suggest supplements for the extra calcium and iron that both you and your baby need. An easier option is just eliminating cow's milk and cow's-milk products, since these are the primary allergenic foods, and also eggs, peanuts, and soy products if someone in your family is allergic to them. General support for this latter option may be growing, with the British government (though not the U.S. government) now recommending that all nursing mothers avoid peanuts.

INSTEAD OF THIS:	TRY THIS:
Cow's milk, cheese, yogurt, and other dairy foods	Multivitamin/mineral supplement (as usually prescribed), calcium supplement (1,000 mg daily), and extra lean meat and poultry
Egg whites and fish	Meat, poultry, and whole grains
Nuts	Meat, poultry, whole grains, beans (not soy), peas, and lentils
Processed and spicy foods	Fresh vegetables and fruit and grains

2. EVERY ALLERGY-PRONE FAMILY NEEDS TO THINK ABOUT SPECIAL FORMULA OPTIONS

Not all women choose to nurse. Even if you are one who does, formula is important when you want or need to stop nursing, because cow's milk should be off-limits until your baby is one year old.

Standard cow's-milk formulas, such as Similac and Enfamil, are certainly better than cow's milk for preventing allergies, but the new generation of hydrolysate and elemental formulas described in Chapter 6 are better still. We do not recommend soy formulas to prevent cow's-milk allergies (except possibly for those that involve only skin reactions) because some research studies have documented that many children who react to cow's milk also react to soy protein. Studies have shown that the risk of allergies when your child drinks a hydrolysate formula is about the same as when she is breast-fed, and lower than for cow's-milk formula.

Probably the best of the widely available hydrolysates for preventing allergies, and unfortunately the most expensive (at about three times the cost of regular formulas), are Alimentum, Nutramigen, and Pregestimil. Good Start, which is marketed as a regular formula (and at about the same price as regular formula), was also originally made for this purpose. Although its proteins are indeed partially hydrolyzed, Good Start is made from milk whey (containing the highly allergenic ß-lactoglobulin), and whether for this reason or because of its only partial hydrolysis, it seems not to give the protection of the full hydrolysates and elementals. Nevertheless, it should be at least as good as the standard cow's milk formulas, and if you find the cost of the hydrolysates prohibitive, it may be worth a try.

Our only caution on the hydrolysates and elementals is a minor one. Because they have become widely available only in the last few years, they have not yet undergone the same level of scrutiny as the standard formulas. We do know that they support normal growth, but they are not yet officially recommended for general use. Thus far, they appear to provide all the key micronutrients as effectively as standard formulas. All that is missing at this point is long-term evidence from testing to show that they are comparable to regular formulas in every way.

3. GO SLOW ON INTRODUCING YOUR BABY TO SOLID FOODS

Babies typically start solid foods at around four months. Simply moving the time you first start solids back to six months rather than four, and then going slowly on introducing some of the foods that have the highest allergenic potential, will give your infant time to become developmentally mature. In addition:

- Cow's milk and dairy products should be rigorously avoided until twelve months. Remember that many, many foods contain dairy products, including some commercial breads, crackers, and cream soups, homemade mashed potatoes (if you add butter or milk), cheeses of all kinds, yogurt, pizza, and ice cream.

- Egg whites, shellfish, regular fish, nuts, soybeans, soy products, citrus fruits, tomatoes, strawberries, and chocolate should also be avoided until twelve months (for less allergenic foods such as rice, follow the guidelines in Chapter 9). This elimination list cannot guarantee that you won't encounter problems, since some people are allergic to the most unusual foods—one baby Mel encountered is allergic to rice cereal, while a man we know is allergic to apples—but at least it will give you the best chance.

- When introducing a food that has higher allergy potential, offer just a teaspoon or two on the first two occasions and avoid giving it within four days of another new potential allergy producer. Then if you have a problem, it will be easier to trace back to the offending food.

WHEN YOUR CHILD DEVELOPS A FOOD ALLERGY OR INTOLERANCE

Food allergies and food intolerances are distressing to both children and their parents. However, the good news is that eliminating the offending foods from your child's diet will stop the problems and let her lead a normal life.

Some studies have found that most allergic symptoms requiring referral to a specialist are traceable to a single food. If this happens to your child, the challenge for you and your physician is to pinpoint the exact food that is the problem. Then you can move on to help your child become symptom-free.

IDENTIFYING AND ELIMINATING PROBLEM FOODS

If you suspect a food allergy or intolerance, your child's primary-care physician will be able to perform several tests to narrow down the exact problem. Unfortunately, not all primary-care providers recognize that food allergies are an important cause of the symptoms we have discussed. In this case, if your child has problems that do not clear up with conventional treatments, you may need to ask for a referral to a specialist.

The doctor you work with will most likely ask you to keep a diary of what your child eats and recommend that you eliminate foods that your child had started eating immediately before the problems appeared. It will take a while to tell whether elimination of recently introduced foods has been successful—typically four to seven days, because the immune response (and the inflammation or tissue injury it causes) takes time to subside. Note that RAST (for radioallergosorbent) and skin patch tests are not considered completely reliable for detecting food allergies (in particular, they sometimes give false positive results).

If removing recently introduced foods from your child's diet doesn't stop the symptoms, your doctor will likely refer you to a specialist for a test called a *double-blind placebo-controlled* (or DBPC) *food challenge.* In this test, suspected allergenic foods are hidden in other foods, so that you and your child and your doctor do not know exactly which ones they are.

Reactions are recorded and the test repeated until it is certain which foods are causing your child's problem. If lactose intolerance is suspected, tests may be performed on your child's breath and stools to help confirm the diagnosis.

Another approach is the *sequential elimination diet,* which can be done at home with you as the administrator and record keeper. In this procedure, your pediatrician instructs you to eliminate each of the traditional allergy-provoking candidates from your child's diet, one by one, each for a period of about one week. As the process goes along, you can reintroduce the foods that don't appear to have any effect on your child's symptoms, so that you don't run the risk of having a diet that is too restricted.

In cases where the problem is an additive or natural component of several different foods, it may be necessary to try a stricter elimination diet. See Chapter 17 for information on multiple-food elimination diets.

Elimination diets can be time-consuming and tedious, especially if the problem food is an unusual one. But studies have shown that children benefit greatly over the long run from decreased symptoms, if patience is taken to get to the root of the problem.

Most often the allergy is to the food itself. Occasionally, however, a food allergy may be more elusive. For example, a test showing an allergy to rice cereal may mean that your baby is allergic to the rice itself, or it could be a reaction to an additive in the cereal. In that case a different brand or type of rice may be fine.

LIVING WITH A FOOD ALLERGY

Once an allergenic food has been identified, total removal of the culprit is generally necessary, because even small amounts will be enough to trigger the same reactions again. The following steps can reduce the risk that your child will consume a dangerous food.

- Minimize eating in restaurants, because you will never know exactly what they are cooking with. When you do eat out, tell your server what symptoms your child will get if he eats the particular items he is allergic to, so that your problem is taken seriously.

- Read labels of everything you buy in the supermarket. Check each item at intervals, especially if the box or package says something like "new recipe." It is quite common for recipe "improvements" to involve adding milk powder, nuts, or other ingredients you are trying to avoid.

- Avoid salad bar items altogether if the problem is sulfites, because they usually contain large amounts and are not labeled. Health food stores are often the best place to shop for products with few additives.

- Try recipe substitutes to make favorite recipes safe. The new recipes may not taste identical, and it might take a few tries to get the proportions right, but often you can end up with a good match. For example, rice and soy beverages can be substituted for milk (Lactaid milk can also be used if the problem is lactose intolerance, though it will not help if the problem is cow's-milk-protein allergy); additional liquid plus ½ teaspoon rising agent can replace egg in some cookie and muffin recipes; corn, rice, and potato flours and gluten-free wheat flours can be used in place of wheat flour; carob powder can replace chocolate (3 tablespoons for 1 ounce).

REINTRODUCTION AT ONE TO THREE YEARS

Because allergies (though not intolerances) to milk, soy products, and eggs usually subside during early childhood, you can eventually try reintroducing these foods in the hope that no bad reaction will occur and that they can become part of your child's normal diet again.

Reintroduction can take place as early as one year of age. If a reaction recurs at that time, the problem food should be stopped and tried again when your child is two or three. In many cases, your child will eventually be able to tolerate the problem food without an adverse reaction. But because you can't know whether a food will still cause an allergic reaction, the reintroduction should be carried out only after you have talked to your pediatrician. In cases where one or more severe reactions have occurred, the reintroduction should actually be performed under the direct supervision of a pediatrician, so that treatment is immediately available in rare cases of shock or respiratory distress.

CELIAC DISEASE

Alex, age two, has been getting thinner and thinner and eats less all the time, although he likes all kinds of foods. In the past year he has also had repeated problems with muscle cramping and mouth sores. His parents are worried and frightened that their once robust, active child has become thin, subdued, irritable, and constantly sick. After several diagnostic tests, their pediatrician identifies celiac disease, or gluten sensitivity. What does this mean?

Celiac disease, also known as celiac sprue, is a lifelong intolerance to gluten, a naturally occurring protein in several cereals (notably wheat, rye, and barley) that gives dough strength and elasticity and helps it rise. Consumption of gluten in susceptible individuals causes an immune reaction that destroys the intestinal villi (fingerlike projections where absorption takes place), leading to diarrhea, malabsorption, and growth failure. Less typical symptoms include general malaise, anemia, dermatitis, and neurological symptoms. About one in two hundred fifty adults and children have celiac disease. Others may have latent sensitivity—meaning that they may potentially develop the disease although it is currently dormant.

Failure to thrive and malnutrition are usual consequences of untreated celiac disease. In addition, celiac disease frequently weakens bones (due to impaired calcium absorption) and increases the risk of intestinal cancers in middle age (due to the chronic inflammatory response of the intestine to gluten).

Diagnosing celiac disease can sometimes take a while, because the symptoms can be caused by several different problems. Blood tests for gluten sensitivity are now available and give a strong indication of whether celiac disease is the problem. However, an intestinal biopsy may also be needed for a conclusive diagnosis because the blood tests are still not 100 percent accurate.

Almost all sufferers of celiac disease can be completely cured of their symptoms by removal of foods containing gluten from their diet. It is important, however, that *all* gluten be permanently removed from the diet—both to prevent a relapse in gastrointestinal symptoms and also to minimize the risk of future intestinal cancers. Because this can require a big effort, consulting an experienced dietitian and enlisting the help of support groups is often very helpful (see page 292).

Wheat, barley, rye, buckwheat, and alfalfa, and all foods made from them, contain gluten. Foods and food components containing hidden gluten include canned soups, hydrolyzed vegetable protein, modified food starch, imitation shellfish, and distilled vinegars. Gluten-free replacement carbohydrates are corn, corn flour, rice, rice flour, tapioca starch, gluten-free wheat flour and bread mix, and lima bean, potato, and soy flours. Oats contain proteins that are similar to gluten; they don't need to be rigorously avoided but shouldn't be a substitute cereal, either. There are several good recipe books to help make gluten-free food enjoyable for the whole family.

FURTHER INFORMATION

Celiac Disease Organizations

Celiac Disease Foundation (818–990–2354)
Celiac Sprue Association (402–558–0600)
Gluten Intolerance Group of North America (206–246–6652)

Books

Me and the Right Food Choices (for ages 5–7). A coloring activity book about food choices for celiac disease. Available from the Gluten Intolerance Group (see above)
The Gluten-Free Gourmet (series). Bette Hagman. Holt, 1995.
Gluten Intolerance. A recipe book available by mail order from the American Dietetic Association (800–877–1600, ext. 5000)

COLIC

Last but certainly not least, a word about food reactions and colic. Colic is a very common problem—about a quarter of all infants suffer from it, and it is terribly distressing to parents and infants alike. There are many definitions of colic, but the most common one is persistent crying at regular times (usually late afternoon) lasting at least three hours a day, several times a week. Colic typically starts at three to six weeks of age and lasts until your child is three to four months old.

There is no general agreement among doctors and scientists about what causes colic and how important food really is. Our opinion, based on evaluating recent research, is that food is important in between 5 and 25 percent of cases.

To combat colic, your first step is to document when your baby cries and how much. This might not seem necessary, and any amount of crying may seem awful, but unless you have a record of how bad the problem was before you started to fix it, it will be hard to tell whether or not you have made progress. You can use the chart on page 293 as a template for a typical day's recording. If the problem is colic, the symptoms—especially crying—should cluster at one or two times a day.

TIME	ESTIMATED MINUTES CRYING	TIME	ESTIMATED MINUTES CRYING
6–7 A.M.	_____	6–7 P.M.	_____
7–8 A.M.	_____	7–8 P.M.	_____
8–9 A.M.	_____	8–9 P.M.	_____
9–10 A.M.	_____	9–10 P.M.	_____
10–11 A.M.	_____	10–11 P.M.	_____
11–12 noon	_____	11–12 midnight	_____
12 noon–1 P.M.	_____	12 midnight–1 A.M.	_____
1–2 P.M.	_____	1–2 A.M.	_____
2–3 P.M.	_____	2–3 A.M.	_____
3–4 P.M.	_____	3–4 A.M.	_____
4–5 P.M.	_____	4–5 A.M.	_____
5–6 P.M.	_____	5–6 A.M.	_____

24-hours total _____ minutes per day

FOOD-BASED COLIC SOLUTIONS

There are four things to try after you have recorded baseline symptoms, depending on whether you're breast- or bottle-feeding. Each method should be tried for a full week to see if it is effective. This may seem horribly slow when what you want to do is help your baby and stop the crying, but a solution that doesn't seem to help on the first day may become more effective a few days later.

- **Burping technique.** Probably the most usual causes of colic are poor burping technique and crying itself. Both cause a lot of air to be swallowed, and that causes pain as the air expands and moves down the gastrointestinal tract. Some parents find an across-the-lap position, with their baby on his tummy, works better than the traditional shoulder position for burping. Gentle patting and stroking for four or more minutes in the middle and at the end of each feeding may be necessary, and even more frequently for very burp-prone babies.

- **Mom's diet.** For breast-fed babies, colic can sometimes result from the mother's diet. A recent study showed that babies whose mothers avoided cow's milk, other dairy products, chocolate, onions, and cruciferous vegetables such as broccoli and cabbage were 50 percent less likely to have colic than babies whose mothers ate these foods.

- **Nursing pattern.** Nursing mothers can also sometimes help a colicky baby by changing the way they nurse. Mothers usually nurse on both breasts at most feeds. But for babies with colic, nursing on a single breast for as long as the baby wants to feed may work better. When you nurse like this, your baby gets less of the watery first milk and more of the fat-rich milk at the end of the feed. It's been suggested that the fat in the hind milk slows the rate at which the milk empties from the stomach, making for more thorough digestion and so less colic. If you go this route, do remember to alternate breasts with each feed, and to feed for the same total amount of time on the one breast as you would if you were offering both breasts, so that your baby still gets all the milk he needs for proper growth and development.

- **Changing the formula.** Formula-fed babies who develop colic may simply be suffering from an undiagnosed reaction to cow's-milk protein in their formula, especially regular formula. Switching to a hydrolysate or elemental formula for seven to ten days will tell you whether this was a problem for your baby.

COMMON PROBLEMS AND FREQUENTLY ASKED QUESTIONS

Rachel, two months, spits up huge amounts of formula after practically every feed. There is nothing her mother has been able to do about this, and no amount of burping seems to help. Her mother is frustrated and wants to know if she should change to a different formula because of a formula allergy.

Spitting up—doctors call it *gastroesophageal reflux*—is quite common and not necessarily a sign of something wrong; some babies are just naturally spitty. Signs of a problem would be spitting up accompanied by a decreased number of wet diapers, respiratory problems such as wheezing or pneumonia, blue spells or difficulty breathing, a skin rash in several areas, irritability combined with a body position that looks consistent with pain, or blood in the spit-up or in the stool. These warrant a call to the doctor.

For simply spitty babies, giving smaller feeds more frequently may help. Rachel's mom should also make sure that her baby is in an upright position during and after feeds, and is placed on her stomach on a firm mattress at night to decrease the risk of aspiration during sleep (in babies who spit up very frequently, the increased risk of SIDS from the tummy-down position is thought to be less than the risk of choking from spit-up). The head of Rachel's bed also should be elevated to keep her more upright during sleep, by placing newspapers, blankets, or pillows *under* the crib mattress (not under her head).

If the spitting persists, Rachel should be taken to her pediatrician, who may recommend trying dry baby rice cereal mixed in every bottle of formula for two weeks (starting as early as three or four weeks if necessary), 1 tablespoon of cereal per 2 to 4 ounces of formula, increasing as necessary to no more than 1 tablespoon per 1 ounce. In this case, the hole in the nipple will have to be enlarged slightly to allow the thicker milk to flow out.

Samuel is four weeks old, and about one week ago started crying every day beginning at about 3 P.M. By the time his father gets home from work, his mother is frustrated, has a headache, and dumps Samuel into his dad's lap. His dad puts Samuel in a Snugli and takes a long walk. Eventually Samuel stops crying and falls asleep. His mother says that Samuel often starts crying right after a feed, is always hungry when he feeds, and will gobble a 4-ounce bottle almost nonstop. She also notes that he passes a lot of gas.

Samuel's problem—colic—can almost certainly be traced back to his swallowing too much air when he feeds. Some babies guzzle their milk, as Sam does, but won't burp up the air that goes along with it. The result is that the air gets down into the gastrointestinal tract and causes distention and cramping. This may not be the whole answer, but trying different nipples to find one that reduces the amount of air Sam swallows should help. Making sure he is gently burped for a few minutes after every ounce of formula should also help ensure that any air that goes down will come back up again in a controlled manner.

Bethany, at eight weeks, has vomiting and diarrhea with a rash on her skin. Her mother has already tried three standard formulas, but nothing seems to make the problem any better.

Bethany's pediatrician needs to be consulted here, as an allergy may be involved. Switching to a hydrolysate formula (see Chapter 6) for seven to ten days to see if that helps will determine whether the first suspicion of a cow's-milk-protein allergy can be confirmed. Occasionally further tests will confirm a cow's-milk-protein allergy that was not alleviated by using a hydrolysate, in which case the elemental formula Neocate is indicated. Because elemental formulas contain no protein (instead they supply amino acids, the simple building blocks of proteins), they are theoretically without any allergy risk, although very rarely an infant may react to other parts of the formula.

It is also possible that Bethany simply has an infection. If so, her symptoms should disappear in a few days. To see whether it was really a formula problem, her parents can try reintroducing a bottle of regular formula again in two weeks, and note whether symptoms come back. If they do not, she can go back to a standard formula.

Mary is breast-feeding five-week-old Michael, who has suddenly developed colic and eczema. His pediatrician recommends that Mary stop breast-feeding and give formula instead, but she is reluctant to take this step.

Eczema and colic are signs that something is certainly wrong and needs to be taken seriously, but Mary is right in being reluctant to give up nursing. It may not be the problem, and even if it is, there may be a solution that does not involve switching to bottle-feeding.

The combination of colic and eczema suggests that Michael is allergic to something in Mary's milk, most likely undigested pieces of cow's-milk protein. Having said this, switching to standard formula is not the right answer, because chances are Michael will react to the cow's-milk protein in formula, too. Mary could try eliminating all cow's-milk products from her own diet and waiting seven days to see if there is an improvement, making sure that she gets enough essential nutrients from other foods and a daily multivitamin/mineral supplement plus a calcium supplement. She has to be 100 percent careful with these dietary changes (including reading all product labels), because even small amounts of a problem protein will be enough to produce the reactions being seen.

If the symptoms persist, Mary can try a stricter diet, removing all soy products, eggs, peanuts, fish, chocolate, and strong spices as well as dairy foods. She can also try feeding from one breast at a time for fifteen to twenty minutes, and may additionally want to avoid cruciferous vegetables such as broccoli. If she still sees no improvement in the eczema or colic after ten days, she should consider switching to a hydrolysate formula for seven days. If she pumps breast milk during this time, she should be able to resume nursing again if the formula does not help.

Angie, age two, has recently been demanding to be carried everywhere, and has been crying when forced to walk herself. In addition, she has been extremely irritable and has less appetite than usual. After several visits to her pediatrician, Angie is diagnosed with juvenile rheumatoid arthritis. What can be done to help her?

Juvenile rheumatoid arthritis is not common (about one in a thousand children develops it) but typically starts between one and three years in susceptible children. It's a serious autoimmune disorder in which a chronic immune response is triggered, in a few cases by repeated shigella infections or by an otherwise silent food allergy. In addition to prescription anti-inflammatory medications, identifying problem foods will help if an undiagnosed food allergy is part of the problem. If this proves to be the case, Angie's parents can design an elimination diet in collaboration with her pediatrician to identify offending foods. Although this will not cure the disease, it may help alleviate some of the symptoms by removing some of the triggers of active disease.

Julie, four years old, has been complaining of stomach aches for the past four months. The pain seems to be worse in the afternoons and evenings, when bloating can be seen, and diarrhea occurs occasionally, too. Julie's parents have discussed the problem several times with the pediatrician. At first the stress of starting preschool was mentioned as a possible cause, but her doctor now thinks that lactose intolerance is more likely and has ordered diagnostic tests to confirm his suspicion.

Julie probably has a typical case of lactose intolerance. If this is confirmed with diagnostic tests, removal of all lactose from Julie's diet (including in milk, yogurt, cheese, other dairy foods, some breads, commercial baked goods, breakfast cereals, margarine, candies, and processed meats) will make the symptoms go away. Julie's mother can then try Julie on small amounts of milk-containing foods to see if small amounts are tolerated even if larger amounts cause problems. Yogurt is often better tolerated than milk by children who are lactose-intolerant, because the lactose in yogurt is already partly fermented in the manufacturing process. In addition, hard cheeses contain lots of protein and calcium but very little lactose, so they can be a valuable dietary component. Enzyme supplements (such as Lactaid), taken with meals or premixed with dairy foods such as milk, can also help keep Julie symptom-free.

---◈---

CHAPTER 17

Food, Hyperactivity, and Attention Deficit Hyperactivity Disorder

Joey was five when his parents finally decided to seek help for his difficult behavior and were told he had attention deficit hyperactivity disorder (ADHD). Luckily, they were referred to a physician who believed that food might be contributing to Joey's problem. With patience the problem foods were identified and removed from his diet. His mother now says, "Joey is a wonderful child, but we suffered so much before we found out what the problem was that it took me two years before I could like him again."

Have you ever wondered whether your child is hyperactive, or might even have ADHD? If so, this chapter is for you. Although food is only one piece of the puzzle, it is one you may be able to use to help you deal with a common and difficult problem.

DOES MY CHILD HAVE A PROBLEM?

Hyperactivity, which is characterized by excessive fidgeting and activity, is one component of the constellation of symptoms that define ADHD.

Around 5 percent of all young children, boys more than girls, have ADHD. Although ADHD is usually very manageable with the right professional help, it is often an emotionally draining disorder for families. As with many other psychiatric classifications, however, the difficult symptoms that sufferers and their families have to face are often balanced by a special energy and vision in these children that their families love, even as they are frustrated by the following common symptoms:

- Unreasonable fidgeting and excessive activity
- Restlessness, irritability, excessive crying, and temper tantrums
- Excessive talking
- Poor sleep with night awakenings, difficulty settling down at bedtime
- Inability to perform simple developmentally appropriate organized tasks
- Inattention when attention is needed
- Out-of-control impulsivity

Before you shout *"Yes,* my child has all of these!" be aware that virtually *all* children display all of these characteristics at one time or another. This is completely normal, and in fact is an important part of children's development. When they are running around the house screeching after dinner, or trying to pick a fight with their siblings or you for no good reason, they are unwittingly following their biological instincts to strengthen their bodies and minds in preparation for the adult world. When you know that this sometimes irritating behavior is subconsciously helping them prepare for their future, it is easier to have the patience that is needed.

So if these "symptoms" can be found in every child, how do you know if yours has a problem? In children under six years of age, psychiatrists diagnose ADHD on the basis of the frequency and extent of the behaviors listed above, and in fact rarely diagnose it before age four, because *normal* behavior up to that time includes many of ADHD's characteristic symptoms. It is essential for an unbiased expert to perform an assessment on your child if you have concerns about ADHD, so the first thing you should do is talk to your pediatrician. You may be right in thinking that something is wrong, but alternatively you may be relieved to find that your child is perfectly normal by the standard of other children of the same sex and age.

DO SOME FOODS AND CHEMICALS IN FOODS CAUSE HYPERACTIVITY OR ADHD?

Food is certainly not the whole problem in the majority of ADHD cases. ADHD is widely considered to be a disease with a strong genetic basis that causes underactivity of the brain neurotransmitter dopamine. Stimulant medications such as Ritalin (methylphenidate) help correct this underactivity and improve symptoms in 70 to 80 percent of affected children.

Nonetheless, food-based research conducted over the last ten years offers the hope that about half of all children with hyperactivity or mild cases of ADHD can be brought into normal behavior ranges with an appropriate diet, and another half of all children with more severe ADHD can experience an improvement in symptoms. What these figures suggest is that some children may be taking drugs when food could help instead, and others who don't respond to medication (or who experience unpleasant side effects) may find food an effective alternative.

Our interpretation of the food-ADHD research is that the results are promising but still in the "not proven" stage. It is possible that there were hidden problems with the design of the research plans and only more research will bring a definitive conclusion. In the meantime, however, a food-based approach is certainly worth considering, with the proviso that in some cases it is possible that the actual foods were not the problem, rather the amount or type of calories that the foods provided was. (We'll talk about the effects of calories when we discuss the controversy over sugar.)

Over twenty years ago Dr. Ben Feingold theorized that food colorings and also salicylates—present in many commercial foods as preservatives and in some fresh fruits and vegetables—were a cause of ADHD. Dr. Feingold saw good success in treating a wide range of patients, and out of these results the Feingold Diet and Feingold Association were born. Unfortunately, research following his original studies did not support Dr. Feingold's conclusions, and many pediatricians and ADHD researchers came to think that food was not the cause of ADHD or the right route to treatment.

More recent research, however, has suggested that individual food chemicals may indeed cause hyperactivity and the other symptoms of ADHD. However, different children appear to be sensitive to different food chemicals and typically may be sensitive to several chemicals at the same time. In one careful research study, thirty-four of fifty children were affected by between two and seven food chemicals, but two children were sensitive to thirty different chemicals! This helps explain why earlier research, most of which tested the effects of just a few foods, was confusing and eventually discounted. For children sensitive to several foods, removing only some of them from the diet will not solve the problem.

Why do some children, but not others, appear to be sensitive to foods in a way that gives them the behavior problems that characterize hyperactivity and/or ADHD? Scientists continue to struggle with this question. It may simply be a general sensitivity to certain foods or substances added to food—a theory favored by some physicians and scientists because it is known that children with hyperactivity and ADHD tend to have more allergies than other children. An alternative explanation is that because of the particular metabolism of these children, they may experience toxic reactions that other children do not have.

Unfortunately, very few children are alike when it comes to the foods that affect them, so the list of implicated items is a long one. Also, some foods that are not on the list may affect your child. Your own observations may be crucial in finding the answer.

---

*Foods That May Cause Hyperactivity/ADHD**

FOOD	PERCENTAGE OF CHILDREN WITH FOOD-SENSITIVE ADHD IN WHOM THESE FOODS APPEAR TO CAUSE PROBLEMS
Artificial colors and preservatives	79%
Soy milk, soybeans, soy sauce, and other soy products	73%
Cow's milk	64%
Chocolate	59%
Grapes	50%
Wheat	49%
Oranges	45%
Hen's eggs	39%
Peanuts	32%
Corn and corn products	29%
Fish	23%
Oats	23%
Melon	21%
Tomato	20%
Ham/bacon	20%
Pineapple	19%
Beef	16%
Beans	15%
Peas	15%
Malt	15%

Apples	13%
Pork	13%
Pears	12%
Chicken	11%
Potatoes	11%
Tea	10%
Coffee	10%
Other nuts	10%

*Modified from Egger et al., *The Lancet*, 1985, vol. i, pp 540–545.

SUGAR AND HYPERACTIVITY

Surprisingly, sugar is one of the few foods for which there is reasonably good scientific evidence that *no* connection exists between it and hyperactivity/ADHD. This is odd, because for decades parents and teachers have looked on sugar as one of the major culprits in the hyperactivity story, and it is hard to believe that they are all completely wrong.

Yet a recent summary of twenty-three research studies in which drinks with sugar were compared to drinks made with a noncaloric sweetener such as saccharin or aspartame reported that sugar is completely harmless. Every study analyzed in the summary tested both sugar and a placebo, and the children (who did not know what they had consumed) were rated for behavior by investigators who also did not know what each child had consumed. An impressive array of neuropsychological and academic tests, as well as teacher and parent ratings of behavior and motor skills, showed no ill effects attributable to sugar.

So what is the real truth about sugar and hyperactivity? There are various possibilities, and getting a definitive answer will take more research. If sugar truly is more important than past research studies have shown, one explanation may be that the placebos used in those studies (aspartame or saccharine) make children hyperactive also, so that both the substance being investigated and the control induced similar results. Another answer may be that children develop a learned association between eating sweet things and feeling hyperactive. If this is the case, it would take time for a child to "unlearn" that behavior. Research studies lasting only a short time might not detect a gradual improvement over time.

Another possibility is that the research indicating that sugar does *not* cause hyperactivity was on target. Instead, it may be that the *calories* in the sweet foods, or rather the particular kinds of calories, that cause the problem.

In my house there is a tongue-in-cheek name for the wild activity and sometimes inappropriate behavior that happens most nights after my daughter (who is not hyperactive) has eaten dinner: "ATP poisoning." ATP is the chemical in the body that makes food energy available to our cells, and you can certainly see its effects in the wake of a good meal. She runs around, creates wild games, becomes generally boisterous, and totally wears my husband and me out. Mel sees precisely the same behavior in his three boys. This happens despite the fact that we don't usually give our children high-sugar desserts or candy. What it looks very much like is that they have been supercharged with energy, which indeed they have, considering all the calories they have eaten. Because most families in America finish meals and snacks with something sweet, blaming the sugar is logical. In families like ours, however, where sugar does not end the meal, the energy surge happens just the same—suggesting that the villain is the calories and not the sugar. This overcharging with calories, when combined with a very active child, may encourage unacceptable behavior.

Not only the amount of calories but also the type of food providing the calories may be implicated in children's hyperactivity. My friend and colleague at Children's Hospital in Boston, Dr. David Ludwig, suspects that some patients who have ADHD improve when they eat a diet consisting largely of foods that have a low glycemic index (foods that are digested and absorbed more slowly, such as high-protein foods, whole grains, and vegetables and fruits) instead of items with a high glycemic index, such as white bread, potatoes, sugary desserts, fruit juices, and sodas. He believes that the reason foods with a low glycemic index help is that they don't provide the same "rush" of blood glucose that high-glycemic-index foods do. Patients put on low-glycemic-index diets to address their weight problem were the key to his observation. You can talk with your pediatrician about the possibility of a low-glycemic-index elimination diet for your child.

VITAMINS AND HYPERACTIVITY

Will vitamins help hyperactivity/ADHD? The short answer is no. There simply isn't any good research showing that adding vitamins will improve the situation. However, it is true that many children with hyperactivity or ADHD are fussy and difficult to feed. This may result in their eating a very restricted diet, putting them at risk of nutritional deficiencies. The complete multivitamin/mineral supplement we recommend for all children up to age six will help prevent shortages of essential nutrients.

Megadoses of vitamins—tablets or capsules that contain doses much larger than the RDAs—don't help treat hyperactivity/ADHD and should be strictly off-limits because all children are at risk of a toxic reaction if large doses of vitamins or minerals are taken.

YOUR DECISION: WILL A SPECIAL ELIMINATION DIET HELP YOUR CHILD WITH ADHD?

If your child is diagnosed with ADHD and is over four years of age, you and your pediatrician may want to try some dietary modifications to see if they help. Children younger than four are rarely diagnosed, but in any case should not be put on limited diets.

There are two main options to try: the *elimination diet* (sometimes called the few-foods or hypoallergenic diet) explained below, or the *modified elimination diet* described in the following section. Because the elimination diet is difficult and restrictive, it is suggested only for children diagnosed with ADHD. If your child is hyperactive but does not have ADHD, you may want to consider the modified elimination diet. Both the elimination diet and the modified elimination diet should be attempted only under the supervision of a qualified physician.

The elimination diet begins with six to ten foods that your child eats exclusively for about two weeks. If the diet improves his behavior, other foods can be added back at a rate of one per week, with your child's behavior monitored to see if the additions have any adverse effect. Eventually, enough foods are added back without adverse behavioral effects so that your child can eat a varied diet while avoiding problem foods.

Working with a pediatrician specializing in allergies or ADHD, you would typically take the following steps to set up an elimination diet for your child.

1. DETERMINE WHAT YOUR CHILD NORMALLY EATS AND WHICH OF THOSE FOODS YOU SUSPECT HE IS SENSITIVE TO

Make a three-day baseline recording of his normal behavior and food intake. To start recording the foods your child eats (types, amounts, times they are eaten), you can simply use a notebook or blank sheet of paper.

A 20-POINT SCALE FOR MEASURING BEHAVIOR

	NOT AT ALL SCORE 0	MILD SCORE 1	MODERATE SCORE 2	VERY SCORE 3	EXTREMELY SCORE 4
1. Irritability/lack of control					
2. Restlessness					
3. Aggression					
4. Poor attention span					
5. Poor sleep					

The chart above is an example of one you can use for behavior.

Use one page like this for each day you record your child's behavior (you can photocopy the page for additional sheets). To use the scale, record your assessment of items 1 through 4 in the evening before you go to bed, and item 5 in the morning. Has your child been irritable or shown lack of control during the day? Grade his response from 0 (not at all) to 4 (extremely). Also grade the day's restlessness, aggression, and lack of attention span, and the night's sleep. For each behavior you will now have a score of 0 to 4. Add up the scores for a maximum of 20. This is your daily score.

2. PLAN AN ELIMINATION DIET WITH YOUR PEDIATRICIAN

An elimination diet begins with a very short list of foods that you will feed your child exclusively for two weeks to see if behavior improves. Two weeks are needed because it takes time for symptoms to subside so that you can see whether the program is helping. It helps to start with a short list of foods and then add foods one at a time (rather than cutting foods out one at a time) because your child may well be sensitive to several foods, and you will likely not see improvements unless you start with a basic diet that does not cause any abnormal behavior.

An elimination diet typically gives you a choice of six to ten foods—two meats (usually lamb and turkey), two carbohydrates such as rice and potatoes, two fruits such as banana and pear, one or two vegetables such as carrots or broccoli, and milk-free, additive-free margarine and/or sunflower oil. Your list should not include any foods that are likely contributors to ADHD—and also no foods that you yourself suspect of causing problems.

GETTING THROUGH TWO WEEKS

Every elimination diet starts with different foods according to what items you believe your child may be sensitive to. However, typically the following are allowed:

Turkey   Rice   Bananas   Carrots   Additive-free margarine
Lamb   Potatoes   Pears   Broccoli Corn oil   Salt

Here are some menu suggestions to help you avoid the monotony.

BREAKFASTS

Plain cooked rice

Rice pudding (boiled rice with
   fruit and margarine)

Raw banana

Fried banana (cooked
   with margarine)

Plain rice with sliced banana or pear

Whole raw pear, cubed as finger food

Any lunch or dinner dish on this
   menu, if desired

LUNCH AND DINNER

Roast turkey with potatoes
   and carrots

Roast lamb with rice and broccoli

Lamb stew

Rice pilaf with carrots, broccoli,
   and turkey

Pilaf with lamb instead of turkey

Stir-fry with lamb or turkey and
   broccoli and carrots over rice

Carrots cooked with a little
   water and oil (see page 168)

Turkey croquettes with mixed
   carrots and broccoli

SNACKS

Banana or pear, cooked or raw

Plain rice cakes

Raw carrots or broccoli "trees"

Leftover breakfast, lunch, or dinner
   dishes, if desired

Potatoes baked or stuffed with
   veggies

Sliced turkey and mashed potatoes

Lamb chops, boiled potatoes dressed
   with margarine, and raw broccoli
   "trees"

French fries with raw carrots and
   broccoli

Pureed carrot and potato soup

Turkey soup with carrots and
   potatoes

FINDING HIDDEN FOOD COLORS AND ADDITIVES

Most processed foods contain additives of some sort. Even basic ingredients such as flour contain whiteners and other chemicals. The easiest way to make sure that the foods you are choosing do not have additives of any kind is to find a store that specializes in organic products. You can then look for labels that say "no additives," "no artificial colors," and so on. Organic fruits and vegetables are also a good idea during a modified elimination diet because this further reduces your child's intake of unknown chemicals.

3. CONTINUE THE DIET UNDER SUPERVISION

You will be asked to keep your child on the elimination diet while you see if symptoms subside, trying not to let your child have other foods (but recording them if she does). This will not be easy, but it's only for two weeks. Elimination diets are boring and difficult, and your child may get frustrated. Be loving and gentle (this diet should never be seen as a punishment, but rather as something that may help you all), and emphasize that it is only for a little while. Counting the days on a calendar may help, as will having everyone in the family eat the same foods, at least and especially when your ADHD sufferer is present. Try to make time to prepare as varied a menu as possible. Even roasted turkey will get terribly boring fourteen days in a row, and simple differences in presentation can help. If your child goes to preschool or day care, you should talk to the caretakers there about what you are doing and ask for their support.

4. KEEP A RECORD

During the two weeks when your child is on an elimination diet, you should make daily assessments of her behavior using the 20-point scale. These will be compared to see if the ratings improve.

5. WHAT IF IT DOESN'T WORK?

If the elimination diet does not seem to improve behavior, take a break for a couple of weeks. Give your child a one-a-day multivitamin during the break to replenish her stores of essential nutrients, and then consider asking your doctor if you can try a different elimination diet for a further two weeks, to see if some of the original list of acceptable foods included items your child is sensitive to.

6. REINTRODUCING FOODS

The exciting part comes once you have a successful elimination diet that has improved your child's behavior. You will look at your charts and realize he hasn't had a bad episode for three or four days, and you'll feel the dawn of hope that a remedy is within reach. At this time you will very slowly start to add foods back into your child's diet and see if they cause problems by going over the daily behavior ratings. The first week, your addition should be a children's multivitamin/mineral supplement approved by the professional who is helping you. The vitamin ensures your child does not lack any of the main essential nutrients on this limited diet. Starting the next week, one food should be added back every seven days. If your child's behavior deteriorates, that food should be removed again and another one tried a week later. Foods that are suspect in this way can be tested a second time at a later date, to see whether or not it was accidental that the behavior worsened.

7. ESTABLISH A WORKABLE DIET

Within six to twelve months, if your child is one of the ones who is sensitive to foods, you can hope to have identified thirty to fifty "safe" foods— enough so that she can eat normal meals without behavioral problems.

This type of elimination diet is a long and difficult project, but happy parents in ADHD research studies testify to the fact that food can make a difference to daily life. In one report, 92 percent of parents felt the study had been so helpful that they voluntarily kept on with a carefully controlled diet after the research ended.

Although this figure is wonderfully optimistic (and may quite possibly include some placebo effect), the process of getting to the right diet can be hard and, as we stressed earlier, can be done only under the supervision of a committed professional who believes that your family is suitable for a food-based approach.

CONSIDERING A MODIFIED ELIMINATION DIET

If you decide that an elimination diet is just too difficult for now, there is another way to see if your child may be helped by diet. This is a modified elimination diet, and the version below is based closely on recent research trials.

If you get good results, you have won with less effort than a classic elimination diet entails. If you don't get good results, you may need to try the more restrictive elimination diet in order to pin down whether or not your child is sensitive to particular foods.

However, remember that all special diets for children should be used only under the supervision of your child's pediatrician and only if your child is four or older. Also remember that this diet—like the classic elimination diet—should be used only for a two-week period. Longer use may deprive your child of some essential nutrients.

A modified elimination diet entails as normal a diet as possible for your child during the two-week test period, but removing a few key suspects. This is done with a series of substitutions as follows:

Modified elimination diet

INSTEAD OF THESE	SUBSTITUTE THESE
All foods with artificial colors, flavors, and preservatives (including MSG)	Home-cooked foods prepared from organic, color-, additive-, and preservative-free ingredients bought in a health food store
Oranges, tomatoes, grapes	Other fruits and vegetables
All refined carbohydrates, such as sugar, white bread, many cereals, bagels, chips, and crackers	Whole-grain products, more allowed fruits and vegetables
Cow's milk and soy milk, cheese and yogurt	A calcium supplement and more of the allowed foods
Chocolate	More whole-grain foods and allowed fruits and vegetables if hungry

All caffeine-containing beverages, including carbonated drinks	Water

As with the classic elimination diet, follow this plan for two weeks under the supervision of your doctor, and record your child's behavior every day. If the hyperactivity improves, you can add back foods one by one and see if the behavior gets worse. Within two to three months you should have a good idea of whether your child can be helped by restricting particular foods.

After settling into a modified diet that eliminates problem foods, many parents also find that the new program becomes routine over time. A few parents have even reported that it resulted in healthier meals overall for the entire family. Our chief hope, however, is that if food indeed proves to have been part of the problem for your child, it can be part of the solution, too.

FURTHER INFORMATION

Further Reading

E. M. Hallowell. *When You Worry About the Child You Love.* Simon & Schuster, 1996.

R. Barkley. *Taking Charge of ADHD.* Guilford Press, 1995.

Web sites

www.mediconsult.com

APPENDIX I

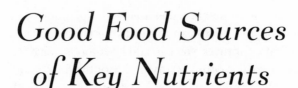

Good Food Sources
of Key Nutrients

RDAs, DRIs, AIs, AND DVs: WHAT ARE THEY?

Nutrient recommendations are revised at intervals so that new scientific information can be taken into account. You may find food values given under any of the following labels. Here's how to crack the code.

- **RDAs** (Recommended Dietary Allowances)—The standard term until 1998. These are currently being reviewed and revised for each essential nutrient.
- **DRIs** (Dietary Reference Intakes)—The new standard term, used when the scientific evidence is good enough to give reliable predictions of requirements. (We cite the new DRIs where available.)
- **AIs** (Adequate Intakes)—Used when recommendations are based on observations of what apparently healthy people eat, because of insufficient laboratory research.
- **DVs** (Daily Values)—The term used on most packaged foods; portions are listed as a percentage of the DV. *DVs are not designed for children.* They are based on the 1968 RDAs for adult men and women (excluding those who are pregnant or lactating). For each nutrient, the DV is the highest amount recommended for any adult group. For example, the current DV for iron, 18 mg, reflects the needs of young women. Because the current RDA for iron in childhood ranges from 6 to 10 mg, the DV incorrectly makes many foods seem like poor iron sources. DVs can help you compare the nutritional value of different items, but you shouldn't use them to work out if your child is eating enough of a particular nutrient.

IRON

RDAs

Under 1 year	6–10 mg
1–3 years	10 mg
4–6 years	10 mg

	mg
Baby rice cereal, dry, ¼ cup	5.2
Product 19/ Total	4.5

Instant oatmeal, fortified, $^1/_2$ packet	2.1
Pumpkin seed kernels, $^1/_2$ oz	2.1
Liver, 1 oz	1.4
Pasta, $^1/_2$ cup cooked	1.3
Cooked white or refried beans, $^1/_4$ cup	1.1
Regular fortified breakfast cereals, $^1/_4$ cup	1.0
Molasses, 1 tbsp	1.0
Egg noodles, $^1/_3$ cup cooked	0.9
Sauerkraut, $^1/_4$ cup	0.9
Dried figs, 2 pieces	0.8
Whole-wheat bread, 1 slice	0.8
Roasted mixed nuts, 1 oz	0.7
Dried apricots or peaches, 4 halves	0.7
Spinach, $^1/_4$ cup	0.7
Snap peas, $^1/_4$ cup	0.6
Sweet potatoes, canned	0.6
Egg, 1 whole	0.6
Bread, white, rye, or oatmeal, 1 slice	0.6
Wheat germ, 1 tbsp	0.6
Lean beef (including lean ground beef), 1 oz	0.5
Peanut butter, 1 oz	0.5
Lean lamb, 1 oz	0.4
Sardines, canned, 1 oz	0.4
Oatmeal, not fortified, $^1/_4$ cup cooked	0.4
Turkey, 1 oz	0.4
Brown sugar, 1 tbsp	0.3
Dried parsley, thyme, $^1/_4$ teaspoon	0.3

CALCIUM

DRIs

Under 1 year	270 mg
1–3 years	500 mg
4–6 years	800 mg

	mg
Yogurt, low-fat plain or w/ fruit, 1 cup	320–400
Milk, 2%, 1 cup	300
Mozzarella, 1 oz	200
Cheddar cheese, 1 oz	200
Calcium-fortified fruit juice, 4 oz	135
Frozen yogurt, $^1/_2$ cup	160–200
Sardines, canned, 1 oz	110
Ice milk, $^1/_2$ cup	105
Molasses, 1 tbsp	137

Tofu, $^1\!/_4$ cup   65
Almond butter, $^1\!/_2$ oz   35
Kale, $^1\!/_4$ cup   25

ZINC
RDAs

Under 1 year	5 mg
1–3 years	10 mg
4–6 years	10 mg

	mg
Product 19 / Total, $^1\!/_4$ cup	3.8
Our oatmeal bread, 1 slice (page 214)	1.5
Lean beef (including lean ground beef), 1 oz	1.4
Lean lamb, 1 oz	1.4
Fortified regular breakfast cereals, $^1\!/_4$ cup	1.3
Roasted mixed nuts, 1 oz	1.3
Crab, 1 oz	1.2
Wheat germ, 1 tbsp	1.2
Dark chicken meat, 1 oz	1.0
Milk, milkshakes, 1 cup	1.0
Pumpkin seed kernels, $^1\!/_2$ oz	1.0
Turkey, 1 oz	0.9
Yogurt, low-fat with fruit, $^1\!/_2$ cup	0.9
Hard cheese such as cheddar, Parmesan, 1 oz	0.9
Lobster, 1 oz	0.8
Peanut butter, 1 oz	0.8
Refried beans, $^1\!/_4$ cup	0.7
Yellow wax beans, $^1\!/_4$ cup	0.6
Cooked white beans, $^1\!/_4$ cup	0.6
Whole-wheat bread, 1 slice	0.6
Egg, 1 whole	0.5
Pasta, $^1\!/_2$ cup	0.5
Peas, $^1\!/_4$ cup	0.4
Pumpernickel, 1 slice	0.4
Rye bread, 1 slice	0.3
Oatmeal, $^1\!/_4$ cup cooked	0.3
Egg noodles, $^1\!/_3$ cup cooked	0.3
Asparagus, $^1\!/_4$ cup	0.3
Okra, $^1\!/_4$ cup	0.3
Spinach, $^1\!/_4$ cup	0.3
Broccoli, $^1\!/_4$ cup	0.2
Corn, $^1\!/_4$ cup	0.2
Dried figs, 2 pieces	0.2

FOLATE

DRIs

Under 1 year	65–80 mcg
1–3 years	150 mcg
4–6 years	200 mcg

	mcg
Spinach, ¼ cup cooked	65
Liver, 1 oz	60
Beans, ¼ cup cooked	60
Honeydew melon, 1 slice	40
Orange juice, ¼ cup	30
Asparagus, 2 spears	30
Brussels sprouts, ¼ cup	25
Broccoli, cabbage, ¼ cup cooked	20
Lettuce, ¼ cup	20
Cauliflower, ¼ cup	15
Peanut butter, ½ oz	15
Bread, 1 slice	10–15
Banana, ½	12
Egg, 1 yolk	12
Milk, 1 cup	12

VITAMIN B_6 (PYRIDOXINE)

DRIs

Under 1 year	0.1–0.3 mg
1–3 years	0.5 mg
4–6 years	0.6 mg

	mg
Liver, 1 oz	0.4
Oatmeal, ⅓ cup cooked	0.3
Banana, ½	0.3
Chicken, ¼ cup light or dark meat	0.2
Spinach, ¼ cup	0.11
Beef, 1 oz lean	0.1
Avocado, ¼	0.1
Cod, baked, 1 oz	0.1
Wheat germ, 1 tbsp	0.1
Prunes, 4 dried	0.1
Sunflower seeds, 1 tbsp	0.1
Milk, yogurt, 1 cup	0.1
Peanut butter, 2 tbsp	0.1
Tomato, 1 medium	0.1

Rice, $1/2$ cup cooked	0.1
Cauliflower, $1/4$ cup cooked	0.07
Egg yolk, 1 large	0.07
Cantaloupe melon, 1 slice	0.06
Broccoli, $1/4$ cup	0.06
Whole-wheat bread, 1 slice	0.05

VITAMIN B$_{12}$ (COBALAMIN)

DRIs

Under 1 year	0.4–0.5 mcg
1–3 years	0.9 mcg
4–6 years	1.2 mcg

	mcg
Liver, 1 oz	32.0
Milk, 1 cup	0.9
Tuna, canned, 1 oz	0.9
Beef, lean, 1 oz	0.6
Egg, 1 whole	0.6
White fish, 1 oz	0.4
Cheese, 1 oz	0.4
Ice cream, $1/3$ cup	0.2
Chicken, 1 oz	0.1

VITAMIN A

RDAs

Under 1 year	375 mcg RE[1]
1–3 years	400 mcg RE[1]
4–6 years	500 mcg RE[1]

	mcg RE[1]
Liver, 1 oz	3,000
Sweet potato, $1/2$ cup small	1,250
Carrots, $1/2$ cup raw	1,000
Spinach, $1/4$ cup cooked	450
Squash, $1/4$ cup cooked	450
Cantaloupe melon, $1/4$ cup	200
Red pepper, $1/4$ cup	145
Milk, 1 cup	140
Dried apricots, 3 halves	100

[1]RE, retinol equivalents, the unit used for Vitamin A requirements

Egg, 1 yolk	100
Cheddar cheese, 1 oz	86
Tomato, 1 medium	75
Papaya, 1/4 cup	71
Broccoli, 1/4 cup cooked	55

VITAMIN C

DRIs

Under 1 year	**30–35 mg**
1–3 years	**40 mg**
4–6 years	**45 mg**

	mg
Kiwi, 1 fresh	74
Orange, 1/3 fresh	30
Orange juice, 1/4 cup	30
Pepper, 1/4 fresh	25
Tangerine, 1 fresh	25
Cranberry juice, 1/4 cup	25
Papaya, 1/4 cup	23
Cantaloupe, 1/4 cup	20
Broccoli, 1/4 cup cooked	20
Strawberries, 1/4 cup	20
Tomato, 1 medium	20
Cabbage, cauliflower, 1/4 cup	17
Mango, 1/3 fresh	15
Potato, 1 small baked	15
Spinach, 1/4 cup	10

VITAMIN E

RDAs

Under 1 year	**3–4 mg**
1–3 years	**6 mg**
4–6 years	**7 mg**

	mg
Milk, whole or 2%, 1 cup	7.6
Corn, soybean oil, 1/2 tbsp	6.0
Sunflower oil, 1/2 tbsp	4.5
Avocado, 1/4 whole	2.0
Macaroni and cheese, 1/2 cup	1.8
Peanut butter, 1/2 oz	0.9
Peas, 1/4 cup	0.9
Olive oil, 1/2 tbsp	0.9

APPENDIX 2

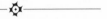

Growth Charts

HOW TO USE CENTILE CHARTS

The following twelve pages show centile charts for comparing your baby's weight and height to expected growth patterns. Use only weight and height values measured by your baby's pediatrician or nurse, because it can be hard to get accurate measurements with a home scale and tape measure.

To use a chart, trace a vertical line from the number on the horizontal axis corresponding to your baby's age. Then trace a horizontal line from the weight or length measurement on the vertical axis. The centile line nearest to where the two lines cross is your baby's current position.

The 50th centile represents typical growth, and the 15th to the 85th centiles show the healthy range for most normal babies. However, your family history and other issues your pediatrician may highlight are important also, since growth depends in part on genetic inheritance as well as on nutrition and lifestyle. If your child's height is on the 10th centile, for example, this is probably normal if you or your husband is short, but a potential concern if you are both tall or of normal height.

Note: There are different charts for babies who start life breast-fed versus formula-fed:

- Use the new World Health Organization charts on pages 319 to 322 (charts A–D) if your baby is under one year and was breast-fed for at least one month. Babies grow quite differently in the first year of life according to whether they started life on breast milk or formula. Using these special charts based on data from the National Center for Health Statistics will help you and your pediatrician avoid misinterpreting your baby's growth pattern.
- Use the standard charts based on data from the National Center for Health Statistics on pages 323–326 (charts E–H) if your child is between one and three years of age, or if she or he was never breast-fed.
- Use the standard charts on pages 327 to 330 (charts I–L) if your child is over three years or if you start using charts only after two years.

318

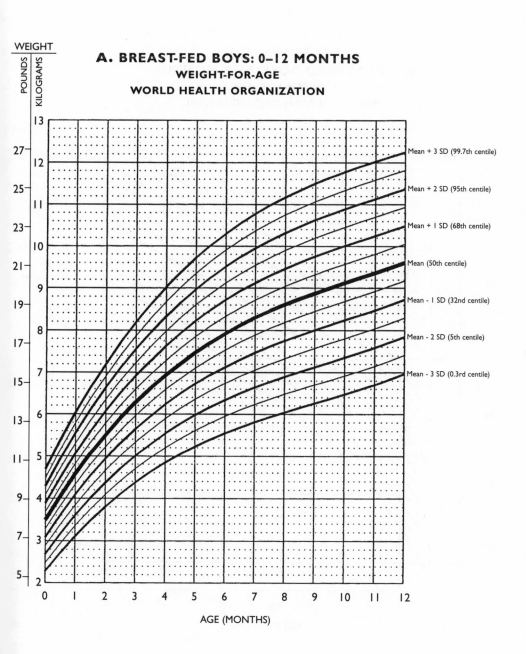

WEIGHT

POUNDS KILOGRAMS

A. BREAST-FED BOYS: 0–12 MONTHS
WEIGHT-FOR-AGE
WORLD HEALTH ORGANIZATION

Mean + 3 SD (99.7th centile)

Mean + 2 SD (95th centile)

Mean + 1 SD (68th centile)

Mean (50th centile)

Mean – 1 SD (32nd centile)

Mean – 2 SD (5th centile)

Mean – 3 SD (0.3rd centile)

AGE (MONTHS)

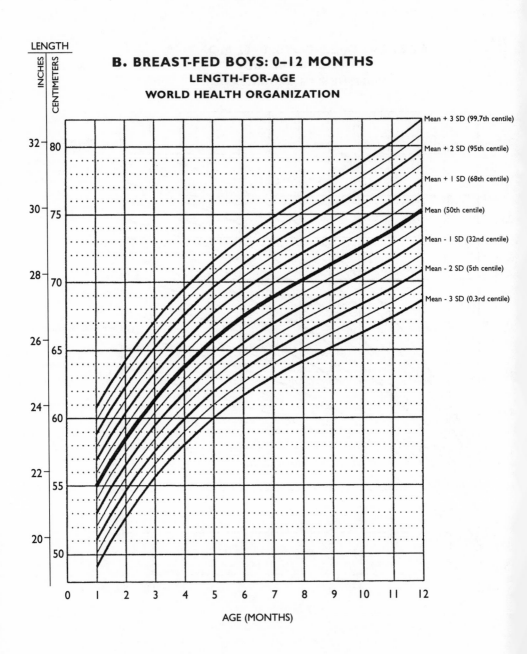

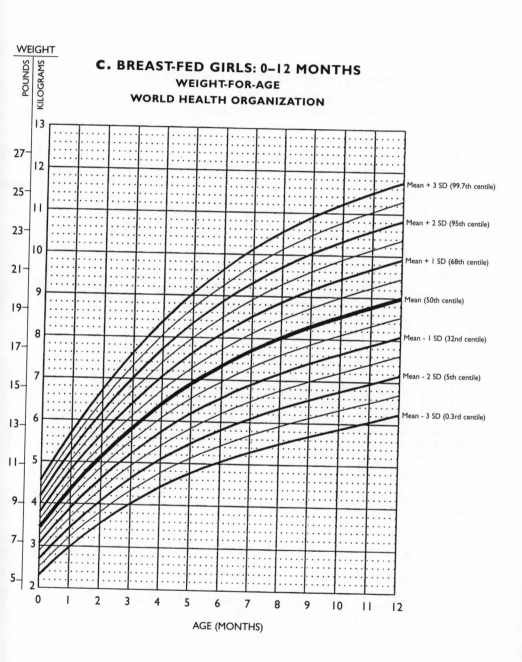

WEIGHT

POUNDS KILOGRAMS

C. BREAST-FED GIRLS: 0–12 MONTHS
WEIGHT-FOR-AGE
WORLD HEALTH ORGANIZATION

Mean + 3 SD (99.7th centile)

Mean + 2 SD (95th centile)

Mean + 1 SD (68th centile)

Mean (50th centile)

Mean - 1 SD (32nd centile)

Mean - 2 SD (5th centile)

Mean - 3 SD (0.3rd centile)

AGE (MONTHS)

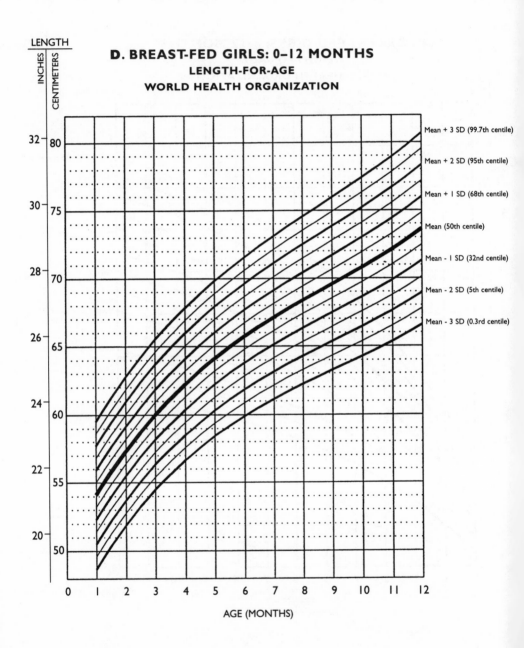

D. BREAST-FED GIRLS: 0–12 MONTHS
LENGTH-FOR-AGE
WORLD HEALTH ORGANIZATION

Mean + 3 SD (99.7th centile)
Mean + 2 SD (95th centile)
Mean + 1 SD (68th centile)
Mean (50th centile)
Mean - 1 SD (32nd centile)
Mean - 2 SD (5th centile)
Mean - 3 SD (0.3rd centile)

AGE (MONTHS)

E. BOYS: BIRTH–3 YEARS
WEIGHT AND LENGTH FOR AGE
NATIONAL CENTER FOR HEALTH STATISTICS

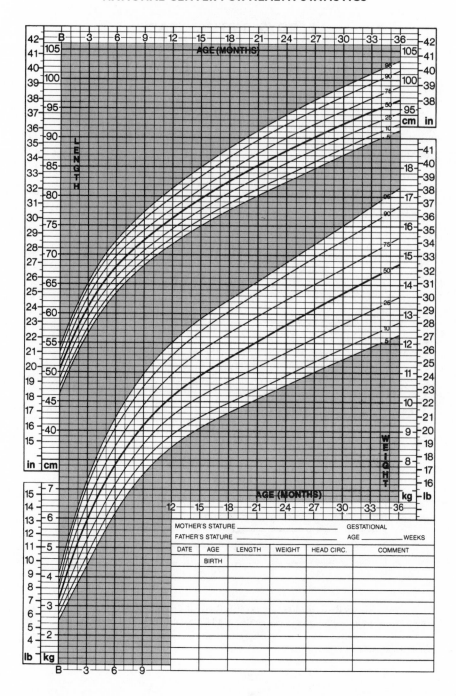

Adapted from: Hamill PVV, Drizd TA, Johnson CL, Reed RB, Roche AF, Moore WM. Physical growth: National Center for Health Statistics percentiles. AM J CLIN NUTR 32-607-629, 1979. Data from the National Center for Health Statistics (NCHS), Hyattsville, Maryland. © 1982 Ross Products Division, Abbott Laboratories.

F. BOYS: BIRTH–3 YEARS
WEIGHT FOR LENGTH CENTILES
NATIONAL CENTER FOR HEALTH STATISTICS

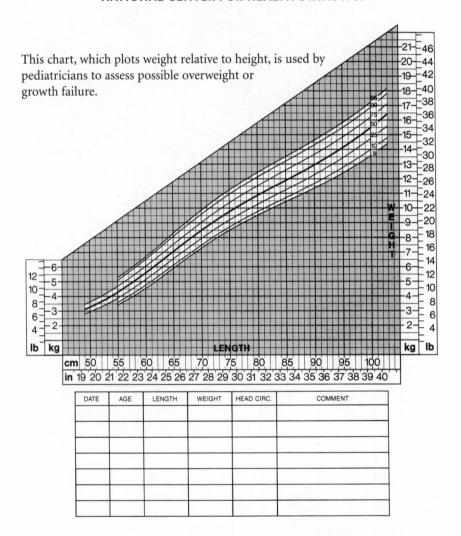

This chart, which plots weight relative to height, is used by pediatricians to assess possible overweight or growth failure.

DATE	AGE	LENGTH	WEIGHT	HEAD CIRC.	COMMENT

Adapted from: Hamill PVV, Drizd TA, Johnson CL, Reed RB, Roche AF, Moore WM. Physical growth: National Center for Health Statistics percentiles. AM J CLIN NUTR 32-607-629, 1979. Data from the National Center for Health Statistics (NCHS), Hyattsville, Maryland. © 1982 Ross Products Division, Abbott Laboratories.

G.GIRLS: BIRTH–3 YEARS
WEIGHT AND LENGTH FOR AGE
NATIONAL CENTER FOR HEALTH STATISTICS

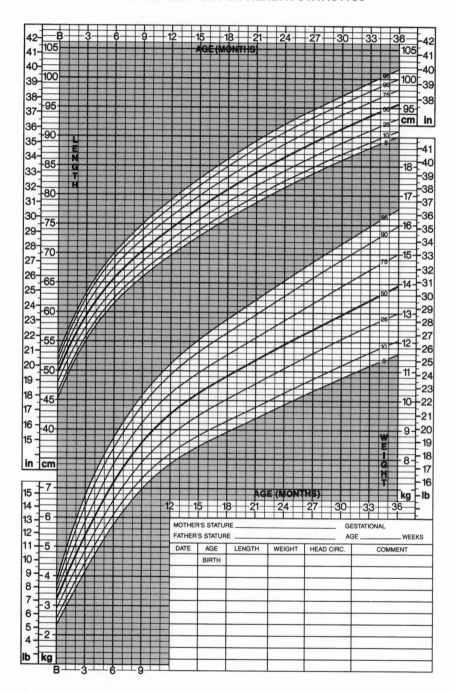

Adapted from: Hamill PVV, Drizd TA, Johnson CL, Reed RB, Roche AF, Moore WM. Physical growth:
National Center for Health Statistics percentiles. AM J CLIN NUTR 32-607-629, 1979. Data from the
National Center for Health Statistics (NCHS), Hyattsville, Maryland. © 1982 Ross Products Division,
Abbott Laboratories.

H. GIRLS: BIRTH–3 YEARS
WEIGHT FOR LENGTH CENTILES
NATIONAL CENTER FOR HEALTH STATISTICS

This chart, which plots weight relative to height, is used by pediatricians to assess possible overweight or growth failure.

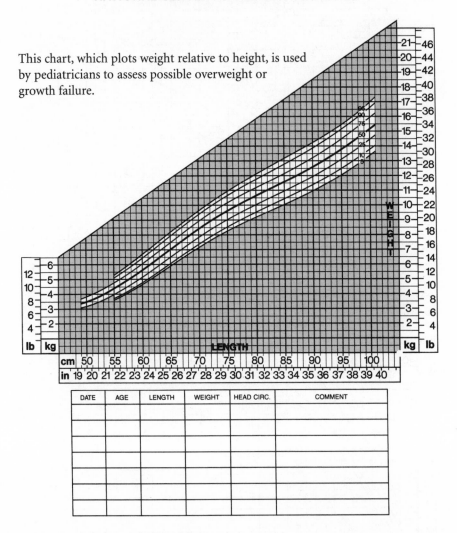

DATE	AGE	LENGTH	WEIGHT	HEAD CIRC.	COMMENT

Adapted from: Hamill PVV, Drizd TA, Johnson CL, Reed RB, Roche AF, Moore WM. Physical growth: National Center for Health Statistics percentiles. AM J CLIN NUTR 32-607-629, 1979. Data from the National Center for Health Statistics (NCHS), Hyattsville, Maryland. © 1982 Ross Products Division, Abbott Laboratories.

I. BOYS: 2–18 YEARS
WEIGHT AND LENGTH FOR AGE
NATIONAL CENTER FOR HEALTH STATISTICS

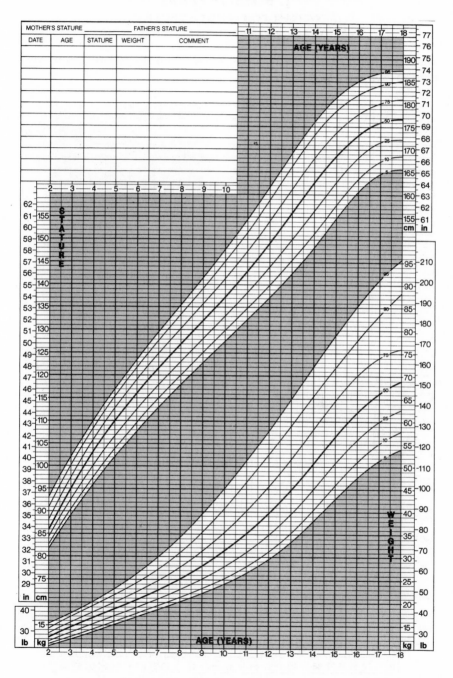

Adapted from: Hamill PVV, Drizd TA, Johnson CL, Reed RB, Roche AF, Moore WM. Physical growth: National Center for Health Statistics percentiles. AM J CLIN NUTR 32-607-629, 1979. Data from the National Center for Health Statistics (NCHS), Hyattsville, Maryland. © 1982 Ross Products Division, Abbott Laboratories.

J. BOYS: 2+ YEARS
WEIGHT FOR LENGTH CENTILES
NATIONAL CENTER FOR HEALTH STATISTICS

This chart, which plots weight relative to height, is used by pediatricians to assess possible overweight or growth failure.

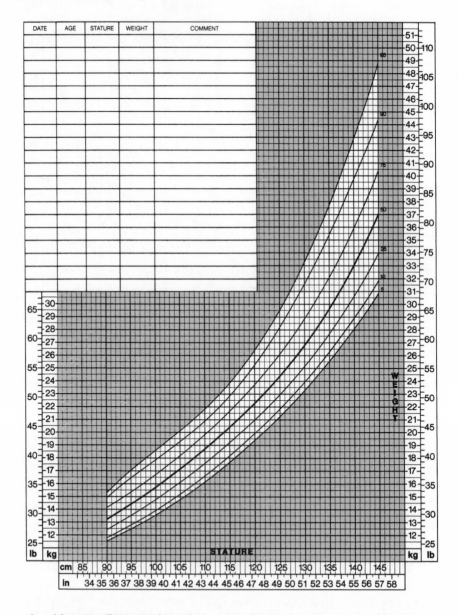

Adapted from: Hamill PVV, Drizd TA, Johnson CL, Reed RB, Roche AF, Moore WM. Physical growth: National Center for Health Statistics percentiles. AM J CLIN NUTR 32-607-629, 1979. Data from the National Center for Health Statistics (NCHS), Hyattsville, Maryland. © 1982 Ross Products Division, Abbott Laboratories.

K. GIRLS: 2–18 YEARS
WEIGHT AND LENGTH FOR AGE
NATIONAL CENTER FOR HEALTH STATISTICS

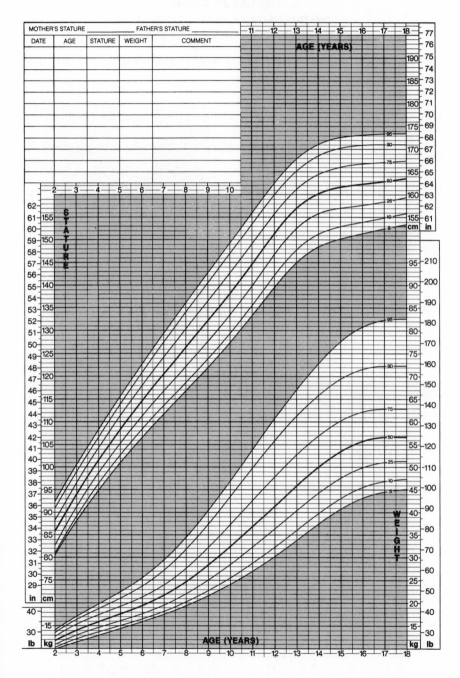

Adapted from: Hamill PVV, Drizd TA, Johnson CL, Reed RB, Roche AF, Moore WM. Physical growth: National Center for Health Statistics percentiles. AM J CLIN NUTR 32-607-629, 1979. Data from the National Center for Health Statistics (NCHS), Hyattsville, Maryland. © 1982 Ross Products Division, Abbott Laboratories.

L. GIRLS: 2+ YEARS
WEIGHT FOR LENGTH CENTILES
NATIONAL CENTER FOR HEALTH STATISTICS

This chart, which plots weight relative to height, is used by pediatricians to assess possible overweight or growth failure.

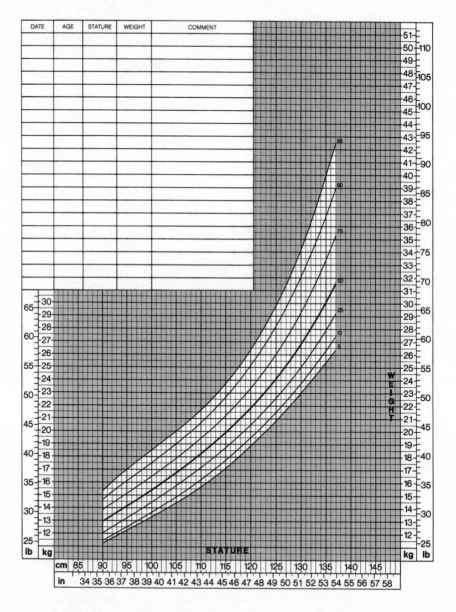

Adapted from: Hamill PVV, Drizd TA, Johnson CL, Reed RB, Roche AF, Moore WM. Physical growth: National Center for Health Statistics percentiles. AM J CLIN NUTR 32-607-629, 1979. Data from the National Center for Health Statistics (NCHS), Hyattsville, Maryland. © 1982 Ross Products Division, Abbott Laboratories.

BIBLIOGRAPHY

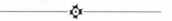

General References

U.S. Department of Agriculture and U.S. Department of Health and Human Sciences. *Nutrition and Your Health: Dietary Guidelines for Americans,* 1995.

National Research Council. *Recommended Dietary Allowances.* Washington, D.C.: National Academy Press, 1989.

Glinsmann, W. H., S. J. Bartholemy, and F. Coletta. "Dietary guidelines for infants: a timely reminder," *Nutrition Reviews,* vol. 54 (1996): 50–57.

Mahan, L. K. and S. Escott-Stump. *Krause's Food, Nutrition, and Diet Therapy.* Philadelphia: W. B. Saunders Company, 1996.

Olson, R. E. "The dietary recommendations of the American Academy of Pediatrics," *American Journal of Clinical Nutrition,* vol. 61 (1995): 271–73.

Shils, M. E., J. A. Olson, and M. Shike. *Modern Nutrition in Health and Disease,* vols. 1 and 2. Philadelphia: Lea & Febiger, 1994.

Suskind, R. M. and L. Lewinter-Suskind. *Textbook of Pediatric Nutrition.* New York: Raven Press, 1993.

Walker, W. A. and J. B. Watkins. *Nutrition in Pediatrics.* Hamilton, Ontario: B.C. Decker, Inc., 1996.

Walker, W. A. and J. B. Watkins. *Nutrition in Pediatrics: Basic Science and Clinical Applications.* London: B.C. Decker, Inc., 1997.

Chapter 1: Metabolic Programming

American Academy of Pediatrics. "Infant feeding practices and their possible relationship to the etiology of diabetes mellitus," *Pediatrics,* vol. 95 (1994): 752–54.

Boulton, L., Z. Lanron, and J. Rey. *Long-term Consequences of Early Feeding.* Philadelphia: Lippincott-Raven, 1996.

Ciba Foundation Symposium. *The Childhood Environment and Adult Disease.* New York: John Wiley & Sons, 1991.

Davis, M. K., D. A. Savitz, and B. I. Graubard. "Infant feeding and childhood cancer," *Lancet,* vol. 2 (1988): 365–68.

Goldberg, G. R. and A. M. Prentice. "Maternal and fetal determinants of adult diseases," *Nutrition Reviews,* vol. 52 (1994): 191–200.

Kretchmer, N., J. L. Beard, and S. Carlson. "The role of nutrition in the development of normal cognition," *American Journal of Clinical Nutrition,* vol. 63 (1996): 997S–1001S.

Kruesi, M. J. P. and J. L. Rapaport. "Diet and human behavior: how much do they affect each other?" *Annual Review of Nutrition,* vol. 6 (1986): 113–30.

Lewis, D. S., H. A. Bertrand, C. A. McMahan, H. C. McGill, K. D. Carey, and E. J. Masoro.

"Preweaning food intake influences the adiposity of young adult baboons," *Journal of Clinical Investigation,* vol. 78 (1986): 899–905.

Lozoff, B., E. Jimenez, and A. W. Wolf. "Long-term developmental outcome of infants with iron deficiency," *New England Journal of Medicine,* vol. 325 (1991): 687–94.

Lucas, A. "Role of nutritional programming in determining adult morbidity," *Archives of Disease in Childhood,* vol. 71 (1994): 288–90.

Lucas, A., M. S. Fewtrell, R. Morley, P. J. Lucas, B. A. Baker, G. Lister, and N. J. Bishop. "Randomized outcome trial of human milk fortification and developmental outcome in preterm infants," *American Journal of Clinical Nutrition,* vol. 64, *(1996): 142–51.*

Lucas, A., R. Morley, T. J. Cole, S. M. Gore, P. J. Lucas, P. Crowle, R. Pearse, A. J. Boon, and R. Powell. "Early diet in preterm babies and developmental status at 18 months," *Lancet,* vol. 335 (1990): 1477–81.

Lucas, A., R. Morley, T. J. Cole, G. Lister, and C. Leeson-Payne. "Breast milk and subsequent intelligence quotient in children born preterm," *Lancet,* vol. 339 (1992): 261–64.

Mayer, E. J., R. F. Hamman, E. C. Gay, D. C. Lezotte, D. A. Savitz, and G. J. Klingensmith. "Reduced risk of IDDM among breast-fed children," *Diabetes,* vol. 37 (1988): 1625–32.

Peters, J. M., S. Preston-Martin, S. J. London, J. D. Bowman, J. D. Buckley, and D. C. Thomas. "Processed meats and risk of childhood leukemia," *Cancer Causes and Control,* vol. 5 (1994): 195–202.

Prentice, A. M., A. Lucas, L. Vasquez-Velasquez, P. S. Davies, and R. G. Whitehead. "Are current dietary guidelines for young children a prescription for overfeeding?" *Lancet,* vol. 2 (1988): 1066–69.

Preston-Martin, S. and W. Lijinsky. "Cured meats and childhood cancer," *Cancer Causes and Control,* vol. 4 (1994): 484–86.

Pugliese, M. T., F. Lifshitz, G. Grad, P. Fort, and M. Marks-Katz. "Fear of obesity—a cause of short stature and delayed puberty," *New England Journal of Medicine,* vol. 309 (1983): 513–18.

Ravelli, G. P., Z. A. Stein, and M. W. Susser. "Obesity in young men after famine exposure in utero and early infancy," *New England Journal of Medicine,* vol. 295 (1976): 349–53.

Roberts, S. B. and R. McDonald. "The evolution of a new research field: metabolic programming by early diet," *Journal of Nutrition,* vol. 128 (1998): 440S.

Sarasua, S. and D. A. Savitz. "Cured and broiled meat consumption in relation to childhood cancer: Denver, Colorado (United States)," *Cancer Causes and Control,* vol. 5 (1994): 141–48.

Sargent, J. D., T. A. Stukel, M. A. Dalton, J. L. Freeman, and M. J. Brown. "Iron deficiency in Massachusetts communities: socioeconomic and demographic risk factors among children," *American Journal of Public Health,* vol. 86 (1996): 544–50.

Waterland, R. A., and C. Garza. "Potential mechanisms of metabolic imprinting that lead to chronic disease," *American Journal of Clinical Nutrition,* vol. 69 (1999): 179–97.

Chapter 2: Inside Your Child's Head

Birch, L. L. "Effects of peer model's food choices and eating behaviors on preschoolers' food preferences," *Child Development,* vol. 51 (1980): 489–96.

Birch, L. L., and J. O. Fisher. "Development of eating behaviors among children and adolescents," *Pediatrics,* vol. 101 (1998): 539–49.

Birch, L. L., S. L. Johnson, G. Andresen, J. C. Peters, and M. C. Schulte. "The variability of young children's energy intake," *New England Journal of Medicine*, vol. 324 (1991): 232–35.

Birch, L. L., D. W. Marlin, and J. Rotter. "Eating as the 'means' activity in a contingency: effects on young children's food preference," *Child Development*, vol. 55 (1984): 431–39.

Birch, L. L., L. McPhee, L. Steinberg, and S. Sullivan. "Conditioned flavor preferences in young children," *Physiology and Behavior*, vol. 47 (1990): 501–505.

Birch, L. L., S. I. Zimmerman, and H. Hind. "The influence of social-affective context on the formation of children's food preferences," *Child Development*, vol. 51 (1980): 856–61.

Fallon, A. E., P. Rozin, and P. Pliner. "The child's conception of food: the development of food rejections with special reference to disgust and contamination sensitivity," *Child Development*, vol. 55 (1984): 566–75.

Gemelli, R. *Normal Child and Adolescent Development.* Washington, D.C.: American Psychiatric Press, Inc., 1996.

Lepper, M. R., G. Sagotsky, J. L. Dafoe, and D. Greene. "Consequences of superfluous social constraints: effects on young children's social inferences and subsequent intrinsic interests," *Journal of Personality and Social Psychology*, vol. 42 (1982): 51–65.

Olson, C. M., D. J. Pringle, and C. D. Schoenwetter. "Parent-child interaction: its relation to growth and weight," *Journal of Nutrition Education*, vol. 3 (1976): 67–70.

Pinker, S. *The Language Instinct.* New York: William Morrow and Company, Inc., 1994.

Chapter 3: The Key Eight Nutrients

"A summary of conference recommendations on dietary fiber in childhood (conference on Dietary Fiber in Childhood, New York, May 24, 1994)," *Pediatrics*, vol. 96 (1995): 1023–28.

American Academy of Pediatrics-Committee on Nutrition. "Statement on cholesterol," *Pediatrics*, vol. 90 (1992): 469–73.

Anonymous. "Trans fatty acids and coronary heart disease risk. Report of the expert panel on trans fatty acids and coronary heart disease," *American Journal of Clinical Nutrition*, vol. 62 (1995): 655S–708S.

Carlson, S. E., M. T. Clandinin, H. W. Cook, E. A. Emken, and L. J. Filer. "Trans fatty acids: infant and fetal development," *American Journal of Clinical Nutrition*, vol. 66 (1997): 717S–36S.

Consensus Panel, 1994. "A summary of conference recommendations on dietary fiber in childhood," *Pediatrics* supplement (1995): 1023–28.

Craig, W. J. "Phytochemicals: guardians of our health," *Journal of the American Dietetic Association*, vol. 97 (Suppl 2, 1997): S199–S204.

Crawford, M. A. "The role of essential fatty acids in neural development: implications for perinatal nutrition," *American Journal of Clinical Nutrition*, vol. 57 (Suppl 5, 1993): 703S–10S.

Dwyer, J. T. "Dietary fiber for chidren: how much?" *Pediatrics*, vol. 96 (1995): 1019–22.

Eaton, S. B., S. B. Eaton, III, and M. J. Konner. "Paleolithic nutrition revisited: a twelve-year retrospective on its nature and implications," *European Journal of Clinical Nutrition*, vol. 51 (1997): 207–16.

Fairweather-Tait, S. J. "Iron-zinc and calcium-Fe interaction in relation to Zn and Fe absorption," *Proceedings of the Nutrition Society*, vol. 54 (1994): 465–73.

Fuchs, G. J., R. P. Farris, M. DeWier, S. Hutchinson, R. Strada, and R. M. Suskind. "Effect of dietary fat on cardiovascular risk factors in infancy," *Pediatrics*, vol. 93 (1994): 756–63.

Gaziano, J. M. "Antioxidants in cardiovascular disease: randomized trials," *Nutrition Reviews*, vol. 54 (1996): 175–84.

Glinsmann, W. H., S. J. Bartholemy, and F. Coletta. "Dietary guidelines for infants: a timely reminder," *Nutrition Reviews*, vol. 54 (1996): 50–57.

Johnston, C. C., J. Z. Miller, C. W. Slemenda, T. K. Reister, S. Hui, J. C. Christian, and M. Peacock. "Calcium supplementation and increase in bone mineral density in children," *New England Journal of Medicine*, vol. 327 (1992): 82–87.

Kelley, D. S., and A. Bendich. "Essential nutrients and immunologic functions," *American Journal of Clinical Nutrition*, vol. 63 (1996): 994S–96S.

Kennedy, E., and J. Goldberg. "What are American children eating? Implications for public policy," *Nutrition Reviews*, vol. 53 (1995): 111–26.

Lifshitz, F., and N. Moses. "Growth failure—a complication of dietary treatment of hypercholesterolemia," *American Journal of Diseases of Children*, vol. 143 (1989): 537–42.

Lloyd, T., M. B. Andon, N. Rollings, J. K. Martel, J. R. Landis, L. M. Demers, D. F. Eggli, K. Kieselhorst, and H. E. Kulin. "Calcium supplementation and bone mineral density in adolescent girls," *Journal of the American Medical Association*, vol. 270 (1993): 841–44.

Massey, L. K., and S. J. Whiting. "Dietary salt, urinary calcium, and kidney stone risk," *Nutrition Reviews*, vol. 53 (1995): 131–39.

National Institutes of Health. "Optimal calcium intake," *NIH Consensus Statement*, vol. 12 (1994): 1–31.

NCEP. "National cholesterol education program (NCEP): highlights of the report of the expert panel on blood cholesterol levels in children and adolescents," *Pediatrics*, vol. 89 (1992): 495–501.

Nettleton, J. A. "Are n-3 fatty acids essential nutrients for fetal and infant development?" *Journal of the American Dietetic Association*, vol. 93 (1993): 58–64.

Prentice, A. "Calcium requirements of children," *Nutrition Reviews*, vol. 53 (1995): 37–45.

Roncagliolo, M., M. Garrido, T. Walter, P. Peirano, and B. Lozoff. "Evidence of altered central nervous system development in infants with iron deficiency anemia at 6 months delayed maturation of auditory brainstem responses," *American Journal of Clinical Nutrition*, vol. 68 (1998): 683–90.

Joint Working Group of the Canadian Pediatric Society and Health Canada. "Nutrition recommendations update: dietary fats and children," *Nutrition Reviews*, vol. 53 (1995): 367–75.

Walravens, P. A., A. Chakar, R. Mokni, J. Denise, and D. Lemonnier. "Zinc supplements in breast-fed infants," *Lancet*, vol. 340 (1992): 683–85.

Yates, A. A., S. A. Schlicker, and C. W. Suitor. "Dietary reference intakes: the new basis for recommendations for calcium and related nutrients, B vitamins, and choline," *Journal of the American Dietetic Association*, vol. 98 (1998): 699–706.

Chapter 4: Food for Thought

Cohen, R. J., K. Haddix, E. Hurtado, and K. G. Dewey. "Maternal activity budgets: feasibility of exclusive breast-feeding for six months among urban women in Honduras," *Social Science & Medicine*, vol. 41 (1995): 527–36.

Cunningham, A. S., D. B. Jelliffe, and E. F. P. Jelliffe. "Breast-feeding and health in the 1980s: a global epidemiologic review," *Journal of Pediatrics*, vol. 118 (1991): 659–66.

Dewey, K. G., M. J. Heinig, and L. A. Nommsen-Rivers. "Differences in morbidity between breast-fed and formula-fed infants," *Journal of Pediatrics*, vol. 126 (1995): 696–702.

Donovan, S. M., and J. Odle. "Growth factors in milk as mediators of infant development," *Annual Review of Nutrition*, vol. 14 (1994): 147–67.

Heinig, M. J., and K. G. Dewey. "Health advantages of breast-feeding for infants: a critical review," *Nutrition Research Reviews*, vol. 9 (1996): 89–110.

Hill, P. D., J. L. Andersen, and R. J. Ledbetter. "Delayed initiation of breast-feeding the preterm infant," *Journal of Perinatal & Neonatal Nursing*, vol. 9 (1995): 10–20.

Littman, H., S. V. Medendorp, and J. Goldfarb. "The decision to breast-feed—the importance of father's approval," *Clinical Pediatrics*, vol. 33 (1994): 214–19.

Shu, X. O., J. Clemens, W. Zheng, D. M. Ying, B. T. Ji, and F. Jin. "Infant breast-feeding and the risk of childhood lymphoma and leukemia," *International Journal of Epidemiology*, vol. 24 (1995): 27–32.

Sullivan, S. A., and L. L. Birch. "Infant dietary experience and acceptance of solid foods," *Pediatrics*, vol. 93 (1994): 271–77.

Varendi, H., R. H. Porter, and J. Winberg. "Does the newborn baby find the nipple by smell?" *Lancet*, vol. 344 (1994): 989–90.

Varendi, H., R. H. Porter, and J. Winberg. "How do newborns find their mother's breast?" *Birth*, vol. 22 (1995): 174–75.

Chapter 5: Breast-feeding Made Easy

"Academy endorses the 10 steps and criteria of the breast-feeding health initiative," *American Family Physician*, vol. 50 (1994): 457–58.

Alexander, J. M., A. M. Grant, and M. J. Campbell. "Randomised controlled trial of breast shells and Hoffman's exercises for inverted and non-practile nipples," *British Medical Journal*, vol. 304 (1992): 1030–32.

Atkinson, H. C., E. J. Begg, and B. A. Darlow. "Drugs in human milk: clinical pharmacokinetic considerations," *Clinical Pharmacokinetics*, vol. 14 (1988): 217–40.

Capretta, P. J., J. T. Petersik, and D. J. Stewart. "Acceptance of novel flavours is increased after early experience of diverse tastes," *Nature*, vol. 254 (1975): 689–91.

Cooper, R. L., and M. M. Cooper. "Red pepper–induced dermatitis in breast-fed infants," *Dermatology*, vol. 193 (1996): 61–62.

Cronenwelt, L., T. Stukel, M. Kearney, J. Barrett, C. Covington, K. DelMonte, R. Reinhardt, and L. Rippe. "Single daily bottle use in the early weeks postpartum and breast-feeding outcomes," *Pediatrics*, vol. 90 (1992): 760–66.

Dewey, K. G., M. J. Heinig, and L. A. Nommsen. "Maternal weight-loss patterns during prolonged lactation," *American Journal of Clinical Nutrition*, vol. 58 (1993): 162–66.

Dewey, K. G., and M. A. McCrory. "Effects of dieting and physical activity on pregnancy and lactation," *American Journal of Clinical Nutrition*, vol. 59 (1994): 446S–53S.

Fitzgerald, E. F., S. A. Hwang, B. Bush, K. Cook, and P. Worswick. "Fish consumption and breast milk PCB concentrations among Mohawk women at Akwesasne," *American Journal of Epidemiology*, vol. 148 (1998): 164–72.

Katan, M. B., P. L. Zock, and R. P. Mensink. "Trans fatty acids and their effects on lipoproteins in humans," *Annual Review of Nutrition*, vol. 15 (1995): 473–93.

Kramer, P. "Breast-feeding of adopted infants," *British Medical Journal,* vol. 311 (1995): 188–89.

Lothian, J. A. "It takes two to breast-feed: the baby's role in successful breast-feeding," *Journal of Nurse-Midwifery,* vol. 40 (1995): 328–34.

Lucas, A., R. B. Drewett, and M. D. Mitchell. "Breast-feeding and plasma oxytocin concentrations," *British Medical Journal,* vol. 281 (1980): 834–35.

Mennella, J. A., and G. K. Beauchamp. "Maternal diet alters the sensory qualities of human milk and the nursling's behavior," *Pediatrics,* vol. 88 (1991): 737–44.

Mennella, J. A., and G. K. Beauchamp. "The effects of repeated exposure to garlic-flavored milk on the nursling's behavior," *Pediatric Research,* vol. 34 (1993): 805–808.

Perez-Escamilla, R., E. Pollitt, B. Lonnerdal, and K. G. Dewey. "Infant feeding policies in maternity wards and their effect on breast-feeding success: an analytical overview," *American Journal of Public Health,* vol. 84 (1994): 89–97.

Rice, D. C. "Neurotoxicity of lead, methylmercury, and PCBs in relation to the Great Lakes," *Environmental Health Perspectives,* vol. 103 (Suppl 9, 1995): 71–87.

Roberts, S. B., T. J. Cole, and W. A. Coward. "Lactational performance in relation to energy intake in the baboon," *American Journal of Clinical Nutrition,* vol. 41 (1985): 1270–76.

Roberts, S. B., A. A. Paul, T. J. Cole, and R. G. Whitehead. "Seasonal changes in activity, birthweight, and lactational performance in rural Gambian women," *Transcripts of the Royal Society of Tropical Medicine and Hygiene,* vol. 76 (1982): 668–78.

Specker, B. L. "Nutritional concerns of lactating women consuming vegetarian diets," *American Journal of Clinical Nutrition,* vol. 59 (Suppl, 1994): S1182–86.

Stintzing, G., and R. Zetterstorm. "Cow's milk allergy, incidence, and pathogenetic role of early exposure to cow's milk formula," *Acta Pediatrica Scandanavia,* vol. 68 (1979): 383–87.

Sullivan, S. A., and L. L. Birch. "Infant dietary experience and acceptance of solid foods," *Pediatrics,* vol. 93 (1994): 271–77.

Victora, C. G., E. Tomasi, M. T. A. Olinto, and F. C. Barros. "Use of pacifiers and breast-feeding duration," *Lancet,* vol. 341 (1993): 404–406.

Wright, A., S. Rice, and S. Wells. "Changing hospital practices to increase the duration of breast-feeding," *Pediatrics,* vol. 97 (1996): 669–75.

Ziemer, M. M., D. M. Cooper, and J. G. Pigeon. "Evaluation of a dressing to reduce nipple pain and improve nipple skin condition in breast-feeding women," *Nursing Research,* vol. 44 (1995): 347–51.

Chapter 6: New Options in Formula Feeding

American Academy of Pediatrics—Committee on Nutrition. "The use of whole cow's milk in infancy," *Pediatrics,* vol. 72 (1983): 253–55.

Hide, D., and B. Wharton. "Hydrolysed protein formulas: thoughts from the Isle of Wight meeting," *European Journal of Clinical Nutrition,* vol. 49 (Suppl 1, 1995): S100–S106.

Innis, S. M., C. M. Nelson, D. Lwanga, F. M. Rioux, and P. Waslen. "Feeding formula without arachidonic acid and docosahexaenoic acid has no effect on preferential looking acuity or recognition memory in healthy full-term infants at nine months of age," *American Journal of Clinical Nutrition,* vol. 64 (1996): 40–46.

Innis, S. M., C. M. Nelson, F. M. Rioux, and D. J. King. "Development of visual acuity in relation to plasma and erythrocyte omega-6 and omega-3 fatty acids in healthy term gestation infants," *American Journal of Clinical Nutrition,* vol. 60 (1994): 347–52.

Lee Y. H. "Food-processing approaches to altering allergenic potential of milk-based for-mula," *Journal of Pediatrics*, vol. 121 (1992): S47–S50.

Makrides, M., M. Neumann, K. Simmer, J. Pater, and R. Gibson. "Are long-chain polyun-saturated fatty acids essential nutrients in infancy?" *Lancet*, vol. 345 (1995): 1463–68.

Makrides, M., K. Simmer, M. Goggin, and R. A. Gibson. "Erythrocyte docosahexaenoic acid correlates with the visual response of healthy, term infants," *Pediatric Research*, vol. 33 (4 Pt 1, 1993): 425–27.

Moran, J. R. "Effects of prolonged exposure to partially hydrolyzed milk protein," *Journal of Pediatrics*, vol. 121 (1992): S90–S94.

Ponder, D. L., S. M. Innis, J. D. Benson, and J. S. Siegman. "Docosahexaenoic acid status of term infants fed breast milk or infant formula containg soy oil or corn oil," *Pediatric Research*, vol. 32 (1992): 683–88.

Redel, C. A., and R. J. Shulman. "Controversies in the composition of infant formulas," *Pediatric Clinics of North America*, vol. 41 (1994): 909–24.

Scott, F. W. "AAP recommendations on cow milk, soy, and early infant feeding," *Pediatrics*, vol. 96 (1995): 515–17.

Van Winkle, S., S. M. Levy, M. C. Kiritsy, J. R. Heilman, J. S. Wefel, and T. Marshall. "Water and formula fluoride concentrations: significance for infants fed formula," *Pediatric Dentistry*, vol. 17 (1995): 305–10.

Wharton, B., and D. Hide. "The role of hypoallergenic formulae in cow's milk allergy and allergy prevention," *European Journal of Clinical Nutrition*, vol. 49 (Suppl 1, 1995): S1–S106.

Chapter 7: Feeding a Premature Infant

Biancuzzo, M. "Breast-feeding preterm twins: a case report," *Birth*, vol. 21 (1994): 96–100.

Bosque, E. M., J. P. Brady, D. D. Affonson, and V. Wahlberg. "Physiologic measures of kan-garoo versus incubator care in a tertiary-level nursery," *Journal of Obstetric, Gynecologic & Neonatal Nursing*, vol. 24 (1995): 219–26.

Dobbing, J., editor. *Developing Brain and Behaviour: The Role of Lipids in Infant Formula.* New York: Academic Press, 1997.

Field, T. M. "Interventions for premature infants," *Journal of Pediatrics*, vol. 109 (1986): 183–91.

Hill, P. D., J. L. Andersen, and R. J. Ledbetter. "Delayed initiation of breast-feeding the preterm infant," *Journal of Perinatal and Neonatal Nursing*, vol. 9 (1995): 10–20.

Hill, P. D., and L. P. Brown. "Initiation and frequency of breast expression in breast-feeding mothers of lbw and vlbw infants," *Nursing Research*, vol. 44 (1995): 352–55.

Lemons, P. K., and J. A. Lemons. "Transition to breast/bottle feedings: the premature in-fant," *Journal of the American College of Nutrition*, vol. 15 (1996): 126–35.

Lucas, A., M. S. Fewtrell, R. Morley, P. J. Lucas, B. A. Baker, G. Lister, and N. J. Bishop. "Randomized outcome trial of human milk fortification and developmental outcome in preterm infants," *American Journal of Clinical Nutrition*, vol. 64 (1996): 142–51.

Mead L. J., R. Chuffo, P. Lawlor-Klean, and P. P. Meier. "Breast-feeding success with preterm quadruplets," *Journal of Obstetric, Gynecologic & Neonatal Nursing*, vol. 21 (1992): 221–27.

Meier, P., and L. P. Brown. "State of the science. Breast-feeding for mothers and low birth weight infants," *Nursing Clinics of North America*, vol. 31 (1996): 351–65.

Roberts, S. B., and A. Lucas. "Effect of two extremes of dietary intake on protein accretion in preterm infants," *Early Human Development,* vol. 12 (1985): 301–307.

Schanler, R. J. "Human milk fortification for premature infants," *American Journal of Clinical Nutrition,* vol. 64 (1996): 249–50.

Walker, M. "Breast-feeding the premature infant," *NAACOG's Clinical Issues,* vol. 3 (1992): 621–33.

Chapter 8: The Family Balancing Act

"Position paper of the American Council on Science and Health: Public health concerns about environmental polychlorinated biphenyls," *Ecotoxicology and Environmental Safety,* vol. 38 (1997): 71–84.

"Tufts University Health and Nutrition Letter," vol. 16 (1998): 1–8.

Ahl, A. S., and B. Buntain. "Risk and the food safety chain: animal health, public health, and the environment," *Revue Scientifique et Technique,* vol. 16 (1997): 322–30.

American Academy of Pediatrics—Committee on Nutrition. "The use of whole cow's milk in infancy," *Pediatrics,* vol. 72 (1983): 253–55.

American Dietetic Association. "Position of the American Dietetic Association: food irradiation," *Journal of the American Dietetic Association,* vol. 96 (1996): 69–72.

Dennison, B. A., H. L. Rockwell, and S. L. Baker. "Excess fruit juice consumption by preschool-aged children is associated with short stature and obesity," *Pediatrics,* vol. 99 (1997): 15–22.

Johnston, P. K. "Vegetarian nutrition, Second International Congress on Vegetarian Nutrition, Arlington, Virginia," *American Journal of Clinical Nutrition,* vol. 59 (Suppl 5, 1994).

Jones, J. M. *Food Safety.* St. Paul, Minnesota: Eagen Press, 1992.

Liebman, B. "Sugar: the sweetening of the American diet," *Nutrition Action,* vol. 25 (1998): 3–7.

Oparil, S. "Dietary sodium and health, Conference on dietary sodium and health, Arlington, Virginia," *American Journal of Clinical Nutrition,* vol. 65 (Suppl 2, 1997).

Prince, D. M., and M. A. Welschenbach. "Olestra: a new food additive," *Journal of the American Dietetic Association,* vol. 98 (1998): 565–69.

Rumm-Kreuter, D., and I. Demmel. "Comparison of vitamin losses in vegetables due to various cooking methods," *Journal of Nutrition Science and Vitaminology,* vol. 36 (1990): S14–S15.

Sanders, T.A.B., and S. Reddy. "Vegetarian diets and children," *American Journal of Clinical Nutrition,* vol. 59 (1994): 1176S–1181S.

Slutsker, L., S. F. Alterkruse, and D. L. Swerdlow. "Foodborne diseases: emerging pathogens and trends," *Infectious Disease Clinics of North America,* vol. 12 (1998): 199–216.

Stevenson, M. H. "Nutritional and other implications of irradiating meat," *Proceedings of the Nutrition Society,* vol. 53 (1994): 317–25.

Tauxe, R. V. "Emerging foodborne diseases: an evolving public health challenge," *Emerging Infectious Diseases,* vol. 3 (1997): 425–34.

Weinberger, M. H. "Salt sensitivity: does it play an important role in the pathogenesis and treatment of hypertension?" *Current Opinions in Nephrology & Hypertension,* vol. 5 (1996): 205–208.

Wender, E. H., and M. V. Solanto. "Effects of sugar on agressive and inattentive behavior in children with attention deficit disorder with hyperactivity and normal children," *Pediatrics,* vol. 88 (1991): 960–66.

Chapter 9: Four to Twelve Months

Barness, L. A. "Bases of weaning recommendations," *Journal of Pediatrics,* vol. 117 (1990): S84–85.

Dusdieker, L. B., J. P. Getchell, T. M. Liarakos, W. J. Hausler, and C. I. Dungy. "Nitrate in baby foods: adding to the nitrate mosaic," *Archives of Pediatric and Adolescent Medicine,* vol. 148 (1994): 490–94.

Heinig, M. J., L. A. Nommsen, J. M. Peerson, B. Lonnerdal, and K. G. Dewey. "Energy and protein intakes of breast-fed and formula-fed infants during the first year of life and their association with growth velocity: the DARLING study," *American Journal of Clinical Nutrition,* vol. 58 (1993): 152–61.

Heinig, M. J., L. A. Nommsen, J. M. Peerson, B. Lonnerdal, and K. G. Dewey. "Intake and growth of breast-fed and formula-fed infants in relation to the timing of introduction of complementary foods: the DARLING study," *Acta Pediatrica,* vol. 82 (1993): 999–1006.

Hendricks, K. M., and S. H. Badruddin. "Weaning recommendations: the scientific basis," *Nutrition Reviews,* vol. 50 (1992): 125–33.

Herschkowitz, N., J. Kagan, and K. Zilles. "Neurobiological bases of behavioral development in the first year," *Neuropediatrics,* vol. 28 (1997): 296–306.

Hervada, A. R., and D. R. Newman. "Weaning: historical perspectives, practical recommendations, and current controversies," *Current Problems in Pediatrics,* vol. 22 (1992): 223–40.

Hide, D. W. The clinical expression of allergy in breast-fed infants. In: *Immunology of Milk and the Neonate* by J. Mestecky. New York: Plenum Press, (1991): 475–80.

Lascari, A. D. "Carotenemia," *Clinical Pediatrics,* vol. 20 (1981): 25–29.

Lucas, A., G. Weing, S. B. Roberts, and W. A. Coward. "How much energy does the breast-fed infant consume and expend?" *British Medical Journal,* vol. 295 (1987): 75–77.

Lukens, J. N. "The legacy of well-weather methemoglobinemia," *Journal of the American Medical Association,* vol. 257 (1987): 2793–795.

Merhav, H., Y. Amitai, H. Paltai, and S. Godfrey. "Tea drinking and microcytic anemia in infants," *American Journal of Clinical Nutrition,* vol. 41 (1985): 1210–13.

Walravens, P. A., A. Chakar, R. Mokni, J. Denise, and D. Lemonnier. "Zinc supplements in breast-fed infants," *Lancet,* vol. 340 (1992): 683–85.

Chapter 10: Twelve to Twenty-one Months

Birch, L. L., D. W. Marlin, and J. Rotter. "Eating as the 'means' activity in a contingency: effects on young children's food preference," *Child Development,* vol. 55 (1984): 431–39.

Centers for Disease Control. "Dietary intake of vitamins, minerals, and fiber of persons ages 2 months and over in the United States: third national health and nutrition examination survey, phase 1, 1998–1991," *U.S. Department of Health and Human Services,* vol. 258 (1994): 1–26.

Fallon, A. E., P. Rozin, P. Pliner. "The child's conception of food: the development of food rejections with special reference to disgust and contamination sensitivity," *Child Development,* vol. 55 (1984): 566–75.

Matkovic, V. "Calcium metabolism and calcium requirements during skeletal modelling and consolidation of bone mass," *America Journal of Clinical Nutrition,* vol. 54 (1991): 245S–60S.

Chapter 11: Twenty-one Months to Three Years

Gelander, L., J. Karlberg, and K. Albertson-Winkland. "Seasonality in lower leg length velocity in prepubertal children," *Acta Paeditatrica,* vol. 82 (1994): 1249–54.

Harvey, J. A., P. Kenny, J. Poindexter, and C. Y. Pak. "Superior calcium absorption from calcium citrate than calcium carbonate using external forearm counting," *Journal of the American College of Nutrition,* vol. 9 (1990): 583–87.

Jarvinen, V. K., I. I. Rytomaa, and O. P. Heinonen. "Risk factors in dental erosion," *Journal of Dental Research,* vol. 70 (1991): 942–47.

Nicklas, T. A., W. Bao, L. S. Webber, and G. S. Berenson. "Breakfast consumption affects adequacy of total daily intake in children," *Journal of the American Dietetic Association,* vol. 93 (1993): 886–91.

VanWinkle, S., S. M. Levy, M. C. Kiritsy, J. R. Heilman, J. S. Wefel, and T. Marshall. "Water and formula fluoride concentrations: significance for infants fed formula," *Pediatric Dentistry,* vol. 17 (1995): 305–10.

Chapter 12: Three to Six Years

Birch, L. L. "Effects of peer model's food choices and eating behaviors on preschoolers' food preferences," *Childhood Development,* vol. 51 (1980): 489–96.

Connor, W. E. "The decisive influence of diet on the progression and reversibility of coronary heart disease," *American Journal of Clinical Nutrition,* vol. 64 (1996): 253–54.

Niinkoski, H., H. Kapinleimu, J. Viikari, et al. "Growth until three years of age in a prospective, randomized trial of a diet with reduced saturated fat and cholesterol," *Pediatrics,* vol. 99 (1997): 687–94.

Shannon, B. M., A. M. Tershakovec, J. K. Martel, C. L. Achterberg, J. A. Cortner, H. S. Smiciklas-Wright, V. A. Stallings, and P. D. Stolley. "Reduction of elevated LDL-cholesterol levels of four- to ten-year-old children through home-based dietary education," *Pediatrics,* vol. 94 (1994): 923–27.

The Writing Group for the DISC Collaborative Research Group. "Efficacy and safety of lowering dietary intake of fat and cholesterol in children with elevated low-density lipoprotein cholesterol: The Dietary Intervention Study in Children (DISC)," *Journal of the American Medical Association,* vol. 273 (1995): 1429–35.

Chapter 13: Feeding Your Sick Child

Acra, S. A., and F. K. Ghishan. "Electrolyte fluxes in the gut and oral rehydration solutions," *Pediatric Clinics of North America,* vol. 43 (1996): 433–49.

American Academy of Pediatrics. *Pediatric Nutrition Handbook.* Elk Grove Village, IL: American Academy of Pediatrics, 1998.

Cohen, M. B., A. G. Mezoff, W. Laney, J. A. Bezerra, B. M. Beane, D. Drazner, R. Baker, and J. R. Moran. "Use of a single solution for oral rehydration and maintenance therapy of infants with diarrhea and mild to moderate dehydration," *Pediatrics,* vol. 95 (1995): 639–45.

Gavin, N., N. Merrick, and B. Davidson. "Efficacy of glucose-based oral rehydration therapy," *Pediatrics,* vol. 96 (1996): 45–51.

Hurtado, E. K., A. H. Claussen, and K. G. Scott. "Early childhood anemia and mild or moderate mental retardation," *American Journal of Clinical Nutrition*, vol. 69 (1999): 115–19.

Pizarro, D., G. Posada, L. Sandi, and J. R. Moran. "Rice-based oral electrolyte solutions for the management of infantile diarrhea," *New England Journal of Medicine*, vol. 324 (1991): 517–21.

Rautanen, T., S. Kurki, and T. Vesikari. "Randomised double blind study of hypotonic oral rehydration solution in diarrhoea," *Archives of Disease in Childhood*, vol. 76 (1997): 272–74.

Reis, E. C., J. G. Goepp, S. Katz, and M. Santosham. "Barriers to use of oral rehydration therapy," *Pediatrics*, vol. 93 (1994): 708–11.

Santosham, M., I. Fayad, M. A. Zikri, et al. "A double-blind clinical trial comparing World Health Organization oral rehydration solution containing equal amounts of sodium and glucose," *Journal of Pediatrics*, vol. 128 (1996): 45–51.

Santucci, K. A., A. C. Anderson, W. J. Lewander, and J. G. Linakis. "Frozen oral hydration as an alternative to conventional enteral fluids," *Archives of Pediatric and Adolescent Medicine*, vol. 152 (1998): 142–46.

Chapter 14: Food, Sleep, and Your Baby

Adair, R., B. Zukerman, H. Bauchner, B. Phillipp, and S. Levenson. "Reducing night waking in infancy: a primary care intervention," *Pediatrics*, vol. 89 (1992): 585–88.

Dahl, R. E. "The impact of inadequate sleep on children's daytime cognitive function," In: *Seminars in Pediatric Neurolgy*, vol. 3 (1996): 44–50.

Ferber, R. "Childhood sleep disorders," *Neurological Clinics*, vol. 14 (1996): 493–511.

Fernstrom, J. D. "Dietary amino acids and brain function," *Journal of the American Dietetic Association*, vol. 94 (1994): 71–77.

Kahn, A., G. Francois, M. Sottiaux, E. Rebuffat, M. Nduwimana, M. J. Mozin, and J. Levitt. "Sleep characteristics in milk-intolerant infants," *Sleep*, vol. 11 (1988): 291–97.

Ma, G., M. Segawa, Y. Nomura, Y. Kondo, M. Yanagitani, and M. Higurashi. "The development of sleep-wakefulness rhythm in normal infants and young children," *Tohoku Journal of Experimental Medicine*, vol. 171 (1993): 29–41.

Oberlander, T. F., R. G. Barr, S. N. Young, and J. A. Brian. "Short-term effects of feed composition on sleeping and crying in newborns," *Pediatrics*, vol. 90 (1992): 733–40.

Pinilla, T. and L. L. Birch. "Help me make it through the night: behavioral entrainment of breast-fed infants' sleep patterns," *Pediatrics*, vol. 91 (1993): 436–44.

Rivekees, S. A. "Developing circadian rhythmicity. Basic and clinical aspects," *Pediatric Clinics of North America*, vol. 44 (1997): 467–87.

Sadeh, A. "Sleep and melatonin in infants: a preliminary study," *Sleep*, vol. 20 (1997): 185–91.

Steinberg, L. A., N. C. O'Connell, T. F. Hatch, M. F. Picciano, and L. L. Birch. "Tryptophan intake influences infants' sleep latency," *Journal of Nutrition*, vol. 122 (1992): 1781–91.

Yogman, M. W. and S. H. Zeisel. "Diet and sleep patterns in newborn infants," *New England Journal of Medicine*, vol. 309 (1983): 1147–49.

Chapter 15: Problems with Weight

Barlow, S. E. and W. H. Dietz. "Obesity evaluation and treatment: expert committee recommendations," *Pediatrics*, vol. 102 (1998): E29.

Birch, L. L., D. W. Marlin, L. Kramer, and C. Peyer. "Mother-child interaction patterns and the degree of fatness in children," *Journal of Nutrition Education*, vol. 13 (1981): 17–21.

Bjorntorp, P., and B. N. Brodoff. *Obesity.* Philadelphia: J. B. Lippincott Company, 1992.

Bruch, H. "Family transactions in eating disorders," *Comprehensive Psychiatry*, vol. 12 (1971): 238–48.

Epstein, L. H., A. M. Valoski, M. A. Kalarchian, and J. McCurley. "Do children lose and maintain weight easier than adults: a comparison of child and parent weight changes from six months to ten years," *Obesity Research*, vol. 3 (1995): 411–17.

Fisher, J. O., and L. L. Birch. "Fat preferences and fat consumption of three- to five-year-old children are related to parental adiposity," *Journal of the American Dietetic Association*, vol. 95 (1995): 759–64.

Ludwig, D. S., J. A. Majzoub, A. Al-Zahrani, G. E. Dallal, I. Blanco, and S. B. Roberts. "High glycemic index foods and overeating," *Pediatrics*, vol. 103 (1999): E26.

Maffeis, C., G. Talamini, and L. Tato. "Influence of diet, physical activity, and parents' obesity on children's adiposity: a four-year longitudinal study," *International Journal of Obesity*, vol. 22 (1998): 758–64.

Maloney, M. J., J. McGuire, S. R. Daniels, and B. Specker. "Dieting behavior and eating attitudes in children." *Pediatrics*, vol. 84 (1989): 482–89.

McCrory, M. A., P. J. Fuss, N. P. Hays, A. G. Vinken, and A. S. Greenberg. "Eating out and overeating in America: association between restaurant food consumption and body fatness in healthy adult men and women aged 19 to 80," *Obesity Research*, vol. 7 (1999): in press.

McCrory, M. A., P. J. Fuss, J. E. McCallum, M. Yao, A. G. Vinken, N. P. Hays, and S. B. Roberts. "Dietary variety within food groups: association with food intake and body fatness in adult men and women," *American Journal of Clinical Nutrition*, vol. 69 (1999): 440–47.

Ogden, C. L., R. P. Troiano, R. R. Briefel, R. J. Kuczmarski, K. M. Flegal, and C. L. Johnson. "Prevalence of overweight among preschool children in the United States, 1971 through 1994," *Pediatrics*, vol. 99 (1997): E1–14.

Roberts, S. B. "Early Diet and Obesity," In: *Nutrition During the Second Six Months.* New York: Raven Press, (1991): 303–16.

Roberts, S. B., and A. S. Greenberg. "The new obesity genes," *Nutrition Reviews*, vol. 54 (1996): 41–49.

Roberts, S. B., F. X. Pi-Sunyer, and M. Dreher, et al. "Physiology of fat replacement and fat reduction and effects of dietary fat and fat substitutes on energy regulation," *Nutrition Reviews*, vol. 56 (1998): S29–49.

Troiano, R. P., K. M. Flegal, R. J. Kuczmarski, S. M. Campbell, and C. L. Johnson. "Overweight prevalance and trends for children and adolescents," *Archives of Pediatric and Adolescent Medicine*, vol. 149 (1995): 1085–91.

Whitaker, R. C., J. A. Wright, M. S. Pepe, K. D. Seidel, and W. H. Dietz. "Predicting obesity in young adulthood from childhood and parental obesity," *New England Journal of Medicine*, vol. 337 (1997): 869–73.

Chapter 16: About Allergies, Food Intolerances, and Colic

"Breast-feeding and avoidance of food antigens in the prevention and management of allergic disease," *Nutrition Reviews*, vol. 36 (1978): 181–83.

Atherton, D. J., J. F. Soothill, M. Sewell, and R. S. Wells. "Double-blind controlled crossover trial of an antigen-avoidance diet in atopic eczema," *Lancet,* vol. 1 (1978): 401–407.

Brown, M. A., M. J. Halonen, and F. D. Martinez. "Cutting the cord: is birth already too late for primary prevention of allergy?" *Clinical and Experimental Allergy,* vol. 27 (1997): 4–6.

Cant, A. J. "Food allergy in childhood," *Human Nutrition: Applied Nutrition,* vol. 39A (1985): 277–93.

Cant, A. J., J. A. Bailes, and R. A. Marsden. "Cow's milk, soya milk and goat's milk in a mother's diet causing eczema and diarrhea in her breast-fed infant," *Acta Pediatrics Scandanavia,* vol. 74 (1985): 467–68.

Chandra, R. K. "Role of maternal diet and mode of infant feeding in prevention of atopic dermatitis in high risk infants," *Allergy,* vol. 44 (Suppl 9, 1989): 135–39.

Chandra, R. K. (1991). "Interactions between early nutrition and the immune system," *Ciba Foundation Symposium,* vol. 156 (1991): 89–92.

De Martino, M., M. Peruzzi, M. deLuca, A. G. Amato, L. Galli, L. Lega, C. Azzari, and A. Vierucci. "Fish allergy in children," *Annals of Allergy,* vol. 71 (1993): 159–65.

Dramer, M. S., and B. Moroz. "Do breast-feeding and delayed introduction of solid foods protect against subsequent atopic eczema?" *Journal of Pediatrics,* vol. 98 (1981): 546–50.

Fergusson, D. M., L. J. Horwood, and F. T. Shannon. "Early solid feeding and recurrent childhood eczema: a ten-year longitudinal study," *Pediatrics,* vol. 86 (1990): 541–46.

Hathaway, M. J. and J. O. Warner. "Compliance problems in the dietary management of eczema," *Archives of Disease in Childhood,* vol. 58 (1983): 463–64.

Hide, D., and B. Wharton. "Hydrolysed protein formulas: thoughts from the Isle of Wight meeting," *European Journal of Clinical Nutrition,* vol. 49 (1995): S100–106.

Hide, D. W. The clinical expression of allergy in breast-fed infants. In: *Immunology of Milk and the Neonate* by J. Mestecky. New York: Plenum Press, (1991): 475–80.

Hill, D. J. "The colic debate," *Pediatrics,* vol. 96 (1995): 165.

Hill, D. J., M. A. Firer, M. J. Shelton, and C. S. Hosking. "Manifestations of milk allergy in infancy: clinical and immunologic fingings," *Journal of Pediatrics,* vol. 109 (1986): 270–76.

Hill, D. J., and C. S. Hosking. "Preventing childhood allergy," *Medical Journal of Australia,* vol. 158 (1993): 367–69.

Hourihane, J. O., S. A. Kilburn, P. Dean, and J. O. Warner. "Clinical characteristics of peanut allergy," *Clinical & Experimental Allergy,* vol. 27 (1997): 634–39.

Hourihane, J.O.B. "Peanut allergy: recent advances and unresolved issues," *Journal of the Royal Society of Medicine,* vol. 30 (1997): 40–44.

Hourihane, J.O.B., S. A. Roberts, and J. O. Warner. "Resolution of peanut allergy: case-control study," *British Medical Journal,* vol. 316 (1998): 1271–75.

Kerner, J. A. "Formula allergy and intolerance," *Pediatric Gastroenterology,* vol. 24 (1995): 1–25.

Kmietowicz, Z. "Women warned to avoid peanuts during pregnancy and lactation," *British Medical Journal,* vol. 316 (1998): 1926.

Lucas, A., O. G. Brooke, T. J. Cole, R. Morley, and M. F. Bamford. "Food and drug reactions, wheezing, and eczema in preterm infants," *Archives of Disease in Childhood,* vol. 65 (1990): 411–15.

Lust, K. D., J. E. Brown, and W. Thomas. "Maternal intake of cruciferous vegetables and other foods and colic symptoms in exclusively breast-fed infants," *Journal of the American Dietetic Association,* vol. 96 (1996): 47–48.

Metcalfe, D. D. "Food allergy," *Current Opinion in Immunology,* vol. 3 (1991): 881–86.

Miskelly, F. G., M. L. Burr, E. Vaughan-Williams, A. M. Fehily, B. K. Butland, and T. G. Merrett. "Infant feeding and allergy," *Archives of Disease in Childhood,* vol. 63 (1988): 388–93.

Nehra, V. "New clinical issues in celiac disease," *Gastroenterology Clinics of North America,* vol. 27 (1998): 453–65.

Noma, T., I. Yoshizawa, K. Aoki, K. Yamaguchi, and M. Baba. "Cytokine production in children outgrowing hen egg allergy," *Clinical & Experimental Allergy,* vol. 26 (1996): 1298–1307.

Perry, C. A., J. Dwyer, J. A. Gelfand, R. R. Couris, and W. W. McCloskey. "Health effects of salicylates in foods and drugs," *Nutrition Reviews,* vol. 54 (1996): 225–40.

Pruessner, H. T. "Detecting celiac disease in your patients," *American Family Physician,* vol. 57 (1998): 1023–34.

Sackier, J. M. "Adverse reactions to antihistamine-decongestant," *Annals of Allergy, Asthma & Immunology,* vol. 74 (1995): 356.

Sicherer, S. H., A. W. Burks, and H. A. Sampson. "Clinical features of acute allergic reactions to peanut and tree nuts in children," *Pediatrics,* vol. 102 (1998): E6.

Stintzing, G., and R. Zetterstrom. "Cow's milk allergy, incidence and pathogenetic role of early exposure to cow's milk formula," *Acta Pediatrica Scandanavia,* vol. 68 (1979): 383–87.

Tariq, S. M. "Allergen avoidance in the primary prevention of atopy," *British Journal of Clinical Practice,* vol. 50 (1996): 99–102.

Vandenplas, Y. "The use of hydrolysates in allergy prevention programmes," *European Journal of Clinical Nutrition,* vol. 49 (1995): S84-91.

Wolke, D. "The colic debate," *Pediatrics,* vol. 96 (1995): 165–66.

Zeiger, R. S., and S. Heller. "The development and prediction of atopy in high-risk children: follow-up at age seven years in a prospective randomized study of combined maternal and infant food allergen avoidance," *Journal of Allergy & Clinical Immunology,* vol. 95 (1995): 1179–90.

Chapter 17: Food, Hyperactivity, and Attention Deficit Hyperactivity Disorder

Atherton, D. J., J. F. Soothill, M. Sewell, and R. S. Wells. "Double-blind controlled crossover trial of an antigen-avoidance diet in atopic eczema," *Lancet,* vol. 1 (1978): 401–407.

Biederman, J. "Attention-deficit/hyperactivity disorder: a life-span perspective," *Journal of Clinical Psychiatry,* vol. 59 (Suppl 7, 1998): 4–16.

Boris, M. and F. S. Mandel. "Foods and additives are common causes of the attention deficit hyperactive disorder in children," *Annals of Allergy,* vol. 72 (1994): 462–67.

Breakey, J. "The role of diet and behavior in childhood," *Journal of Pediatric Child Health,* vol. 33 (1997): 190–94.

Carter, C. M., M. Urbanowicz, R. Hemsley, L. Mantilla, S. Strobel, P. J. Graham, and E. Taylor. "Effects of a few food diet in attention deficit disorder," *Archives of Disease in Childhood,* vol. 69 (1993): 564–68.

Egger, J., P. J. Graham, C. M. Carter, D. Gumley, and J. F. Soothill. "Controlled trial of oligoantigenic treatment in the hyperkinetic syndrome," *Lancet,* vol. 1 (1985): 540–45.

Feingold, B. F. "Hyperkinesis and learning disabilities linked to artificial food flavors and colors," *American Journal of Nursing,* vol. 75 (1975): 797–803.

Findling, R. L., and J. W. Dogin. "Psychopharmacology of ADHD: children and adolescents," *Journal of Clinical Psychiatry,* vol. 59 (Suppl 7, 1998): 42–49.

Goldman, L. S., M. Genel, R. J. Bezman, and P. J. Slantez. "Diagnosis and treatment of attention-deficit disorder/hyperactivity disorder in children and adolescents. Council on Scientific Affairs, American Medical Association," *Journal of the American Medical Association,* vol. 279 (1998): 1100–107.

Greenhill, L. L. "Diagnosing attention-deficit/hyperactivity disorder in children," *Journal of Clinical Psychiatry,* vol. 59 (Suppl 7, 1998): 31–41.

Kanarek, R. B. "Does sucrose or aspartame cause hyperactivity in children?" *Nutrition Reviews,* vol. 52 (1994): 173–75.

Kapla, B. J., J. McNicol, R. A. Conte, and H. K. Moghadam. "Dietary replacement in preschool-aged hyperactive boys," *Pediatrics,* vol. 83 (1989): 7–17.

Perry, C. A., J. Dwyer, J. A. Gelfand, R. R. Couris, and W. W. McCloskey. "Health effects of salicylates in foods and drugs," *Nutrition Reviews,* vol. 54 (1996): 225–40.

Rowe, K. S., and K. J. Rowe. "Synthetic food coloring and behavior: a dose response effect in a double-blind, placebo-controlled, repeated-measures study," *Journal of Pediatrics,* vol. 125 (1994): 691–98.

Schahill, L., and A. deGraft-Johnson. "Food allergies, asthma, and attention deficit hyperactivity disorder," *Journal of Child & Adolescent Psychiatric Nursing,* vol. 10 (1997): 36–42.

Wolraich, M. L., S. D. Lindgren, P. J. Stumbo, L. D. Stegnik, M. I. Appelbaum, and M. C. Kiritsy. "Effects of diets high in sucrose or aspartame on the behavior and cognitive performance of children," *New England Journal of Medicine,* vol. 330 (1994): 301–307.

Wolraich, M. L., D. B. Wilson, and J. W. White. "The effect of sugar on behavior or cognition in children," *Journal of the American Medical Association,* vol. 274 (1995): 1617–21.

Zametkin, A. J., and W. Liotta. "The neurobiology of attention-deficit/hyperactivity disorder," *Journal of Clinical Psychiatry,* vol. 59 (Suppl 7, 1998): 17–23.

INDEX

Additives, food, 76, 281, 290, 308
AIs (Adequate Intakes), 312
Alar, 119
Alcohol, 75, 125
Allergies, 275-98
    causes of, 278
    cow's milk and, 245–47
    diagnosis/treatment of, 288–89
    versus food intolerances, 277–82
    frequent questions about, 294–98
    hydrolysate formula and, 87, 100
    living with, 289–90
    prevention of, 144, 282–84
    protection from, 8–9, 54, 144
    recognizing, 276–77
    strategies for, 285–88
    twenty-one months to three years and, 189
Alpha-linolenic acid, 32, 90
Anemia. *See* Iron
Antibiotics in meat, 120–21
Antioxidants, 10–11, 30, 46–48, 47, 122
Arachidonic acid, 90
Artificial sweeteners, 129
Attention deficit hyperactivity disorder
    (ADHD), 299–311
    diagnosis of, 299–300
    diet and, 300–302, 305
    foods that may cause, 302–3
    sugar and, 303–4
    vitamins and, 304–5

B vitamins, 30, 44–46, 314–16
Babies. *See* Newborns; Premature infants;
    specific ages for
Baby food, commercial, 148–49, 150–51, 171
Baby-sitters, family meals and, 129–30
Bacteria, intestinal, 34
Balanced diet, 6, 20, 188–89, 208
    for family meals, 113–18
Benzoic acid, 281
Bilirubin. *See* Jaundice, breast milk
Bioflavinoids, 48
Body image, 223–24, 251
Bone, development of, 9, 41–42
Boredom, variety instinct and, 19–21
Bottle(s), 78, 93–94, 182–83
    cleaning, 122
    milk teeth and, 166

    transition to cup from, 139, 164–65, 182
Botulism, honey and, 145
Bowel movements, 84–85, 98. *See also*
    Constipation, Diarrhea
Brain development, 9–10, 31–32, 53–54
Breakfast(s), 174, 176
Breast infection, 83
Breast milk, 32, 43–44, 60–61, 63. *See also*
    Expression, breast milk
    for first year, 134–35, 138
    versus formula, 55, 138
    jaundice and, 85
    measuring baby's intake of, 107
    taste, 74
Breast shields, shells. *See* Nipple shield
Breast size, nursing and, 81–82
Breast-feeding, 10, 59–85. *See also* Colic;
    Let-down reflex; Premature infants
    adequacy of, 72–73
    advantages of, 53–56
    allergy protection and, 9, 54, 282–83, 285–86
    baby's bowel movements and, 84–85
    baby's cavities and, 166
    baby's diarrhea during, 83
    baby's growth pattern during, 77
    breast infection during, 83
    burping skills and, 69
    comfort during, 68
    cow's milk allergy and, 284–85
    duration of exclusive, 77
    duration of sessions for, 66–67
    engorgement problems and, 68, 82
    from four weeks on, 77–81
    frequency of, 66–67
    frequent questions about, 81–85
    growth spurts and, 70, 72, 84
    harmful substances and, 75
    inadequate milk for, 72–73, 84
    introducing solid food and, 80, 109
    mother's diet for, 75–76, 294
    mother's exercise during, 79–80
    mother's health and, 56
    nutrition, milk supply and, 73–74
    on-demand *versus* scheduled, 69–70
    one *versus* two breasts for, 72
    pain, 64
    positioning for, 62–64, 65
    premature infants, 101–2
    in public, 79

reducing nighttime, 242–44
separations and, 78–79
sleep latency and, 244–45
starting, 60–67
stopping, 80–81, 84, 156
supplemental bottles during, 78
from three days to four weeks, 67–76
transition to cow's milk and, 164
Bridge of familiarity, 22–23, 27, 271
for twelve-to-twenty-month olds, 177–78
for two-year-olds, 199–200
Burns, 170
Burping, 69, 93, 97–98, 293

Caffeine, 75, 76, 125, 245
Cakes, 127
Calcium, 9, 30, 41–42, 313
for non-milk-drinkers, 202–3
for three-to-six-year-olds, 208
for twelve-to-twenty-month olds, 182
Caloric density, 256, 258
Calories, 6, 9, 30, 36–37
hyperactivity and, 303–4
Campylobacter jejuni bacteria, 121
Cancer prevention, 10–11
Candy, 126, 256
Cavities, baby bottle, 166
Celiac disease, 290–92
Cereals, nighttime sleeping and, 244
Chemicals in foods, 118–21
hyperactivity/ADHD and, 301
Child's diet perspective, 14–28
control instinct and, 16–18
hunter-gatherer instincts and, 26, 27, 186–87
imitative behavior and, 23–24, 27, 155, 180
love and, 27–28
on new foods, 21–22
research on, 15–16
resistance in, 24–26
similars and, 22–23
sucking reflex and, 18–19
variety instinct and, 19–21
Chinese food, 212
Choking, 143, 144, 170, 189
Cholesterol, 186–87
Clostridium botulinum, 145
Cobalamin, 315–16. *See also* B vitamins
Cod fried (recipe), 172
Colds, 238
Colic, 6, 83, 292–94, 295, 296–97
formula and, 87, 96–98
Colostrum, 60, 61
Conservatism instinct, 186
Constipation, 36, 85, 200–201, 203, 225
formula feeding and, 98
Control instinct, 16–18, 27
Convenience foods, 127–28

Cookies, 127, 191
recipe for, 193
Cooking. *See* Food preparation
Cow's milk, 32
sensitivity to, 245–47, 284–85
transition to, 161, 163–65, 182–83
Crackers, whole-wheat sesame (recipe), 193
Cradle (nursing) position, 63, 65
Cup feeding, 138–39, 164–65, 182–83, 225
Cyanide, 280

Dairy products, 32, 240. *See also* Milk
Day-care centers, 131–32
DDT, 119
Decosahexaenoic acid (DHA), 90
Dehydration, 232, 234, 236, 239–40
Desserts, 20, 127, 226, 254, 261
DHA. *See* Decosahexaenoic acid
Diabetes
adult-onset, 250
juvenile onset, 282
Diaper rash, 141
Diarrhea, 83, 231–37, 239–40, 295–96
formula feeding and, 98
fruit juice and, 183, 240
toddler, 204–5
Dieting, 251. *See also* Menus
eating disorders and, 270
nursing and, 73, 76
Discounting principle, 25–26, 177, 179–80, 219–20
Double-blind placebo-controlled food (DBPC) challenge, 288–89
DRIs (Dietary Reference Intakes), 30–31, 312
Drugs during delivery, 66
DVs (Daily Values), 312

E. coli bacteria, 121, 123
Eating, strategies for, 11
Eating disorders, 250, 269–70
Eating out
food allergies and, 289
with four-to-twelve-month-olds, 191
limiting, 265
with three- to six-year-olds, 211–12, 217
with twenty-one months to three-year-olds, 191
Echinacea, 239
Eczema, 275, 276, 296–97
Eggs, 34, 115, 117, 122–23
Electrolyte solutions, oral, 233, 235, 236, 237
Elemental formula(s), 86, 88, 91, 286–87
Elimination diet, sequential, 289, 297
changing, 308–9
hyperactivity and, 305–9
menus for, 307
modified, 309–11

planning, 306
  recordkeeping for, 305–6, 308
Encouragement, resistance to, 24–26, 27, 194
Engorgement problems, 68, 82
Enjoyment of food, 16
Example, parental, 23–24, 27, 155, 180
Exclusive nursing, 77
Exercise, 42, 266–67
  during nursing, 79–80
Expression, breast milk, 71, 73, 78, 79
  premature births and, 103, 104–5, 107
Extrusion reflex, 133

Failure to thrive, 8, 183–84, 203–4, 273, 291
Familiarity, bridge of. *See* Bridge of familiarity
Family day care, 131–32
Family meals, 28, 113–32
  artificial sweeteners and, 129
  baby-sitters, others and, 129–32
  desserts/cookies/cakes and, 127
  fast food/convenience foods and, 127–28
  fat-free/lite foods and fat substitutes, 128
  foods to avoid/limit, 124–26
  irradiated foods and, 121–24
  kitchen safety guidelines and, 122
  nutritional requirements for, 116–17
  pesticide/chemical concerns and, 118–21
  practical steps for, 117–18
  strategies for, 114–17
  vegetarian/macrobiotic, 124
Family medical history, 115, 161, 186–87, 251
Fast food, 127–28, 154
Fat(s), 30, 31–34, 114, 188, 259
  brain development and, 10, 31–32
  breast-feeding and, 53
  caloric density and, 258
  formulas containing, 90
  heart disease and, 186–87, 207
Fat substitutes, 128
Fat-free foods, 128, 258
Feeding skills, fostering age-appropriate, 17–18
Feingold, Ben, 301
Ferber, Richard, 247
Fever, 231–37
Fiber, 30, 34–36, 114, 189, 208
Fifteen, rule of, 21–22, 27, 177, 196, 271
Fish, 75, 125, 172
Flat nipples, breast-feeding and, 63, 107. *See
  also* Inverted nipples
Fluoride, 181
  formula feeding and, 95
  for nursing babies, 80
  for six-months and older, 149–50
  for twelve-to-twenty-three-month olds, 166,
    181
Folate, 30, 44–46, 314–15
Follow-up formula, 88, 92
Food groups, portions by age, 116

Food intolerance(s), 275–98
  causes of, 278
  colic and, 292–94
  diagnosis/treatment of, 288–89
  of food additives/contaminants, symptoms
    of, 281
  versus food allergies, 277–82
  formula and, 87
  frequent questions about, 294–98
  to gluten, 290–92
  of natural foods, symptoms of, 280–81
  recognizing, 276–77
Food opportunities, 25
Food preferences. *See also* Child's diet
    perspective
  determining future, 12
  imitation and, 23–24, 27, 155, 180
  similars and, 22–23
Food preparation, 115, 117, 196–97, 213
Food shopping, 26, 118, 216
Food tricks, 200
Football (nursing) position, 65
Fore milk, 60
Formula(s), 86–100
  amount to feed, 94–95
  for allergy prevention, 286–87
  colic and, 294
  elemental, 86, 88, 91
  essential fatty acids in, 32
  follow-up, 88, 92
  hydrolysate, 86, 87, 88, 91
  hypoallergenic, 9, 86
  lactose-free, 88, 91–92
  for premature infants, 107–108
  sleep latency and, 244–45
  soy, 89, 91–92
  standard, 86, 87, 88, 89–90
  tryptophan levels in, 245
  types of, 87–92
  zinc in, 43–44
Formula feeding, 86–100
  baby's disdain for, 100
  first feedings of, 92–94
  frequent questions about, 96–100
  introducing after breast feeding, 156
  milk intolerance and, 100
  on-demand, 94–95
  for premature infants, 107–8
  safety procedures for, 96–97
  solid foods and, 137
  types of, 87–92
Fortifier formulas, 108
Four-to-twelve-month olds, 133–58
  balancing solid foods/milk for, 143–44
  breast milk for, 138
  commercial baby food, 148–49, 150–51
  cup feeding for, 138–39
  eating out with, 149
  first spoonfuls, 136–37

foods to avoid, 144–45
formula for, 138
frequent questions about, 155–58
menus and schedules for, 146–48
milk's place in meals for, 139
multivitamin/mineral supplements for, 149–50
new foods for, 141–42
opportunities/goals for, 134–35
solid foods for, 135–37, 140–41
strategies for feeding, 150–55
time-frame for new foods for, 142–43
Free radicals, 46
Friends, family nutrition and, 130–31, 217
Fruit(s), 42, 178, 188
  antioxidants and, 46–47
  child's weight gain and, 252, 261, 263
  premature heart disease and, 187
Fruit drinks, 126, 236, 255, 261
Fruit juice(s), 152, 183, 240, 255
Fussy eaters, 199, 224–25, 270–71

Galactosemia, 92
Garage hazards, 170
Gardening, 26, 196–97
Gastroesophageal reflux. See Spitting-up,
  Vomiting
Glycemic index, 256, 259, 260, 271, 304
Grazing versus scheduled meals, 157
Growth failure. See Failure to thrive
Growth patterns, 72, 155, 163, 183, 203–4
  centile charts and, 318–30
  formula feeding and, 99
  nursing and, 70, 72, 84
  weighing to measure, 107

Habits, eating, 176, 189
Heart disease, premature, 33, 186–87
Herb teas, 76
Hind milk, 60, 294
Histamine, 280
Holiday food, 220
Home food versus outside food, 24, 27, 218–19,
  224, 256
Homocysteine, 45
Honey, botulism and, 145
Horizontal (nursing) position, 65
Hormones in meat, 120
Housekeepers, family meals and, 129–30
Hunger signals, recognizing, 133, 151–53, 195–96
Hunter-gatherer instincts, 21, 26, 27, 186–87
Hydrolysate formula(s), 86, 87, 88, 91, 286–87
  cow's milk sensitivity and, 246
Hyperactivity, 299–311
  diagnosis of, 299–300
  diet and, 300–302
  foods that may cause, 302–3
  modified elimination diet for, 305–9

substitutions for modified elimination diet
  for, 309–11
  sugar and, 303–4
  vitamins and, 304–5
Hypoallergenic formula(s), 9, 86

Illness, nursing and, 70, 105
  breast infection, 83
Imitation, food preferences and, 23–24, 27, 155,
  180
Immune system, 8–9
  breast-feeding and, 54
Impacted stools, 225–26
Inducements, for eating, 24–26, 27, 194, 204
Insects, 119
Instincts, children's diet, 16–27
Intelligence. See Brain development
International Lactation Consultants
  Association, 59–60
Inverted nipples, breast-feeding and, 63, 81, 107
Irradiation, foods, 121–24
Iron, 30, 38–40, 135, 138, 188, 208
  brain development and, 9–10
  dangers of excess, 40
  sources of, 39, 312–13

Jaundice, breast milk, 85
Juice(s), 152, 171, 271–72
  citrus and teeth, 166
  fruit and vegetable, 152
  unpasteurized, 123
Juvenile rheumatoid arthritis, 297

Kangaroo care, 103, 104
Kitchen accidents, 170

La Leche League, 60
Lactation consultant/counselor, 59–60, 71, 102–3
Lactose intolerance, 279–82, 297–98
Lactose-free formula, 88, 91–92
Lead in drinking water, 75
Leakage, breast milk, 63, 68
Let-down reflex, 61, 68–69, 71
  baby's aversion to, 82–83
Linolenic acid, 32, 80
Lipoprotein lipase enzyme, 253
Listeria monocytogenes (bacteria), 125
Lite foods, 128
Love, food and expressions of, 27–28
Ludwig, David, 304

Macrobiotic diets, 124
Malnutrition, 4, 291
  accidental, 8, 203–4

Marmite, 45–46
Marx, Groucho, 25
Meat(s), 115, 122, 125
Medical history. *See* Family medical history
Memory, childhood, 12
Menus
    for breast/formula-fed eleven-month-olds, 148
    for breast/formula-fed six-month-olds, 146
    for formula-fed eleven-month-olds, 147
    for four-to-twelve-month-olds, 146–48
    for modified elimination diet, 309–11
    snack substitutes for weight control, 262–63
    for twelve–to–twenty–month–olds, 173
    for twenty–one months to three–year–olds, 190
Mercury, nursing mothers and, 75
Messy eaters, 155–56
Metabolic programming, 3–13
    for allergy protection, 8–9
    for bone and tooth development, 9
    for brain development and IQ, 9–10
    calcium and, 41–42
    for cancer prevention, 10–11
    definition of, 5, 7–8
    eating strategies and, 11
    future food preferences and, 12
    for weight, 8
    weight problems and, 252
Metoclopromide, 105
Milk. *See also* Breast milk; Cow's milk; Formula(s)
    child's weight gain and, 255, 263
    colds and, 240
    constipation and, 201
    essential fatty acids in, by type, 32
    exceptions to whole-milk rule, 165
    fat requirements and, 33–34
    for four-to-twelve-month olds, 134–35, 143–44
    intolerance for, formula feeding and, 100
    for three-to-six-year-olds, 207–8
    transition to cow's milk, 163–65
    for twelve-to-twenty-one month olds, 161, 182
    for twenty-one months to three years, 188, 205
Milk teeth, 166
Mineral supplements. *See* Multivitamin/ mineral supplements
Minerals, 30, 37–44; *Also see* Calcium, Iron, Zinc
Mold on food, 123
Monosodiumglutamate (MSG), 281
Mucus, dairy foods, 240
Multivitamin/mineral supplements, 48, 116–17, 149, 176, 268, 271, 274
    for colds, 238–39
    formula feeding and, 95

    for four-to-twelve-month olds, 149–50
    for fussy eaters, 225
    myths about, 6
    for nursing babies, 80
    for nursing mothers, 76
    phytochemicals and, 11
    for twelve-to-twenty-month olds, 176–77
Myelination, 32, 45

Nannies, family meals and, 129–30
New foods, 18, 21–22, 27, 271
    similars and, 22–23
Newborns, 53–58
    breast-feeding advantages, 53–57
    harness instincts, 57
    parental instincts in, 57–58
Nibblers (nursing), 70
Nicotine, nursing mothers and, 75
Nipple confusion, 71, 105
Nipple shield, 81, 107
Nipples, bottle, 93–94, 122
Nipples, breast, 63, 68, 81, 82, 107
Nitrates, 141, 145
Nitrites, 10, 47, 76, 125, 144
Nursing. *See* Breast-feeding
Nursing bras, 63
Nutritional requirements, 6, 29–50
    for antioxidants, 46–48
    eight key nutrients, 30
    family, 116–17
    for fat, 31–34
    for fiber, 34–36
    for folate and B vitamins, 44–46
    for minerals, 37–44
    multivitamin/mineral supplements and, 48
    for nursing mothers, 73–74
    portion goals for, 31
    recommendations for, 46
    for water, 48–49
Nutritional supplements. *See* Multivitamin/mineral supplements

Oat pancakes (recipe), 175
Oatmeal bread (recipe), 214
Obesity, 8, 210, 249–74. *See also* Weight
Olestra, 128
On-demand feeding, 69–70, 107, 146–47
    formula and, 94–95
    grazing and, 157
One-year-olds. *See* Twelve to twenty-one months
Oral electrolyte solutions, 233–37
Oral maintenance solutions. *See* Oral electrolyte solutions.
Organic foods, 118–21

Outside food *versus* home food, 24, 27, 218–19, 224, 256
Overeating, 99
Overweight. *See* Weight

Pacifiers, 66, 95
Pain, breast, 64, 71
Paleolithic nutrition. *See* Hunter-gatherer instincts
Parental role model for food, 23–24, 27, 155, 180
Parmesan dressing and dip, creamy, 198
Peanut allergy, 283
Pediatrician, signs for calling, 234
Persuasion, resistance to, 24–26, 27
Pesticides, 118–21
Phenylethylamine, 280
Physical activity, 42, 266–67
Phytochemicals, 11, 48
Pizza, 214–15, 259–60
Poisoning, 169–70, 171
Polychlorinated biphenyls (PCBs), nursing mothers and, 75
Portions, 31, 192, 194, 264–65
Pregnancy, allergy prevention and, 285–86
Premature infants, 101–9
  breast milk expression for, 103, 104–5, 107
  breast-feeding and, 54, 102–7
  formula options for, 107–8
  at home, 108–9
  kangaroo care for, 103
  supplemental nursing systems and, 106, 107
Preschool, 220–22
Processed foods with additives, 76
Produce
  chemical residues on, 120
  kitchen safety guidelines for, 123
Progesterone, 60
Projectile vomiting, 99
Prolactin, 60
Protein, 30
Pumpkin muffins, Kathleen's, 198
Pumps, breast milk expression, 71, 79
Pyridoxine, 315. *See also* B vitamins

Rashes, skin, 141, 143
RDAs (Recommended Dietary Allowances), 30–31, 312
Recipes
  for children's and adults' meals, 115
  for chocolate or vanilla cookies, 193
  for cod fried, 172
  for cooking with children, 198, 214–15
  for food allergies/intolerances, 290
  for oat pancakes, 175
  for oral electrolytes, 237
  for roll-ups, 211
  for whole-wheat sesame crackers, 193

Reflux, gastroesophageal. *See* Spitting-up, Vomiting
Refused food, 180, 192, 204, 205
Relatives, family nutrition and, 130–31
Repetition of foods, 154, 177–78, 196. *See also* Rule of fifteen
Resistance, 24–26, 180
Reverse psychology, 25–26
Role models, 180, 217
Roll-ups (recipe), 211
Rooting reflex, 64, 93
Roughage. *See* Fiber
Rule of fifteen, 21–22, 27, 177, 196, 271

Saccharin, 129
Safety, 169–70
  baby food jars and, 149
  formula feeding procedures for, 96–97
  kitchen guidelines for, 122–23
Salmonella bacteria, 121, 122
Salt, 42, 126, 187
Saturated fats, 33, 186
Scheduled feeding, 69–70, 146–48, 161, 174–75
Self-feeding, 161, 179
Self-regulation, 135, 153, 154–55, 161, 179–80
  eating disorders and, 269
Shigella bacteria, 121, 297
Sick children, 231–40
  appetite reducing illnesses in, 238
  dehydration and, 232, 234, 239–40
  diarrhea in, 231–33
  early refeeding for, 237
  fever in, 231–33
  fluids for, 234–36
  frequent questions about, 238–40
  vomiting in, 231–33
Sippy cups, 139, 225
Sleep, 241–48, 300
  all-night, 242–44
  breast-feeding *versus* formula for, 244–45
  cow's milk sensitivity and, 245–47
  eating and, 247–48
Snack foods, 20, 191, 256, 259, 262–63
Sodas, 125–26, 236, 263
Solid foods, 135, 136, 140–41, 143, 150–51, 155
  allergy protection and, 9, 283–84, 287–88
  milk and, 143–44
  for premature infants, 109
Soy formula, 89, 91–92
Spicy foods, 212
Spitting-up, 99, 294–95
Sports drinks during childhood illness, 236
Standard formula, 86, 87, 88, 89–90
  for premature infants, 108
Stunting, nutritional, 4, 203
  weight control and, 256–57
  zinc and, 43

Sucking, non-nutritive, 66, 95
Sucking reflex, 18, 27, 67, 93, 94, 106
Sugar, 126, 171–72, 303–4
Sulfites, 281, 290
Supermarkets, 26, 195, 197, 217
Supplemental nursing systems for premature
   infants, 106, 107
Supplements. *See* Multivitamin/mineral
   supplements
Swallowing reflex, 46

Table-clearing after eating, 194
Tartrazine, 281
Tea, 145
Teeth
   brushing, 157
   diet and, 41, 166–67
Teething, 133, 156, 157–58, 162
Television and food, 219, 265, 267
Temper tantrums, 195
Three to six years, 206–27
   body image of, 223–24
   books for, 216–17
   control instinct of, 18
   cooking with, 213, 216
   discounting principle and, 25, 219–20
   feeding, 208, 210
   frequent questions about, 224–26
   gardening with, 216
   home food versus other food for, 218–19
   menus for, 209, 222
   movies for, 217
   negative outside influences on, 218–19
   nutrition/health discussions with, 221, 223
   opportunities/goals for, 207–8
   positive outside influences on, 216–17
   preschool and, 220–21
   social inclinations of, 206–7
   strategies for feeding, 213, 216–20
   strongly flavored/spicy foods and, 212
   traveling/eating out with, 210–13
Thrive, failure to. *See* Failure to thrive
Toddler diarrhea, 204–5
Trans fatty acids, 32, 33, 145, 186
Transitional formulas for premature infants, 108
Tryptophan, 244–45
Twelve to twenty-one months, 159–84
   average daily intake for, 161–63
   everything into mouth by, 18–19, 133–34
   fluoride and, 181
   food traps to avoid, 171–72
   foods to try for, 165–68
   frequent questions about, 182–84
   menus/schedules for, 172–75
   multivitamin/mineral supplements for,
      176–77
   new foods for, 27
   opportunities/goals for, 160–61

safety concerns in feeding, 169–70
strategies for feeding, 177–80
transition to cow's milk, 163–65
Twenty-one months to three years, 185–205
   consistent responses for, 194–95
   constipation and, 200–201, 203
   control instinct of, 18, 192, 194–96
   cookies/snack foods for, 191
   cooking with, 196–97
   eating inducements and, 194, 204
   eating patterns of, 192
   feeding, 189
   food jags/fussiness for, 199–200
   food tricks and, 200
   frequent questions about, 203–5
   gardening with, 196–97
   menus for, 190
   mistakes and, recovering from, 197, 199
   opportunities/goals for, 188–89
   portion sizes for, 192, 194
   refusals by, 192
   strategies for feeding, 191–99
   table-clearing after eating and, 194
   temper tantrums and, 195
Tyramine, 280

Vacations and food, 210–12
Vaccinations, nursing and, 70
Variety principle, 19–21, 27, 47, 154, 177–78, 196
   for balanced family diet, 114
   grazing and, 157
   weight control and, 261
Vegetable(s), 42, 46–47, 142, 168–69, 177, 178,
      188
   child's weight gain and, 252, 261
   frozen, canned, 115
   premature heart disease and, 187
Vegetable juices, 152
Vegetarian diets, 124
Vitamin supplements. *See* Multivitamin/
   mineral supplements
Vitamins, 30
   A, C, and E, 46–48
   cancer prevention and, 10–11
   colds, 238–39
   hyperactivity and, 304–5
   irradiation and loss of, 122–24
   sources of, 47, 316–17
Vomiting, 231–37, 295–96. *See also* Spitting-up
   formula feeding and, 98
   projectile, 99

Water, 48–49, 76, 126
   nitrates in, 145
   switching from juice to, 271–72
Water intoxication, 67
Watermelon cooler (recipe), 215

Weaning, 6, 61, 84, 135
  allergy prevention and, 284
Weight, 8, 210, 249–75. *See also* Growth patterns
  adult dieting and, 270, 272–73
  eating disorders and, 269–70
  eating out and, 265, 268
  emotional hunger and, 265–66, 268, 271
  factors in problems with, 254–56
  food choices and, 256–64, 268, 273
  food restrictions and, 264–65, 268, 273–74
  frequent questions about, 270–74
  goals for, 254, 268
  identifying problems with, 250–51
  marking loss of, 268
  multivitamin/mineral supplements and, 268, 274

physical activity and, 266–67, 268
premature heart disease and, 187
recording child's daily intake, 254, 255, 268, 272
strategies for normalizing, 253–68
susceptibility to problems with, 251–52
Well-baby check-ups, 29
Whole-wheat flour, 210
Window of opportunity, 18–19

Yard hazards, 170–71

Zinc, 9, 30, 42–44, 238–39, 313–14

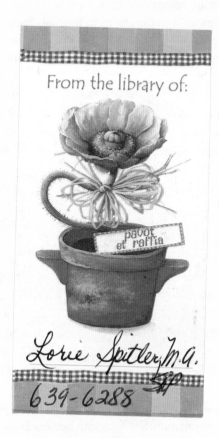

ABOUT THE AUTHORS

———————◈———————

SUSAN B. ROBERTS, Ph.D., is Chief of the Energy Metabolism Laboratory at the Jean Mayer USDA Human Nutrition Research Center on Aging at Tufts University, Professor of Nutrition at the Tufts University School of Nutrition Science and Policy, Scientific Staff Member in the Department of Pediatrics, and Associate Professor of Psychiatry at Tufts University Medical School. She is an internationally-recognized expert on infant and adult nutrition, with more than 100 research publications in journals including the *New England Journal of Medicine, JAMA,* and *The Lancet.* Her publications are on topics including the long-term effects of childhood nutrition, infant nutrient requirements, infant and adult obesity, breast-feeding, nutritional needs of premature infants, and nutrition and aging. She also chairs national meetings on metabolic programming and dietary prevention of obesity, and sits on international committees for evaluation of nutritional requirements. She lives in Newton, Massachusetts, with her husband and daughter.

MELVIN B. HEYMAN, M.D., M.P.H., is Professor of Pediatrics and Chief of the Division of Pediatric Gastroenterology, Hepatology, and Nutrition at the University of California in San Francisco (UCSF), and Director of the NIH-funded Combined Fellowship Training Program in Pediatric Gastroenterology and Nutrition at UCSF and Stanford University. He directs and is internationally recognized for his expertise in an active clinical program for nutrition and gastroenterology disorders (including inflammatory bowel diseases) in childhood, and is developing a comprehensive pediatric nutrition center for patient care, education, and research. He also has published over 100 research papers on pediatric nutrition and gastroenterology. He lives in San Francisco with his wife and three sons.

LISA TRACY is a senior editor with *The Philadelphia Inquirer* and author of two previous books on nutrition. She lives with her son in Moorestown, New Jersey.